FOR YOUR BODY ONLY

Discover The Diet
You Were Born to Eat

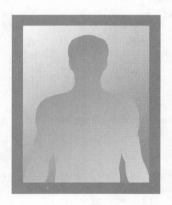

Dr. Gregory H. Tefft
America's Leader in Personalized Nutrition

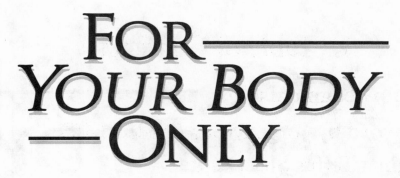

FOR YOUR BODY ONLY

Discover The Diet You Were Born to Eat

Dr. Gregory H. Tefft

FOR INFORMATION CONTACT:

Published in the United States by:
Dragon Door Publications, Inc
P.O. Box 4381, St. Paul, MN 55104
Tel: (651) 487-2180 • Fax: (651) 487-3954
Credit card orders: 1-800-899-5111
Email: dragondoor@aol.com • Website: www.dragondoor.com

ISBN 0-938045-41-5

Book design, Illustrations and cover by Derek Brigham
Website http//www.dbrigham.com
Tel/Fax: (612) 827-3431 • Email: dbrigham@visi.com

Manufactured in the United States
First Edition: May 2002

DISCLAIMER

Table of Contents

Chapter One

How the One-Size-Fits-All Mindset Is Wrecking Our Health

The Phenomenon of *Biochemical Individuality*...the breakthrough science of *Metabolic Typing*...why the 40-30-30 Zone recommendations are fundamentally unsound...the three primary characteristics of the one-size-fits-all mindset...the Way of the *Piecemealer*—a little bit of this, a little bit of that...the Way of the Shotgunner—if a little is good, more is better...the Way of the *One Sizer*—glib know-it-all demands respect... will the real nutritionist please stand up?

Chapter Two

Exposing the Fraud of One-Size-Fits-All Nutrition

Simple logic shows why one-size-fits-all doesn't cut it...research statistics and implications...expert research queries safety of one-size-fits-all diet...the good news.

Chapter Three   35
You Are 100% Unique—
The Health Implications of Biochemical Individuality
Why RDA's are not adequate for most individuals...why no two diet patterns can ever be quite the same...the Achilles heel of popular diet systems...what is Metabolic Typing?...where do metabolic types come from and what are their implications?...religious and evolutionary perspectives on metabolic types...a contemporary message about evolution and genes...the truth about allergies...do we really need Metabolic Typing?...the historic origins of metabolic typing...some ancient metabolic typing systems...Chinese typing...Ayurvedic typing ...Greek typing...modern Metabolic Typing and Profiling...historical overview...the landmark systems...the Sheldon system...the Bieler system...the D'Adamo system...the Watson system...the Kelley system...the Power system...the Tefft system...Metabolic typing—the process...a word about tribes...the Eskimo versus the Indian...the death of soil quality ..."good" foods, "bad" foods, and "compatible" foods—how to know what is what for you...*Forced Feeding Incompatibility Syndrome* (FFIS).

Chapter Four   81
Personalized Nutrition—
The Next Megatrend
The limitations of pseudo-individualized supplements...the fatal flaw of the "Body Type" diet...if you were my patient...Step 1: Quantification and Qualification—computing calories and food patterns...the quantifying process...the energy usage of physical activity...specific dynamic activity...dangerous territory...the qualifying process...the protein-carb-fat connection...Step 2: Pure Metabolic Typing...metabolic typing procedures...metabolic typing in practice...the adrenal type...physicality...personality...metabolic and dietary factors...the diet connection...the adrenal type...putting it together...Step 3: Laboratory Assessment, aka Profiling...the four factors of metabolism...the four metabolic factors under the microscope...Factor One—digestion...Factor Two—absorption... Factor Three—assimilation...Factor Four—elimination (excretion)...

Step 4: Diet and Supplement Customization...Part 1...Part 2...Step 5: The Final Step—Re-Evaluation...typing process overview...typing: the eicosanoid connection...the fat solution...typing and the athlete...typing in action: two case studies...metabolic maps—a new diagnostic frontier...summation.

Workbook 227

Step 1: Compute Calories...how to quantify and qualify your diet...estimating your BRM... calculating your Daily Physical Activity Need (DPAN)...your Specific Dynamic Activity (SDA)...your true energy need per day...your Target Calorie Level (TCL)...computing your macronutrient balance....how to obtain the right amount of protein, carbohydrate, and fat from "real foods."...best protein sources...best carbohydrate sources...best fat sources...food exchanges...sample diet worksheets...correct food preparation... RDA's...Step 2: Quick Check —Pure Metabolic Typing...the Super Quick Check...dead giveaways...Typing at a glance...the Super Duper Quick Check...rules...the metabolic types...extra guidelines for accurate metabolic typing...mixed types...Step 2A: Quick Check Zone...diet patterns...supplemental augmentation...Step 3: how to use this workbook...nutritional stereotyping out—biochemical individuality in...Part I: what's wrong with my body?...Metabolic Typing theory vs. Metabolic Profiling science...pretesting Metabolic Genetics with Quick Check...the nutrition testing/profiling procedures...Part II: repairing your body with perfect nutrition...food patterns and nutrient zones...balance mineral ratios...synergize vitamin proportions...equalize protein intake...proportion fats ...the sugar equation...food rotation and detoxification...hormone maximization.

Appendicies

Appendix A 333

Psychological Typing Combined with Body Typing
Ectomorphy, esomorphy and endomorphy... temperaments... ectotonia, mesotonia and endotonia...examples.

Appendix B 341

Five Examples of Blood Type Diet Categories
Omnivore diet for blood types B and AB...carni-vegan diet for blood type O...pesca-vegan diet for blood type A1 (Asian descent)...pesca-

lacto-vegan diet for blood type A1 (European descent)...semi lacto-vegan diet for blood type A2.

List of Tables

Acknowledgments

I would like to thank my dear mother, Dorothea S. Tefft, for raising me with a strong belief in the value of good nutrition and to my late father, George Tefft, for always believing in me. I also want to thank my dearest wife, Lindy, for her unfailing devotion, and for making *For Your Body Only* possible. Her support has made my life the most fulfilling and complete experience that I could have ever hoped for.

Foreword

By Jorge Monastersky, M.D.

Our contemporary world of medicine is a very dynamic, highly complex, and exceedingly sophisticated arena. The forces that shape and mold it are in a constant state of change, which is subject to an array of both positive and negative influences. On the one hand, you have those who only desire to provide mankind with the most efficient and effective healing methodologies. On the other hand, we have those dedicated to maximizing profits with little regard for the human condition. A constant struggle between these two opposing forces incites an atmosphere of turmoil, which is politically weighted in favor of the special interest groups who truly control the overall profit factor and therefore have an agenda to strenuously maintain the status quo. Because of this, bigger profit margins have become a higher priority than healing successes. The current U.S. health statistics speak for themselves . . . more money spent on healthcare than ever before, yet a greater incidence of degenerative disease (and especially heart disease) than ever in our history! Now it's time for a change!

My professional specialization as a cardiologist affords me a very special perspective on the diet-disease connection. Heart disease is the number one killer of all humans and represents the primary degenerative disease that is most easily improved upon with proper nutrition. In fact, optimum nutrition, regular exercise, and effective stress management dramatically reduces its incidence. If each of us practiced the right lifestyle, this disease process (and the majority of other ones present in society) would be overwhelmingly diminished. But this is not where the money is being spent!

Instead, we're putting trillions of dollars into quick fixes and after-the-fact crisis intervention some of which may be more health risky than the disease process itself . . . none of which eradicates the true cause of the disease in the first place! So, in frustration, I tell my patients: "eat right, exercise regularly, and try to reduce stress." This helps the most under any and all conditions of your treatment. I also tell them that there is no "magical pill" that can cure them, so forget that notion. But I ask you—is this enough? No . . . there's much more.

For Your Body Only takes you to that special place where the root cause of degenerative disease is found. It takes you deep into the realm of the diet-wellness connection where each uniquely different human being is treated, precisely and naturally. For Your Body Only shows you what modern nutritional medicine is truly capable of once you bypass the fallacy of "one-size-fits-all."

Interestingly, ancient healers developed much of the philosophy behind our highly evolved modern-day individualized nutritional sciences, believing too that each of us is unique and must be treated accordingly. Thankfully, modern metabolic science allows us to put each body "under the microscope" and accurately match nutrition to each person's needs synergistically combining the most beneficial practices of the ancients together with the advanced thinking of modern researchers and therapists. Going back to a naturally healthy way of life was never so easy!

Dr. Tefft brings us to the final frontier of nutrition where complete wellness and greater longevity are the status quo . . . where diet related disease is absent . . . where each and every one of us can be our healthiest, our fittest—our best! For Your Body Only gives new meaning to your doctor's advice to eat right by replacing this "one size fits all" mega-generality with scientific precision on an awe inspiring level of order of which few of us are aware. The process of Metabolic Typing once again puts human needs ahead of capitalistic priorities. It allows each of us to actively participate in our own wellness success instead of being coerced by an unsympathetic healthcare system into becoming just another bleak medical statistic.

I recommend this book for you to read before delving into indiscriminate and ineffective diet and supplement practices. *For Your Body Only* will give you the much-needed insights you'll require to solve the nutrition—wellness puzzle. This is a book that occupies a place in my office and in my heart. I have always believed in the power of personalized nutrition—so should you!

Gregory Tefft's Story
and His Vision for You

I became excited about nutrition and exercise as early in my life as age seven when I became a champion swimmer. At this time, I discovered the principles of "cause and effect". I developed the notion that if "cause and effect" were really true, I could **custom design my own body** to have a one-of-a-kind body of which I was the sole architect and builder. So, at this early age, I set out on the course to prove the principles of "cause and effect" either as erroneous or as a true fact of life. This process was very exciting!

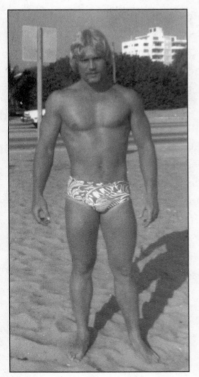

I began applying these principles. My first series of achievements included multiple swimming victories leading to local, county, state, and national rankings and a fifth placing in a pre-Olympic track and field meet. I missed the Olympic team qualifying cutoffs for both sports but I still felt glorious. Imagine—"cause and effect" enabled me to excel in two completely different sports and others as well.

1973—one year after missing the Olympic Team cutoff for 1972 Olympics in Munich, Germany. Age 19.

I became very ambitious with my new found success and decided to establish as my next goal the attainment of powerlifting successes— something that is even more opposite than swimming and track are to each other.

I began my powerlifting campaign by gaining thirty pounds in six weeks which doubled my initial strength levels overall. I used no drugs or steroids just diet and supplements. Then…all of a sudden one afternoon I couldn't breathe! I started gasping for air and felt like I was going to suffocate. A friend rushed me to the hospital and I ended up in the emergency room. My diagnosis was given as a severe case of asthma of unknown origin. The doctors loaded me up with

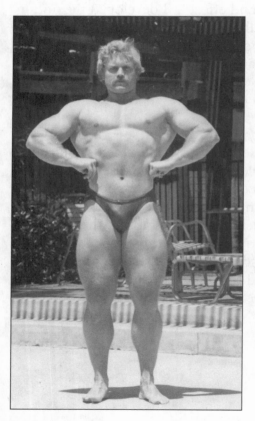

drugs, which helped me to breathe a little easier. I still had a hard time climbing up a flight of stairs without having to stop to catch my breath. I fell from what seemed "super health" to "super illness" literally in one afternoon. The medical doctors said that there simply was no cure for this condition—just symptom reduction with drugs. I was completely devastated by this and began losing my lust for life. Realizing that this illness was my greatest challenge ever, I decided not to accept my fate. My only recourse was to implement "cause and effect" to save my life.

Bulked up to 273 lbs. from powerlifting and preparing for World's Strongest Man Contest which I never entered due to an accidental injury.

Without the help of any doctors, except for the advice of Dr. Carlton Fredericks, a nutrition oriented physician, I systematically implemented "cause and effect" using alternative nutritional medicine and within one and a half years from my original attack, I overcame this devastating disease of asthma. I was ecstatic! "Cause and effect" really worked—it saved my life!

So, with unbridled and eternal enthusiasm (and a freely breathing respiratory system), I applied the principles of "cause and effect" to bring my powerlifting achievements to the Master's Class attainment

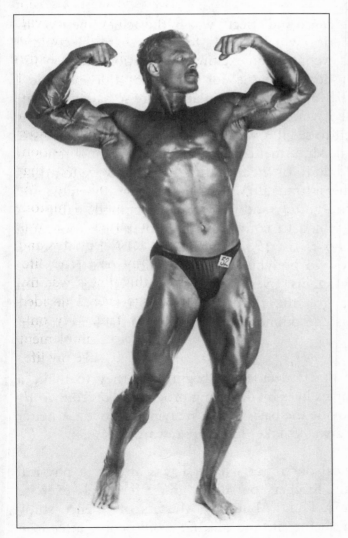

My best shape at bodyweight 216 lbs., bodyfat 3%.

level and then further excelled in the bodybuilding world by placing first in three Natural Mr. America bodybuilding competitions. (Natural means tested for steroids and other drugs)

Then, I thought, "Wow, I really do control the destiny of my body! These principles of nutrition and exercise are more than just something to read about, they are dynamic forces of life". These principles have taken me from my youth through countless athletic achievements and completely through a terrible disease that literally wouldn't allow me to catch my breath.

The ultimate test of "cause and effect" was in the achievement of my first Natural Mr. America win in 1981, four years after I couldn't catch my breath. This event was an exciting competition between 150 men who were in a dogged battle for this great title. While I understood that properly applied nutrition and exercise had gotten me to first place, this time I wondered if maybe I was just lucky. So I set another goal for myself to see if it would work again. It did! In 1982, I received the Natural Mr. America crown for the second time. I reasoned that if I could do it for the third time, I could prove to myself and thousands of others from all walks of life, that nutrition and exercise is *For Your Body Only* and that it would be undeniable and irrefutable data with which to convince others that they too could have the body they chose. In 1982, during the NBA Mr. America competition (there are two bodybuilding associations, the NBA and the NBBA) competing against over 160 participants, I was crowned Natural Mr. America for the third time. At six feet tall, my competitive weight was 216 pounds, which put me in the heavyweight class.

It was at this point that I decided to begin a journey to make a difference in other peoples lives by designing programs *For Your Body Only* which would provide the basis for a satisfying lifestyle. A better body and good health always makes life more rewarding.

Do I become a medical doctor or what? I was already a physical education and health teacher pursuing graduate level exercise physiology to become a Ph.D. But, my Masters of Science study program, all that came before it, and all that would come after it in my pursuit of a Ph.D. was not truly "hitting the spot" where I could clinically implement "cause and effect" for each person with whom I would come in contact. I couldn't really help people to design each of their unique bodies one at a time from start to finish.

Since I knew that nutrition and exercise was the basis for a good body and optimum health, I researched the data available to determine the best study program which in turn would give me the most complete professional academic credentials based upon nutrition and exercise. It would take forty-two hundred classroom hours to become a medical doctor with fifteen hours devoted to nutrition and exercise. In contrast, it would take forty-four hundred hours to become a chiropractor with **more than** *seven hundred hours* **devoted to nutrition and exercise** not to mention the thousands of hours devoted to the science and art of drugless healing. Yes, it was a longer trip, but, chiropractic being the largest licensed drugless healing profession in the world, had the studies and training for which I was looking in order to have the academic, clinical, and legal credentials with which to professionally guide people through the process of designing **your body only.** In 1986 I received my Doctorate of Chiropractic and state license. I'd already passed my federal boards in 1984.

I had no idea about all the wonderful things that would happen to me because of the attainment of these objectives. I was elected as a member of the Sports Medicine Staff of the U.S. National Swim Team, Race Across America, Olympic Team, and other sports organizations. I also received the Reader's Digest Health Awareness Award. Weider publications (Muscle and Fitness, Flex, etc.) ordained me as the "Mind-Body Connector" due to the combination of my academic and athletic achievements. Many celebrities have graced my clinics and at the Malibu Health and Rehabilitation Center in Malibu, California, I became known as "the lifestyle practitioner". I received an endorsement from the World Academy of Personal Development and have acted as a teacher, lecturer, inventor, author, researcher, and technical consultant to many health, nutrition, and rehabilitation and fitness companies and organizations. In fact, I was the first Doctor of Chiropractic to speak before the Orange County division of the California Medical Organization when I was featured in it's 28th Annual Symposium on Sports Medicine. I have been featured on television numerous times from QVC to CBS This Morning to the Orange County News and more. Orange County News TV actually ordained me "America's Leader in Personalized Nutrition". You may even have spotted me on televised body building shows or even some commercials that I've been asked to appear in.

Who would have guessed that all these wonderful things would have happened to me just from choosing this profession? It must be "cause and effect" working again. Then I went one step further and attained my second doctorate as a board certified Naturopathic Physician. Naturopathy is the second largest medical profession in the world and what medical doctors were automatically considered to be before the "drug revolution". It embodies all natural wellness wisdom from ancient to modern times. The forces of nature—air, sunshine, water, food, herbs, movement, and all naturally occurring health-building phenomena, are the medicines used.

I have helped a countless number of patients in practice and always prioritize only natural and conservative healing methods over artificial symptom relief quick fixes and health risky practices. Put yourself in my shoes for a moment. When you are responsible for the healthy livelihood of others, it puts a tremendous amount of pressure on you to be a thorough researcher, an effective listener, a precise diagnostician, a highly skilled clinician, poignant teacher, and intensely committed to practicing natural medicine and individualized body design on your patients as well as yourself. You must be up to the task from every body design principle and healing dimension to serve others well. Narrow-mindedness has no place in the clinical picture.

I have always found that in the final analysis, experience is the best teacher. Formal schooling opens up your mind, fine tunes your thought processes, and solidly structures your fundamental knowledge parameters. However, school is only the beginning. Using school-derived knowledge and then applying it **to yourself** is the first truly significant step in fully comprehending and actualizing the deepest meaning of formal schooling. Learning from your own personal successes and mistakes first, before ever instructing a client or treating a patient, strengthens your convictions to and expertise in precisely fulfilling the needs of patients.

This introspective process of self-discovery deeply reinforces and expands formal knowledge parameters with actual true-to-life experience that subsequently makes it more difficult to forget or overlook the finer points of the entire body design and natural healing process for others, as well as yourself. The continuous self-application of healing knowledge increases your inherent ability to relate to yourself and most importantly to your patient. Know yourself and you will know your patient better! The worst position a practitioner can be in is when a patient fails to respond optimally to instructions or treatment. As clinician, it's your fault for whatever reason—most likely because you didn't fully understand what specifically needed to be done or didn't relate to the patient properly, all of which really is a matter of self-directed experience, experimentation, and follow through. To truly be an effective healing professional and not merely a shallow technician, you must closely embody, self-apply, and experience through yourself and others all that you have learned.

Don't miss a thing! Don't leave your work just in the office! You must be "on the job" at all times, ready to capture the essence of healing at every given opportunity. It's not enough just to be a good student, a competent researcher, to be healthy yourself, to have a good bedside manner or have good technical skill in and of itself. Instead it's imperative to synchronize all of these qualities to achieve the bottom line—complete therapeutic wellness for the patient. A lack of accomplishment in any one of these professional and personal qualities or their combined synergy seriously compromises your effectiveness as a healer for yourself, your patients, and in the indirect contribution to the wellness objectives and healing skills of others who learn from you. Throughout life you must commit to these ways of being in order to fully optimize your potential for all to benefit, otherwise you are not a true professional. This is my mind set as a devoted health practitioner. I encourage other health practitioners and those who wish to be body design and health care practitioners to think this way otherwise they will become detached from their work, their clients, and their patients.

I have always stated that I **PRACTICE WHAT I TEACH** and strive to maintain the best health and fitness levels out of respect for myself and as an inspiration to others' in their personal achievement. My proven commitment has intensely motivated clients and patients to challenge themselves and succeed. I want them to know that I'm not just an "armchair expert" when it comes to fully understanding the human body and that I am right there with them looking for the same answers they're seeking. I want to be super healthy just as much as they do! I don't want to personally suffer from disease as much as I don't want them to. I've always used all that I've learned, formal and informal, as a weapon against disease and improper body design for myself and to benefit others.

I am deeply frustrated about our current health and body trends. As a society we are wholeheartedly accepting natural health and body design advice from so-called "experts," some of whom have never treated a patient in their lives and others who have never practiced a word of what they've preached, others who have no formal education in their claimed specialties, and still others who will say anything to make a few dollars. The net result of all of these self-proclaimed "experts" is highly fragmented and very one-sided information, some valid and some not, and many books written on just one minor piece or another of the overall wellness puzzle. These books are routinely touted as the all-in-one— *"one-size-fits-all"*— "silver bullet" solution when they're not even close to the real truth of the matter. This conventional literary mentality reinforces the magic bullet concept of *"one-size-fits-all"* and all other "one shot" or quick fix erroneous healing philosophies which, all in all, inhibits our battle against disease and improper body design both in thought and deed.

There is simply no *one-size-fits-all* magic bullet! One usable health clue out of thousands of healing variables cannot fulfill our complete wellness or body design needs by itself. The only viable solution to this one-sided "perspective and fragmentation dilemma" is to properly connect the fragmented bits of valid health information which can help us for the directed purpose of attaining complete wellness and successful body design without leaving any aspect overlooked. This mentality is the true key to Holistic Health. Putting all the pieces together will always solve the puzzle, but each piece in and of itself does not complete the puzzle—and never will!

As you will see, "typing" and "profiling" comprehensively connects the dots of the total health puzzle on a practical and scientific level never before accomplished. It measures human needs on a precise

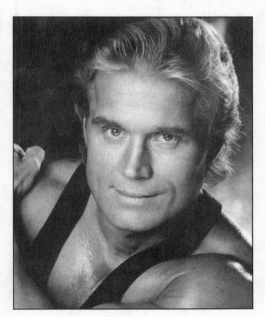

level and leaves nothing to chance. I have never seen such a powerful and all encompassing healing and body design tool. I've searched throughout my lifetime for this solution to so many of my own questions and those of my clients and patients. I feel honored to introduce "typing/profiling" to you through *For Your Body Only*—it will allow you to be what you've always wanted to be!

So let's begin this journey *For Your Body Only....*

Ten Things to Know
Before You Read This Book

1. **All disease manifestation** within the body is nutrition-related. This includes infectious disease, and in particular genetic disease.

2. **Nutrition** is defined as the food we eat, air we breathe, water we drink, supplements we ingest, and all that we do that literally "feeds" or nourishes the body for its own health benefit. This includes exercise, positive thought, and deepened spirituality.

3. **Toxin** is any chemical substance found inside the body that results from improper nutrition, poisonous accumulation, or negative energy, which undermines the body's proper function in any way.

4. **Genes** are the cell and body architects that are derived from protein particles, which have set the body design at its most ideal level and is absolutely unique to each individual. They can be damaged by improper nutrition, toxic accumulation, or unbalanced metabolism.

5. **Metabolism** is the expression of the genes through the chemical factors that convert food, air and water into life and energy. It can be changed for the better or worse by nutrition.

6. **Deficiency** is anything chemical, mechanical, or energetic that the body hasn't enough of for optimum health. "Excess" is the opposite of deficiency. "Perfect Balance" equals the exact fulfillment of the body's chemical, mechanical, and energetic requirements as determined by the genes.

7. **Biochemical uniqueness** is the phenomenon whereby we possess matter and energy distinctions that make us different from one another: No two people are alike.

8. **You are** what you eat, drink, breathe, absorb, and do, whether right or wrong for your genetic design. Right choices create wellness.

9. **The body** is a mechanism of adaptation to bad stress *(distress)*, and good stress *(eustress)*. Too much stress of any kind can undermine it.

10. **When** it comes to good health, "there is always more than what meets the eye!" Adopting the guidelines for health found in *For Your Body Only* will ensure that you never take your health for granted. Read on if you value your health.

Overview

For Your Body Only, The Final Breakthrough:
A Scientific Way to Everlasting Health

Beyond Modern Nutrition

We have witnessed the phenomenon again and again in the fight against fat and the pursuit of optimum wellness. First it was Dr. Atkins, who said "Carbohydrates are bad—eat protein." Later, everyone thought carbohydrates of any kind were the miracle food: "Eat as much as you like and cut out protein and fats." Then it was the Scarsdale Diet, which again extolled the virtues of fat and protein. Next came the Grapefruit Diet, in which a fruit was heralded as the "magic bullet." Following this discovery, doctors effused about oat bran, then, for a brief, happy moment, red wine was determined to be the cure-all. More recently, the antidote of choice was FenPhen . . . until it started killing people. The massive infusion of nutritional supplements into the wellness market today provides a mind-boggling array of wellness solutions.

All these miracle cures, supposed to be great for everybody, yet over 60 percent of all Americans are still overweight and over 80 percent of the disease considered epidemic in the most civilized countries is diet-related. What is really going on?

Put simply, each person is a biochemically unique individual and requires a personally designed diet for optimum health. In this book, readers are inspired to turn their backs on such "one-size-fits-all," "it'll-work-for-you-too" diets and medical philosophies of modern times, and to start exploring their own "one-of-a-kind" bodies and minds for the true secrets of everlasting health.

The philosophy of individualization is the new medical model for the next century, a compilation of all that has come before and the seed of all that will be. It is the center point of all nutritional and health research, and the wave of the future. This is the cherished secret, the final answer—there is nothing after.

For Your Body Only shows that although there have been some truly amazing, life-saving medical breakthroughs in this century, not much in the way of applied nutrition has really been accomplished for the masses. In fact, wellness statistics for the United States reveal a progressive epidemic of degenerative diseases swamping our peace of mind and body. Arthritis, anemia, cancer, heart disease, obesity, diabetes, osteoporosis, allergies, fatigue syndromes, immune dysfunction, and many other disorders head the list of society's contemporary ills. And, these conditions all have one common denominator—nutrition.

Our current nutritional dilemma is simple. Those of us who do watch our diets routinely apply either a one-size-fits-all, or a shotgun ("all or nothing"), or a piecemeal ("a little bit of this, a little bit of that") approach. The same is true for supplementation. This nutritional stereotyping does not work at all; in fact, it is killing people every day.

Further aggravating this situation, the prevailing practice among physicians—and the prevailing expectation of patients—is toward superficial symptom relief instead of true cause relief. Instead of changing diet and lifestyle to eliminate or diminish these conditions, doctors and patients prefer the immediate and less life-altering course of symptom relief—drugs.

However, a significant part of the U.S. population is pushing society into a more natural and conservative approach to common illness, by helping to improve our combined health statistics overall, instead of worsening our position. Unfortunately, when it comes to proper nutrition—the absolute foundation of overall wellness—we are simply not achieving the beneficial results we would expect. This book pinpoints clearly the problems lurking in the dominant one-size-fits-all approach.

Research shows unequivocally that one-size-fits-all nutrition will eventually be completely replaced by highly scientific individualization in accordance with each person's biochemical uniqueness. As scientific individualization permeates our society and the healthcare industry, we will experience a progressive shrinking of diet-related disease and a profound upsurge of wellness advances in both the quality and longevity of life.

As demonstrated in *For Your Body Only*, "dis-ease" at its very source can be eliminated from the body. All readers must do is precisely identify the uniqueness of their own bodies, then begin feeding and treating them based on their own genetic and metabolic requirements. "You are what you eat," and with the proper testing, readers will uncover all their personal nutritional disorders in an absolutely foolproof manner! Uncovering our biochemical individuality allows us to fully commit to completely personalized nutrition-mediated wellness. Individualized nutrition is the final megatrend of health—our only alternative, the silver bullet revealed.

Metabolic Typing and Metabolic Profiling

We can identify our personal nutritional needs through a revolutionary two-step evaluation process. The first step is called Metabolic Typing. This process interconnects genetically predisposed human patterns that divide everyone into one of eight distinct physiological categories. These are based on similar characteristics such as blood type, nervous system characteristics, endocrine gland balance, oxidation patterns, body shape, body composition, personality, hair and facial features, and much more. From these eight genetic groupings, we can match seven theoretical food and supplement patterns. This classification process is then differentiated and refined further with actual nutrition tests known by scientists as metabolic profiling.

"Profiling" reveals the nutrient and toxin composition of the body at a given moment in time regardless of, but in conjunction with, theoretical genetic design. Using the idea of "you are what you eat," one's time-accumulated nutritional biochemistry must be precisely measured, vitamin by vitamin, mineral by mineral, etc., so that we can know exactly what we're dealing with as scientific truth—not theory (as in Typing). By eliminating guesswork about one's nutritional needs, we can customize a nutrition program precisely for each individual, including a list of the exact foods and supplements a person should take in the proper synergistic proportions and amounts that really work!

Where do metabolic types come from? Quite simply, they come from human genetic "pools." Our genetic makeup is a result of more than 40,000 years of evolution. The geographical location of humans' origins has had a profound effect on what they should feed their bodies and how they should live today. The food chain, climate, and topography have shaped our DNA very specifically. Whether a person's ancestors were hunter-gatherers, farmers, fishermen, warriors, peace mongers, lived in cold or warm climates, at high, medium, or low altitudes, all circumstances have affected them as individuals, specifically in what they require from the environment to be at their healthy best.

If a person remains within the path of their genetic origins and antecedent environmental patterns, they will thrive physically and mentally. The Hunzas, Soviet Georgians, Abcasians, and many other unchanged primal societies demonstrate this clearly with sickness-defying health and amazing longevity. The rest of us are at a severe loss in technologically advanced one-size-fits-all "melting pot" societies. Metabolic Typing and precisely individualized nutrition are not new ideas. Hippocrates, the father of medicine, introduced the concept when he held that different types of people have different maladies; his favorite motto was "Thy food shall be thy remedy." The ancient Chinese, Egyptians, Buddhists, and Hindus were also "body-typers."

Modern Typing—and its new lab-tested counterpart, Profiling—began in 1904 when Carl Landsteiner discovered the different blood types. In 1935, Dr. M. Kretschmer established three basic body types, determined by "derm distribution." Four years earlier, Dr. Cary Reams, a medical student of Albert Einstein, had developed the "Theory of Biological Ionization," in accordance with $E=MC^2$. The 1940s and early 50s gave rise to research in Germany linking the ABO blood types to diet, and research by Dr. Charles Stockard connected hormone balance to body and personality patterns. Dr. Sheldon refined Kretschmer's system into the meso-, ecto-, and endomorphs widely used today.

In 1956 the "godfather" of Metabolic Typing and Profiling, Roger Williams, Ph.D., published *Biochemical Individuality* and *Nutrition Against Disease*, which dramatically expanded this body of scientific knowledge. Many followed, including Henry G. Bieler, M.D., who developed the first complete endocrine typing system based on glandular balance and respective nutritional therapies, and the D'Adamos' (James and grandson Peter) blood typing system. Dr. George Watson created the first oxidation typing system utilizing five psychological types, pH ranges, and psychochemical odor-analysis (the forerunner of modern aromatherapy). The Kelley System was the first complete nerve typing system, while the Powers' provided logical combinations of the other systems, with over eight metabolic/body types. Mein catalogued over 25 endocrine/exocrine/constitutional body types. Pottenger further connects structure to function on a body-by-body basis.

Major research efforts have accelerated at a blistering pace. On the cutting edge, the Tefft Alternative Nutrition System combines the most pertinent of these projects, simplifies the information, and then takes the process several steps further. This system recognizes eight different body types, utilizing laboratory and self-tests to refine Metabolic Typing theory many quantum leaps further with the aid of Profiling science. The overall process entails categorizing individuals on the basis of a number of factors, including:

- blood type
- height
- weight
- pulse rate
- blood pressure
- hair characteristics
- skin traits
- muscle size, shape, and tone
- bone factors
- overall shape
- head and face shape
- personality
- ethnicity
- intelligence factors
- dream states

The findings are further refined with easy access (non-medical) laboratory tests that reveal extremely specific information about every pertinent metabolic and nutrient function we can scientifically measure and understand. Properly typed and profiled people will *never* have to guess what foods and supplements they need to live exactly how they were genetically designed to live—and feel great all the while. Just ask any Biosphere I or II researcher, whose UCLA computer predictions for human longevity indicate the capacity for 166 years of disease-free life.

The Future of Typing and Profiling

When Galileo postulated that the world was round, not flat, humankind shuddered and discounted his ideas as stupid and blasphemous. When Jules Verne predicted that man would walk on the moon, the powers-that-be considered this science fiction at best. However, the world's leading scientific minds came to see the sense in both of these ideas.

Metabolic Typing and Profiling has a basis in scientific knowledge light years beyond Galileo's and Verne's at the time of their (apparently) confounding statements. Based on the time lapse between the publication of their ideas and their realization in the scientific community, Typing and Profiling should have been put to widespread use at least 30 years ago. But according to the pervasive one-size-fits-all philosophy, a symptom—instead of its cause, the sickness—is treated. Rather than wellness-dependent healthcare, our system employs a "quick, fix it at all costs" approach, with no priority on health gain. With its commercialization of the fitness and wellness markets, which leads to the rape of the natural world in a quest for more and cheaper treatments, the healthcare industry's eye on the bottom line drives our pursuit of ineffective practices that should have been left behind decades ago. If history does repeat itself, then it is conventional wisdom that has seriously undermined the advancement of holistically integrated, individually based wellness science into the mainstream—in other words, Typing and Profiling have been left on the shelf in favor of "quick fix" techniques. This has been happening despite enlightening breakthroughs in functional nutrition medicine and holistic practices—and dramatic failures in conventional medicine—of such overwhelming magnitude that they can no longer be ignored.

The holistic and medical communities are finally recognizing Metabolic Typing and Profiling as the ultimate wellness miracle. The implicit crime here is that it has taken so much more time to push this optimum wellness technique to the forefront, more than the outright majority of scientific breakthroughs since the beginnings of humankind. This "awareness lag" continues despite the explosive growth of Profiling both inside and out of the doctor's office. We can wait no longer! It is time for each and every one of us to explore the miracle that is Metabolic Typing and Profiling.

Preface

- Why is the one-size-fits-all world of nutrition severely undermining our health?

- Why does your best friend's weight loss diet work for her and not for you?

- Why can't you take off those unwanted pounds or feel your best no matter how hard you try?

- Did you know that almost all diseases are diet-related? What can you do about this?

- Why do you come down with one type of disease and your friend suffers from another?

- Are you aware that your chosen foods and supplements, even when considered healthy, may actually be harming you rather than helping you?

- Why is it that today, with all the books published on health, nutrition, and fitness, with trillions of dollars spent on our healthcare system, and with modern diet and fitness breakthroughs everywhere, we are still unable to overcome fat problems, degenerative diseases, and fatigue syndromes? Why do these problems continue to plague us on the largest scale man has ever experienced in the history of mankind?

The answer to all of these questions is this: because our highly touted modern-day contemporary solutions to these problems are based on one-size-fits-all! This is the belief that what's good for your particular health and well-being is right for everyone else.

This scientifically invalid philosophy is far too generalized to work properly; it totally ignores the fact that each one of us has our own biochemical uniqueness. No two people are exactly alike! How can you determine what's so different about you and your specific nutritional needs? How can you use your individuality as the most potent weapon against being sick, fat, or fatigued ever again?

The rapidly expanding and highly sophisticated science of Metabolic Typing and its lab-tested counterpart Profiling actually originated with the ancients thousands of years ago! In its present state, Metabolic Typing and Profiling determines both biological and biochemical individuality on a precise level never before possible! Every vitamin, mineral, amino acid, fatty acid, sugar, genetic tendency, toxin, and hidden sensitivity within your unique body is measured precisely so that nutritional remedies can be synergized effectively.

This exciting information has never been brought out in all its fascinating detail . . . until now. The concepts contained in this book obliterate overwhelmingly any beliefs you may now have about the crop of current best sellers. 40/30/30, Vata, Pitta, Kapha, Yin Yang, Ancestral Profile, Blood Type, or Metabolic Rate classification cannot stand alone. These techniques have little place in the world of Metabolic Typing and Profiling and individualized nutrition, other than as examples of completely obsolete and/or incomplete lifestyle approaches.

The long awaited and desperately needed science of Metabolic Typing and Profiling represents what is fast becoming the final megatrend of nutrition. Its scientifically applied customized nutrition process is our only hope for optimal wellness in a New World where one-size-fits-all just doesn't work and conventional attempts at individualization are meager at best. With Metabolic Typing and Profiling everyone can finally stop guessing about his or her true nutritional needs!

Come with me on the most fascinating journey you will ever take into the world of eternal wellness. There is no place to go but to the universe within ourselves, where all the answers can now be found—for your body only.

How To Use This Book

Dear Reader:

This book is designed to meet your needs on a most personalized level. Its content is not a gimmick, a fad, or a "generic" approach to wellness. Instead, you will find a poignant scientific truth in its conceptual entirety with nothing left out. No other text is required for you to perfect your innate health; all readers can truly benefit from the knowledge found here, applicable to their highly unique perceptions and physical profiles.

Some chapters have been designed to simply help you understand important ideas. Other chapters are presented in workbook form so that you can start designing your own program immediately. Additionally, the chapters have been divided to meet the needs of those who like to browse, as well as for those who must have every detail, and those who just want to get started as quickly as possible.

For "doers," the Workbook Section is set up in sequential, baby steps, which you can follow in order to develop your own program, step by complete step (there is also an "expanded workbook" that you can order from the publisher). Detail-oriented readers will find *For Your Body Only* written in short subchapters, "thesis style," progressing smoothly so that the material does not become overwhelming; at the same time, the reader will find answers to every logical question, and each concept is systematically made easy to follow.

The book's structure will help you to mentally program yourself for a new (and needed) way of looking at the nutrition-disease connection. For best results, read each chapter at a leisurely pace and don't rush the thought. Browse if you're in a hurry, but come back for the details later.

I, Dr. Tefft, have written this book for "you"—it is addressed to "you" throughout. This approach personalizes the text further and is a style of writing I favor because of its directness.

The first three chapters address what's wrong with our bodies nowadays, and why true wellness is hard to come by our time. The remaining chapters, the Workbook, and the Appendices show each and every one of us how to repair any (or all) of the 223 current diet-related diseases, as well as how to prevent new problems, obliterate fatness, and increase life expectancy dramatically. When you've completed the genetically corrected, metabolically measured nutrition process presented herein, you'll finally take control over your personal wellness destiny.

Consider this book as the last text you'll ever have to read about eliminating nutrition-related disease, which compromises approximately 80% of all disease present in the United States and a progressively larger percentage of disease in other countries. Once and for all, the answers are here—for yourself.

Warning

This book is not meant to be read cover to cover and then simply cast aside. The simplified information found in *For Your Body Only* represents over 60 million pages of research documents dedicated to guaranteeing our wellness, culled from the works of scientists such as Wiley, Einstein, Williams, Riddick, Reams, and many others, all of whom have tapped the only scientifically, schematically valid solutions to our current wellness dilemma. The only reason this body of knowledge (that is, Metabolic Typing and Profiling) is not in conventional use today is because the health and wellness market has exploded in its production of quick fixes and symptom cover-ups, before orthomolecular nutritional science has had a chance to reach the mainstream.

It is up to each and every one of us to use this breakthrough information, not only to successfully overcome our own personal wellness issues, but also to let others know about "Typing and Profiling" as quickly as possible. When more people know about this precise wellness process and start applying it, we can place this most powerful medicine all the more swiftly into the mainstream of life, as a conventional option for one and all.

Billions are being spent to inform you about drugs and quick fixes. Now it's time for the real truth to be told! Please help us to enlighten others so that, someday soon, those resources will be spent on the only scientifically valid process, to defeat disease at its very root. We need not suffer anymore! Help yourself and you'll help us all.

INTRODUCTION

The Circle of Medicine: Where We've Been And Where We're Going

The doctor of the future will give no medicine but will interest his patients in the care of the human frame, in diet, and in the cause and prevention of disease
—Thomas A. Edison

Every day, we are bombarded by the latest U.S. health statistics, which continue to demonstrate just how seriously ill we have become as a nation. Whether it's rampant obesity, the latest "flesh-eating" bacterium, or young children suffering from diseases traditionally signifying advanced age (such as arthritis), the picture seems rather bleak. Is modern medicine failing us, or is there something else afoot? Maybe the answer is, a little of both.

When it comes to modern medicine, there are most decidedly a handful of medical procedures that undoubtedly save lives during crisis or emergency situations. America's diagnostic technologies and surgical methodologies are the best in the world. So why are our general health statistics depressingly poor in comparison to most other countries'? Why are we still suffering from so many degenerative and infectious conditions which continue to plague us? Why are we hooked on so many drugs?

The answer is simple: true and lasting wellness is not found in our ability to save a life in the middle of a catastrophic emergency, but in our ability to create and preserve healthy bodies before a crisis develops that would require emergency help. It's important to save a life whenever possible in a moment of crisis . . . but how can you learn to swim after you've already drowned? It makes more sense to learn how to swim before going near the water unprepared. An ounce of prevention—or natural cause relief correction—is worth a megakiloton of quality life and a quintuple megakiloton of cure!

Other than some truly amazing life-saving medical breakthroughs that we now possess, not much else has been accomplished overall to correct society's ills, besides successfully containing some rampantly infectious diseases. Many of our uncorrected and persistent ills are reflected in U.S. wellness statistics that represent what most authorities refer to as an epidemic of degenerative diseases. Arthritis, anemia, cancer, heart disease, obesity, diabetes, osteoporosis, allergies, fatigue syndromes, digestive disorders, immune dysfunction, and many other disorders fill this disease category and head the list of society's most contemporary ills.

These conditions all seem to all have one common denominator—nutrition. In fact, most authorities acknowledge our current and intensifying epidemic of degenerative disease as truly an epidemic of diet-related disease, to the point where more than 80% of all disease is considered diet-related.

All conscientious health professionals—and most laypeople—are well aware of this "disease-nutrition" connection. Consequently, I believe that most health-conscious people are hoping and pushing for more elaborate information about how to *use nutrition as a successful weapon against disease*. This is the direction that our overall scientific and philosophic emphasis finally seems to be moving towards—away from just symptom-relief drug technology and into the most formidable anti-disease weapon of all—*nutrition*. It is unfortunate that there already exists a huge wealth of information contained within the sciences of natural medicine—and especially nutrition—that has been almost entirely overlooked by modern medicine and mainstream wellness philosophies. Why?

In his book, *Dr. Braly's Food Allergy and Nutrition Revolution*, Dr. James Braly states that ". . . even the best-read physician misses 90–95% of what is published." Imagine what the rest of us miss—it's overwhelming! It is very difficult to keep up with the information explosion we are experiencing in our time. Coupled with this situation are a lot of misdirected politics afoot, especially in the world of the medical profession. According to Dr. Braly,

". . . only about 10% of what is published (about health) is included in the computer stores, and 10% is chosen by review boards of very prominent but very traditional physicians. So, most of the information available through such services follows the established line of prejudice. Because these doctors don't consider the latest nutritional findings important, they don't include them in the material selected for the information bank. Instead, their prejudices cause them to opt for publications on the latest drugs and up-to-date surgical procedures. Even though the last decade or so has produced an abundance of scientific study in the fields of nutrition, fitness, and allergy, little of it makes it's way into mainstream channels."

Dr. Braly also brings out another very important point when he observes there is a double standard when it comes to research. Though only a small percentage of commonly accepted medical procedures and techniques have been subjected to the rigorous scientific testing and double blind studies that traditional medicine advocates, established medicine expects an extraordinarily high level of study and research for even the most innocuous procedures and treatments of alternative medicine.

In fact, the Library of Congress backs Dr. Braly's statement in its study *Assessing the Efficacy and Safety of Medical Technology*. This study found that only 10–20% of all procedures used in present day medical practice have been shown to be of benefit by scientifically controlled clinical trials. It was concluded that the vast majority of medical procedures now being utilized routinely by physicians are "unproven" when subject to the same rigid standards these same orthodox physicians are demanding of alternative, nutritional practitioners.

No wonder, then, that nutrition and natural medicine have been left "out in the cold" when it comes to mainstream U.S. health consciousness until only very recently. Now things have really begun to turn around, and even "deprioritized information" about nutrition and disease is starting to be brought out publicly and even emphasized. As a society, we are finally starting to look for the answer to wellness in the right places. But this progress is only just beginning.

In light of the ever-rising costs of healthcare—and considering that the WHO (World Health Organization), FAO (Food and Agricultural Organization), and other health authorities rate the average U.S. health status so poorly (anywhere from 24th out of 25 countries to 138th out of the healthiest 150 countries in the world), despite the largest health—care budget in the world—it's about time that things changed drastically. Must we occupy the worst epidemiological categories in the world for diseases like cancer, heart disease, osteoporosis, arthritis, obesity, allergies, etc.? Does the U.S. have to go financially bankrupt from the maintenance of ineffective healthcare philosophies? I believe not, especially with people like you and I advocating for change! (It is heartening to learn that the new Bush administration in the White House considers healthcare reform its third highest priority.)

With rampant over-the-counter and illegal drug use, a PDR *(Physician's Desk Reference)* containing over 3,000 pages describing nearly 2,900 prescribable drugs—and with the majority of these pages devoted to explaining contraindications and often lethal side effects—the U.S. is considered by the WHO as the most drug-laden society in the world. Hence, we have a (so-called) "war on drugs" and their abuses. We are finally getting the picture! Symptom-relief drugs aren't the answer! It's not too late! All we have to do is get "back to the basics," and travel full circle in our wellness philosophies—away from crisis medicine and toward a "natural medicine" or "naturopathic" orientation. Let's de-emphasize the use of all drugs in favor of natural cause-relief medicine.

Historically, this is exactly what seems to be happening. All of the previously overlooked "old-fashioned information" about cause-relief natural medicine (widely considered "alternative medicine") is progressively gaining popularity over symptom-relief (i.e., modern) medical practices. And this is exactly what must happen if we are going to get to the very core of what guarantees wellness and longevity for each and every one of us.

TABLE 1

FULL CIRCLE OF WELLNESS PHILOSOPHY

(Natural ➡ Symptom—Relief ➡ Natural)

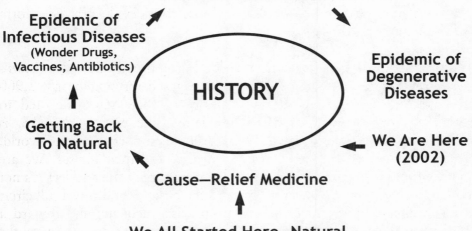

Symptom—Relief Drugs
Wellness Emphasis On: Sophisticated Medical Technologies
Crisis Intervention Medicine

Epidemic of Infectious Diseases
(Wonder Drugs, Vaccines, Antibiotics)

HISTORY

Epidemic of Degenerative Diseases

Getting Back To Natural

We Are Here (2002)

Cause—Relief Medicine

We All Started Here—Natural
(Ancient Times)
Clean Air, Water, Environment
Proper Nutrition, Regular Exercise
Prevention and CAUSE—RELIEF Medicine
(Diet, Genetics, Lifestyle)

The U.S. model of wellness has historically traveled from its natural medicine origins and philosophies into the allopathic, "modern medicine" era, and is now finally headed back into a renewed natural medicine megatrend, as Table 1 demonstrates. Wonder drugs (vaccines, antibiotics) were created to combat infectious disease (polio, small pox, septicemia, etc.), which plagued us through the turn of the century. Freed from the grip of these diseases, our society then moved into a wellness orientation based on symptom-relief drugs and technologies. Now we are headed into a new, "natural medicine" orientation to offset the epidemic of degenerative disease, the root causes of which our present day technologies and drugs can't overcome.

TABLE 2
CONTEMPORARY MEDICAL COMMUNITY

Traditional Medicine aka Allopathics aka Mainstream Medicine	Alternative Medicine aka Natural Medicine
Established conventional "politically correct" medicine operating on the premise that germs cause disease and must be dealt with using anti-germ and anti-symptom drugs. Consists of primarily M.D.'s. (the "charmed circle"*)	Generic term that falls outside of the "establishment" or "charmed circle." Practitioners subscribe to the philosophy that you treat the body to strengthen it against the germ. These Natural Medicine specialties include: Chiropractic, Acupuncture, Sports Medicine, Nutrition, Clinical Ecology, Preventive Medicine, Orthomolecular Medicine, Naturopathy, Homeopathy, Iridology, Reflexology, etc., or any discipline that predominantly relies on nutrition, exercise, and self care rather than physician managed drugs and surgery.
Emphasis on post-crisis medicine focusing on drug-oriented "symptom-relief" surgical procedures and highly infectious diseases. Conventional physicians treat symptoms.	*Emphasis* on prevention, cause-relief, and non-surgical therapies. Natural orientation physicians treat the cause.
Benefits "Wonder Drugs" like antibiotics and vaccines, life-saving surgeries, and elaborate diagnostic techniques.	*Benefits* naturopathic therapeutic approach to all disease treating its underlying causes in the body but especially effective for degenerative, diet-related, and neuro-musculoskeletal disease. (80% of all disease is diet-related.)
Shortcomings No deep or lasting therapeutic impact on the majority of disease endemic to the U.S. Contributes multiple side-effects and after effect syndromes in patients.	*Shortcomings* some infectious diseases and life-threatening crises this type of medicine is not appropriate for.
Origins Allopathy has been around for approximately one century in its present drug-medicine, and surgery-dependent form. Should really be called Alternative Medicine due to its lack of long term roots in history. In fact, most (if not all medical practitioners prior to the1900s relied completely on "natural remedies. There weren't many synthetic drugs at that time.	*Origins* many thousands of years of folk medicine, Chinese Medicine, Egyptian Medicine, Ayurvedic/Seyurvedic Medicine, Greek (Hippocrates) Medicine, etc., combinedwith modern Naturopathy and drugless healing techniques. Should really be called Traditional Medicine not Alternative Medicine.

*A term used by Dr. James Braly to reflect the political union of modern medical practitioners.

Notable Quotables From Our Top Trendsetters

The following quotes represent what many of our society's trendsetters are saying about the direction wellness must take. These trendsetters are helping us to move more quickly through the Circle of Wellness back towards the natural origins of healing and health.

Modern medicine is already in its twilight years. It is about 40 or 50 years old and by now there's been a chance for the ill effects to catch up with the originally heralded benefits. The breakthroughs have turned out to be breakdowns and most of the shiny metal has turned out to be tarnished.
—Robert Mendelson

Western scientific medicine is largely concerned with objective, non-personal, physiochemical explanations of disease as well as its technical control. In contrast, many traditional systems of healing are centered on the phenomenon of illness, namely the personal and social experience of disease . . . . Where Western scientific medicine focuses on curing the disease, traditional medicine aims primarily at healing the illness—that is managing the individual and social response to disease.
—David S. Sobel

It's more important to know what kind of patient has a disease than what kind of disease a patient has.
—Hippocrates

Never let a surgeon take out a functionless organ unless it is really diseased. Functionless organs have a way of turning into very useful ones as soon as researchers admit the possibility of function and try to document it.
—Andrew Weil, M.D.

A doctor is a person who still has his adenoids, tonsils, and appendix.
—Lawrence J. Peter

God heals and the doctor takes the fee.
—**Benjamin Franklin**

The placebo is the doctor who resides within.
—**Norman Cousins**

Although analytical approaches to the body and its intake and surroundings have provided much useful information, such fragmented investigations have also obscured dynamic interrelationships which have an important bearing in medicine.
—**Theron Randolph, M.D.**

The whole imposing edifice of modern medicine, for all its breathtaking successes is, like the celebrated Tower of Pisa, slightly off balance.
—**Prince Charles**

The problem here is that the practice of the art of medicine has now developed into what is called "the delivery of healthcare". Health care is a commodity and falls under as it were, the laws of "Caesar." Caring for the sick is not and cannot be entirely a commodity for it requires of man faculties that are aspects of the movement toward inner consciousness, a movement that obeys other laws than the laws of rationalistic, societal order. It requires a non-egoistic attention in a non-egoistic intellect. The practice of medicine, therefore, places the physician between the two worlds, and it does so far more obviously and inescapably than any other profession in our culture.
—**Jacob Needleman**

One of the things the average doctor doesn't have time to do is catch up with the things he didn't learn in school and one of the things he didn't learn in school is the nature of human society, its purpose, its history, and its needs . . . . If medicine is necessarily a mystery to the average man, nearly everything else is necessarily a mystery to the average doctor.
—**Milton Mayer**

The realities of medical economics encourage doctors to do less listening to, thinking about, sympathizing with and counseling of patients—what doctors call "cognitive services." Instead the doctor is encouraged to act, to employ procedures.
—David Hillficker

The art of medicine consists of amusing the patient while nature cures the disease.
—Voltaire

The mechanistic view of the human organism has encouraged an engineering approach to health in which illness is reduced to mechanical trouble and medical therapy to mechanical manipulation.
—Fritjof Capra, M.D.

Health is not so much the absence of disease as it is the presence of an optimal healing process.
—M. Scott Peck

The more I have studied the medical literature the harder it has gotten for me to listen to the dairy industry's promotion of "milk for strong bones." In spite of its high calcium content, milk, because of its high protein content appears actually to contribute to the accelerating development of osteoporosis. The occurrence of this condition has reached truly epidemic proportions in the United States and the promotion of dairy products as an answer to the suffering of millions seems to me to be not only self-serving, but even criminal.
—John Robbins

We appear to be individual bodies, but this individuality is also in a constant state of equilibrium between a true personal authenticity and a continuous participation with the collective energy of all humanity and all existence.
—Richard Moss

The human organism is much larger than we imagined, for as a living entity it is inseparable from a "personal ecology," its working balances with the world. The body is also a much more porous entity than we see, through which millions of microorganisms and foreign molecules circulate, these cohabitors and invaders are held in check by the body's homeostatic, immunological, and detoxification systems and by the benign flora of the gut and other ecological forces.
—Joseph D. Beasley, M.D.

The human body is the universe in miniature. That which cannot be found in the body is not to be found in the universe. Hence, the philosophers' formula, that the universe within reflects the universe without. It follows, therefore, that if our knowledge of our own body could be perfect, we would know the universe.
—Mahatma Gandhi

The mainstream of medicine cannot be identified with any one medical system; rather the mainstream is formed by all the tributaries. Is it even right to assume that there should be a mainstream at all? Perhaps we need to keep the natural rivers running freely rather than dammed and confined.
—Ted Kaptchuk

Even your body is really not your own. It belongs to life, and it is your responsibility to take care of it. You cannot afford to do anything that injures your body, because the body is the instrument you need for selfless action.
—Eknath Easuaran

Be careful about reading health books. You may die of a misprint.
—Mark Twain

I have finally come to the conclusion that a good reliable set of bowels is worth more to a man than any quantity of brains.
—Henry Wheeler Shaw

The person who is afraid to alter his living habits, because he is afraid that other persons may regard him as queer, eccentric or fanatic forgets that the ownership of his body, the responsibility for its well-being belongs to him, not them.
—**Paul Brunton**

Now good digestion wait on appetite. And health on both!
—**William Shakespeare**

To eat is human, to digest, divine.
—**Charles Townsend Copeland**

You can only cure retail but you can prevent wholesale.
—**Brock Chisholm**

The environment is a candidate for healing along with the individual person.
—**David J. Hufford**

Drugs and surgery are all too often given as substitutes for understanding and changing what I believe are the primary underlying causes of coronary heart disease: harmful responses to emotional stresses, a high fat, high cholesterol diet primarily based on animal products and cigarette smoking.
—**Dean Ornish, M.D.**

As to diseases, make a habit of two things: to help or at least do no harm.
—**Hippocrates**

All you have to do is rest. Nature herself, when we let her, will take care of everything else. It's our impatience that spoils things. Most men die of their cures, and not of their diseases.
—**Jean Molière**

Health is the normal and harmonious vibration of the elements and forces composing the human entity on the physical, mental, and moral (emotional) planes of being, in conformity with the constructive principle (great law of life) in nature.
—Henry Lindlahr

To wish to be healthy is part of being healthy.
—Seneca

He is the best physician who is the ingenious inspirer of hope.
—Samuel Taylor Coleridge

Every part of a bone she (nature) makes bone, every part of the flesh, she makes flesh, and so with fat and all the rest; there is no part she has not touched, elaborated, and embellished.
—Galen

Even as the wise physician takes full armamentarium available to him, he never misses the opportunity to educate the patient to the truth that drugs aren't always necessary and that the human body is its own best drug store for most symptoms.
— Norman Cousins

Medical doctors to whom we have entrusted our health because we have not yet learned to care for ourselves, studied disease rather than health in medical school.
—Udo Erasmus, Ph.D.

Half of what we have taught you is wrong. Unfortunately, we do not know which half.
—Dean Burwell

M.D. does not stand for medical deity.
—Bernie Siegel, M.D.

Healthcare should be about health instead of disease. It should be about being as well as you can be, and not just free of symptoms for the moment. It should be about "How healthy can I become?" instead of "oh, good, I don't have any symptoms today." It should be about prevention rather than cure, and about having sufficient vitality to run in road races at age 85, rather than being frail, sickly, and debilitated (or dead). Healthcare should actually be about dying of old age—at 100 or older—instead of from a disease induced and nurtured by the very system that professes to be interested in our health. And finally, healthcare should be a cooperative effort of dedicated physicians from all health disciplines, rather than a political prizefight in which the championship belt is the marketplace. You deserve so much more than you are getting.
—Richard E. DeRoeck, D.C.

A recent government statistic reflected that approximately five times more patients have sought "alternative healthcare" (from practitioners without M.D.'s) than ever before. Compound this statistic with the mammoth growth of the nutrition, exercise, and motivational industries, and you have a new (yet ancient) megatrend of wellness consciousness permeating the U.S., completely centered on "natural" medicine and a self-help emphasis.

There is, however, something that is complicating this scenario, especially with regard to the science of nutrition and its controlling forces. In fact, the latest megatrend of utilizing nutrition to affect wellness is already passé, obsolete in the face of the next (and final) megatrend of nutrition-oriented wellness. This next megatrend represents the "final frontier" of applied nutritional science and is the main focus of this book.

It will come as a surprise that many of the ancient medicine systems originated certain premises and principles highly characteristic of this final megatrend toward natural wellness. A large amount of new information has systematically been compiled over the last 100 years to strengthen its scientific validity and therapeutic applications beyond the wisdom of the ancients. Even the mainstream magazine *Life* made special note of this. In his September 1996 cover story, "The Healing Revolution," George Howe Colt makes the following point: "Surgery or acupuncture? Antibiotics or herbs? Both are better. More and more M.D.'s are mixing Ancient Medicine and New Science to treat everything from the common cold to heart disease."

It's interesting to note that, just when our values toward and application of nutrition in wellness has come full circle, the leading scientific authorities now demonstrate that our generalized nutritional approach is built on a fallacy! Scientific proof is continually compounding to this effect, giving birth to the final megatrend of applied nutrition—the missing link in the way we view wellness and our world, the "final frontier."

Our current nutritional dilemma is quite simple. We routinely apply nutrition on a one-size-fits-all basis, through the "shotgun approach" (all-or-nothing), or via the "piecemeal" philosophy (a little bit of this or a little bit of that) when it comes to our diets and supplements. This simply does not work!

You can be truly healthy when you know how to work with your own uniqueness. *For Your Body* Only will take you where you've never been before—beyond *Perfect Health, The Zone, Blood Type Diet*, and the rest of the bestsellers on nutrition, fitness, and health! You are now entering the final frontier of wellness! It's truly a sad commentary when you consider that most of this insightful information has actually been at our fingertips all along. If only our scientific contemporaries had prioritized this wellness wisdom over the last 100 years, we would not be suffering from our current epidemic of diet-related disease.

Allow me to show you how and why these nutritional practices simply do not work, and what you can do to change—right now! Let me reveal to you the secret of the ancients (and scientific contemporaries). Let me show you why "one-size-fits-all" is now extinct and how the next and final megatrend of nutrition, exercise, and motivation will achieve the balance of wellness you've sought for so long! Let me bring you into a world of individualization you never dreamt possible!

CHAPTER ONE

How the *One-Size-Fits-All* Mindset Is Wrecking Our Health

Progress can only be made by ideas which are very different from those accepted at the moment.
—**Hans Selye**

Nutrition is like a chain in which all of the essential items are the separate links. If the chain is weak or broken at any point, the whole chain fails. If there are 40 items that are essential in the diet, and one of these are missing, nutrition fails just as truly as it would if half the links were missing. The absolute lack of any one item (or several items) results in ill-health and eventually death. An insufficient amount of any one item is enough to bring the stress to the cells and tissues, which are most vulnerable to this particular lack . . . . The links in the nutrition chain are chemical; salt is a chemical, sugar is a chemical, bread and milk are chemicals.
—**Arthur J. Vander, M.D.**

One-size-fits-all nutrition is the basic philosophy of choosing our foods and nutrition supplements on the premise of "what's good for you must be good for me." You see the application of this nutritional philosophy everyday in health food stores, supermarkets, on television, at fitness centers, at home, and in most nutrition and wellness books. The neighborhood health food store salesperson, your favorite celebrity, your workout partner, your family members, and your best friends all love to tell you about their favorite vitamin or food that they swear will work for you because it works for them. They advise you to take the vitamin they are taking, eat the foods they are eating, based on a scientifically unfounded assumption that, first of all, this product is actually good for them—something that is very difficult to prove—and second of all, that this product is right for you as well. This may be even harder to prove.

The Phenomenon of *Biochemical Individuality*

The fact is, science has thoroughly demonstrated that "no two people are exactly alike" in the way their bodies and minds function, and in the precise needs of their minds and bodies for overall wellness. Scientists refer to this phenomenon of personal uniqueness as biochemical individuality.

No two people have the same fingerprint. Most people know this but our individual differences go much deeper. You may recall the movie True Lies, where Arnold Schwarzenegger and Tom Arnold play secret agents. In the movie, an optic reader (computerized opthamalascope) identifies their retinal image before they are allowed to enter their maximum-security headquarters. The obvious (and accurate) inference here is that no two people have the same retinal image. The way we look on the outside (face shape, nose, all body characteristics) provides only minor clues to the very complex differences on the inside of our bodies. No two bodies inside or out are exactly alike. Even identical twins have external and internal differences which can become greater with age. And, of course, everyone who followed the O. J. Simpson case in the summer of 1995 knows that no two blood samples are exactly the same either.

In 1956, Roger Williams published the book *Biochemical Individuality* in which he presented scientific evidence demonstrating the true uniqueness of our bodies. From a biochemical and physiological standpoint, our bodies vary widely from person to person to person. Through hundreds of varied research studies, Dr. Williams presented evidence that everyone is biochemically unique in both external and internal anatomy, and in our chemical composition which is the very essence of our life.

The Breakthrough Science of
Metabolic Typing

Much more research has been accomplished in this area of "biochemical uniqueness" which has led to an entire science of Metabolic Typing, Patterning, and/or Profiling (these terms can be used interchangeably), which continuously reinforces the universal phenomenon that no two people are alike. We do not look the same, act the same, or require the same things for our daily survival. This is especially true when it comes to nutrition.

The next three chapters of this book, along with Table 3—"Categories of Human Uniqueness," will give you a more in-depth look at biochemical individuality and its true implications for each of us. In lieu of this, we can accurately assume that there is overwhelming scientific information establishing that we are each unique.

This chapter will focus on a definitive answer to the question: why does the one-size-fits-all nutritional philosophy persist? From a simple logical standpoint, it doesn't make sense.

If we are all different,

Why do we all strive to eat the same food, take the same supplements, and go on the same lifestyle programs?

Why do we listen to our favorite celebrity, our brother or sister, our brother or sister, our workout partner, personal trainer, and even a doctor that pushes this philosophy?

Why do we strive so much to cut out red meat, or fat, or salt, or whatever from our own diet, in order to fit ourselves into the latest trend, fad, or social movement?

Putting logic aside, the answer is simply that we don't know any better.

"Quick fixes, magical drugs, and ignorance-generated profitability dominate the marketplace"

In the first place, we are not generally aware of Metabolic Typing and Profiling science with its tried and tested implications. In the second place, we are part of a society geared to mass production, oriented toward quantitative results. In this environment, there is a prevailing medical atmosphere of dependence on symptom-relief medicine, instead of on cause-relief, person-specific naturopathic qualitative intervention. Our society's mindset has been turned away from encouraging the acceptance of our metabolic differences in order to expedite more person-specific approaches for nutrition-mediated wellness. Instead, "quick fixes," "magical drugs," and "ignorance-generated profitability" dominate the marketplace.

Our current generic societal mindset is based on special interest wellness politics, and to some extent on the "so-called" sociocultural lag in research where "cutting edge" information is politically delayed or manipulated before being released to the public. These political manipulations and information delays keep us focused away from the realities of wellness to keep profits up for certain groups. The books, *Good Intentions*, by Bruce Nussbaum and *Innocent Casualties* by Elaine Feuer can help you to better understand this situation.

Our society offers what is currently most profitable to the status quo of those political powers governing wellness. This situation is not just observable in the halls of modern medicine—where drug dependence abounds—but within your average health food store as well. As you walk into a typical health food store, you are bombarded by shelves and shelves of one supplement after another, along with many a salesperson eager to sell you "one of each" with no relevant scientific basis for product discrimination. Your invitation for being sold a given supplement is something like "it's the hottest right now," "it works for me," or "most customers really like this one," etc. This kind of philosophic persuasion reinforces one-size-fits-all notions . . . and worse. You'll routinely end up spending more money on items that you actually don't need.

In this scenario, there's really no true person-specific measure of the success these wellness products may have in actually helping you. And, of course, the health food store makes more money on your gullibility and confusion as a consumer. That's all part of the plan to get your money! A former vice president of one of the largest U.S. health food store chains once told me "there's greater profitability in ignorant customers." Isn't that the truth? So don't automatically expect "natural-conscious" industries to tell you much about human individuality either—it's not in their best interest for moneymaking (you won't buy as much).

On the contrary, those "natural wellness" industries "train" you with one-size-fits-all information strategically designed to make you interested in more products so that their profits will soar. As you can see, even the anti-traditional, anti-drug, "rebel" nutritional industries should be seen as guilty for their fostering of one-size-fits-all mentalities; yet, in an apparent paradox, they are helping to move us away from modern medicine's unnatural philosophies by promoting natural products and alternatives. The good news for "capitalists" is that Metabolic Typing and Profiling will ultimately improve business for health food stores. The good news for "health fanatics" is that Metabolic Typing and Profiling will help health food stores to assist you better than ever before.

Why the 40-30-30 Zone recommendations are fundamentally unsound

The Zone, by Barry Sears, Ph.D., is considered by some to be a breakthrough in nutrition science. In this book, the notion is put forth that we are each fundamentally alike metabolically, and that we therefore require daily macronutrient proportions of 40-30-30 (carbohydrates-protein-fat) for optimum metabolism. This could not be further from the truth, given our inherent biochemical uniqueness. Due to differences in our oxidation rates and oxidation amounts, endocrine balance, nerve types, physical characteristics (muscles, bones, shape, etc.), personality patterns, blood types, activity patterns,and many biochemical constituents, our optimum macronutrient ratios (and micronutrient ratios) vary from person to person.

(By the way, the concept of increasing protein intake while decreasing carbohydrate intake to speed up metabolism, help decrease body fat, and reduce water retention (as touted in The Zone) has been understood and practiced for many years, and is nothing new to anyone well versed in human biochemistry and physiology. Most bodybuilders are aware of this technique as well, and manipulate these food proportions to aid in the reduction of body fat and water retention. In fact, many bodybuilders will use a 50 (protein), 30 (carbohydrate), 20 (fat) zone to optimize leanness and hardness in their physiques. For most competitors it works better than 40-30-30 to peak, although again this varies from person to person.)

The one-size-fits-all nutrition research of Dr. Sears typifies much of the nutritional and medical research to which we continually subscribe. Research subjects are routinely studied on a given nutritional protocol, drug or exercise regimen, with little if any differentiation between subjects other than age, weight, sex, and ethnicity. Further metabolic and body type distinctions and differentiations must be made on subjects before including them in research studies. Further "human uniqueness" differentiations will greatly increase the accuracy of research conclusions and add many more dimensions to its implications.

Because of the scarcity of this type of research approach, where human uniqueness is closely differentiated, is it any wonder that one given study will extol the cancer-fighting virtues of betacarotene, for example, while another repeat study condemns the use of betacarotene to prevent cancer and actually concludes that it may cause cancer? This "research conflict" and many more might be discontinued if the study subjects were better differentiated, in accordance with their biochemical individuality. (It just so happens that in the case of betacarotene supplementation some metabolic types will absolutely thrive, while too much betacarotene will be harmful for other metabolic types.)

Your doctor too, is just guessing most of the time

It should be evident that one-size-fits-all research contributes to our one-size-fits-all notions about health and nutrition. Even your family doctor experiments or guesses about what drug he or she prescribes for you, basing the decision on one-size-fits-all perspective with perhaps a little more differentiation (hopefully). Your doctor will be quick to change prescriptions if you don't react favorably, however— he or she is merely guessing about what's right for you in the first place! Imagine if your doctor could differentiate human uniqueness better from the start and prescribe a drug perfectly matched to you. Patients would respond faster, with far fewer side effects.

Unfortunately, our modern medical system is far too engrossed in a one-size-fits-all philosophy, in much the same way as our drugless and preventive medicine practices. Societal emphasis on the one-size-fits-all mindset is reinforced by the practices of both modern medicine and alternative medicine; society's rigidity on this point has ultimately gotten us into a health rut (more about that in Chapter II). As it stands today, we duplicate one-size-fits-all practices habitually without giving it a second thought.

The Three Primary Characteristics of The One-Size-Fits-All Mindset

For now, let's simply acknowledge the existence and practice of one-size-fits-all, especially in relation to nutrition and health (in general). There are three primary characteristics of the one-size-fits-all mentality, which further complicate this erroneous philosophy.

The Way of the *Piecemealer*—
A Little Bit of This, A Little Bit of That

The first practice within the scope of one-size-fits-all nutrition is known as piecemealing or the piecemeal approach to nutrition and health. This is the practice whereby one chooses (supposedly) to complete their nutrition and health program in unconnected bits and pieces. "I'll have that vitamin C . . . I hear that's good . . . perhaps a green drink, and maybe some whitefish today" is what a piecemealer may think. Piecemealing is the art of picking and choosing nutritional components on the basis of guesswork related to what an individual superficially "thinks" they need. Today it's betacarotene, tomorrow it's the grapefruit diet.

This "art" of self-prescription is a manifestation of one-size-fits-all with no scientific foundation, strategy, or philosophy that can impart a meaningful validity. In other words, it is simply a practice of haphazard, non-analytical experimentation without any connection to the reality of what one's actual nutritional needs are, in part or in their entirety. I've seen piecemealers pick various foods and supplements like vitamin E, selenium, broccoli, or tofu without any rhyme or reason other than the following rationale: "the topsoil lacks selenium," "vitamin E is an antioxidant," "broccoli is considered a cancer preventative," and "tofu is better for you than red meat." These piecemeal bits of information are tidbits picked up from various generic sources (friends, media, etc.), but they really have no direct connection to the specific needs of any particular individual.

It should be obvious that the "art" of piecemealing is totally inadequate when it comes to precisely accounting for the 76-plus minerals, 17 vitamins, 5 macronutrients, 40 amino acids, 43 essential fatty acids, and the thousands of vitamin-like substances and phytonutrients your particular body needs in varying degrees for optimum health and well-being.

Few people (in modern society) are able to even come close to choosing the entire optimum eating regimen their bodies need in actuality without a profound nutritional background combined properly with rigorous lab-mediated metabolic testing; there are also 400 measurable toxins to consider as well.

Maybe that's why the HANES (Health And Nutrition Examination Survey) I and II government-sponsored studies found that, of the people tested, over 81% demonstrated profound deficiencies in nutrients—this statistic included supplement takers and people on special diets. Independent lab studies show upwards of 94% of those tested with deficiencies and overloads present. You cannot simply guess your way to a non-deficiency/overload, non-toxic metabolic status—excess nutrients can be as bad for you as deficiencies and can also act as toxins "to boot".

The Way of the *Shotgunner*— If a Little Is Good, More is Better

The "Shotgun Express" is another offshoot of one-size-fits-all nutritional philosophy. This is the phenomenon characterized by the old adage "if a little is good, more is better." Shotgunners simply megadose on foods and supplements that they perceive as good for them. Not satisfied with a little of one thing or another, because somehow they believe that smaller amounts are not adequate for them, shotgunners tend to take the largest individual dosages and the greatest quantity of differing supplements overall.

Shotgunners typically consume nutritional supplements in extreme excess of the recommendations of the RDA, DV, MDR, or other standards-setting organization, in an effort to "absolutely make sure" they are getting enough of what they think they need to achieve whatever health and fitness objectives they have in mind. They assume categorically that even if they do consume too much of a given nutrient or other, the body will simply use what it needs and excrete the rest—with no harm done. In actuality, too much of one nutrient or other can do more damage than good to the body. Excess nutrients can be as bad as deficiencies.

To top it all off, shotgunners demonstrate the same profound imbalances as other subjects in nutrition studies. (More about the risks of shotgunning in later chapters).

The Way of the *One Sizer*—
Glib Know-It-All Demands Respect

The last manifestation of the one-size-fits-all nutritional philosophies are what I term the "I know it all" syndrome. Many one sizers tend to think that they know much more about nutritional sciences than they actually do. A one sizer typically may have picked up a few tidbits of information from one source or another, and perhaps has learned something from an actual experience they've had with diet or supplements (for good or bad). Suddenly, they think they are a nutrition expert, or what I term a pseudo-nutritionist. Yes, this one sizer now "knows it all" because they've read Fit or Fat, lost three pounds, and possesses an autographed picture of Deepak Chopra, M.D. They can now determine what's good for you and what you're doing wrong . . . and may God be with you if you disagree with them, because they "know it all."

After all, they've carefully memorized the antioxidant cofactors and can quote their functions word for word, while you don't even know what a cofactor is. Or maybe they'll tell you you're a Vata, Pitta, or Kapha type (per Dr. Chopra's classifications), when in actuality you have one of eighteen other body types with other discernible metabolic inconsistencies not accounted for in ancient Ayurvedic religious practices. Or perhaps your informed pseudo-nutritionist has more hair on their head, or larger biceps, or better complexion—watch out! Prepare to be put in your place! My overall analogy here is that a little knowledge in the hands of unqualified people can be very dangerous to your health (and sometimes your feelings).

Unfortunately, the "I know it all" syndrome only intensifies within the group of self-proclaimed nutritionists who have actually taken a nutrition course or two along the way. These "nutritionists" believe themselves to be professionals, when nothing could be further from the truth. Some within this group may actually have an unaccredited correspondence degree in nutrition and believe themselves to be nutrition experts. In fact, these people are what I term novice nutritionists.

Will the Real Nutritionist Please Stand Up?

A true professional nutritionist, also known as a clinical nutritionist, will have a high school degree, at least a Bachelor's degree (hopefully in health science, biology, chemistry or physical education), optionally a Master's degree within areas related to nutrition, biology or physiology—maybe an R.D. (Registered Dietitian)—and either an M.D., D.O., D.C., D.D.S. or N.D. and/or some type of Ph.D.'s (although a Ph.D. cannot legally treat a patient) with some specialization in nutrition. A clinical nutritionist will have had thousands of hours of basic and clinical sciences including every knowledge parameter from cadaver dissection to treating diet-related illnesses in a clinical environment. Such professionals vigorously subscribe to the tenets of orthomolecular, molecular, quantum, and functional medicine along with anti-aging medicine. They are addressed as "Doctor."

A novice nutritionist, in contrast, falls short of these criteria and cannot possibly understand enough about the human body's inner workings and the clinical application of precise nutritional science protocol to optimize the body's functions. Neither do they have the license nor the proper tools to treat patients nutritionally or legally— so watch out!

The point here is that the novice nutritionist, because of a lack of educational and clinical background, is prone to duplicate the one-size-fits-all mindset without understanding the concept of biochemical individuality.

Furthermore, the novice nutritionist usually has an even more profound ego than the pseudo-nutritionist does because he or she really "knows it all." (Just ask one!)

I must say that doctors are largely to blame for the overabundance of pseudo- and novice nutritionists among the public. If every doctor paid more attention to the role of applied nutrition in wellness, there would be fewer of these unqualified people advising us. Sadly, most consumers don't know just how much further a tried-and-true, nutrition-oriented M.D., D.O., D.C., D.D.S., N.D., or Ph.D. can take them towards perfect health, as opposed to the attempts at help offered by novice and pseudo-nutritionists.

Clinical nutritionists who practice Metabolic Typing and Profiling, using proven biochemical individuality differentiations, represent the most supreme heights within the field of professional nutritionists. They routinely will use "pure" body typing science combined with the specialized analysis of blood, urine, saliva, hair, and fecal samples to precisely determine your body's nutrient needs, and will be able to fully customize diet and supplements specific to these measured needs.

Conclusion

One-size-fits-all nutrition is a way of life for the majority of people who really don't question or aren't taught to question its validity. Even in light of the profound scientific evidence demonstrating that each of us has our own biochemical individuality with specific nutrient needs that differ from person to person, little attention has been paid to this topic overall by health authorities.

CHAPTER TWO

Does One-Size-Fits-All Nutrition Work?

United States of health are, at heart, the organisms success or failure at adapting to environmental challenges.
—**Renee Dubos**

Health and disease just don't happen to us. They are active processes issuing from inner harmony or disharmony profoundly affected by our states of consciousness, our ability or inability to flow with experience.
—**Marilyn Ferguson**

In the final analysis, the survival and health of the individual and (the) species may depend not so much on further developments and technologies as on the collective application of common sense.
—**S. Bryan Furness**

Use the light that is within you to regain your natural clearness of sight.
—**Lao Tzu**

No, no, no!! One-size-fits-all nutritional practices have got to be history's greatest fraud to be perpetrated on the masses, as you will plainly see in this section.

In light of my own academic achievements, clinical experiences, and real life practices, I must say that the one-size-fits-all "malpractice" is my greatest pet peeve . . . it should become yours as well by the end of this book.

I've grouped the reasons one-size-fits-all does not work into 2 categories: Simple Logic and Research Statistics and Implications.

Simple Logic

The discussion of this first category will appeal to you on a "gut level," because it truly connects with your philosophical and intellectual essence. When compared to animals, we, as humans, have an inherent ability to reason things out far beyond any intelligence factor we have ever measured (so far) in the animal kingdom. Each of us progressively builds up an expansive knowledge base, inherently capable of deducing needed information from that base. This process occurs as a direct result of maturing through society's educational and conditioning processes, in combination with our own uniquely personal self-discovery patterns.

Logic is a primary characteristic of our reasoning capabilities. There are two ways to reason things out: *Inductive Reasoning*—where we draw a conclusion about all the members of a class from examination of only a few members of the class or in simpler terms reasoning from the specific to the general. Then there's *Deductive Reasoning*—where we draw a conclusion about a few members of a class after examination of the entire class or reasoning from the general to the specific.

The one-size-fits-all philosophy is an extrapolation of both reasoning systems.

One-size-fits-all thinking assumes as a premise that "if it works for me, it's right for you" (or right for anyone else, for that matter—specific to general; that is, Inductive Reasoning). One-size-fits-all thought assumes as another premise that "if it's good for everyone else, it must be good for me" (general to specific; i.e., Deductive Reasoning).

To better illustrate this point, let's take vitamin A as an example, from a one sizer's point of view. Numerous research studies have demonstrated the need by all humans for vitamin A. So, the deductive inference is that I as an individual must need vitamin A. Because of this, I'll take my dose as determined by the government, according to the recommended daily allowance or RDA.

Now, because I'm taking the RDA for vitamin A, you should take it as well (as should everyone), because if it's good for me it is good for you. This is an inductive inference. Okay, I'll buy that! This logic has you coming and going as regards Vitamin A, from both an inductive and deductive standpoint that meets, somewhat, in the middle.

What happens when you add to this logical formulation that no two people are the same and therefore have many differing needs? Uh-oh—now we can't be sure if one person needs the same amount or type of vitamin A or not, because now we see how false is the assumption that we humans are simply one class of generic bodies, cast from exactly the same mold.

In fact, when it comes to RDA's for vitamin A and all other vitamins and minerals, the Food and Nutrition Board qualifies its RDA data by stating "RDA's should not be confused with requirements for a specific individual. They are not guidelines for formulating diets nor assessing the nutritional status of individuals." Given this information—in order to be logical—we're going to have to go on a case-by-case basis when it comes to nutrition and *deductively* reason specifically for each individual. Maybe along the way we can find subclasses of humans with similar categorizable physiological traits, where more logical assumptions can be made specific to that particular category of humans. Then perhaps we can make some "partially" accurate deductive and inductive inferences for that human subclass only.

Purely on the "gut" level, one-size-fits-all thinking doesn't make logical sense, given the scientific premise that we are each biochemically unique and therefore have different nutritional needs. Yes, all humans need vitamin A, but that's really all we can safely assume. One-size-fits-all does not give you any qualitative parameters, because it falsely deals with humans as one class of physiological beings. It presumes that we're all made from the same mold, when in fact the quality (as well as quantity) of our needs is directly specific to the individual. *Viva la difference!* One-size-fits-all is not logical! It is therefore an invalid philosophy.

Research Statistics and Implications

The effects of our general inattention to nutritional needs, the one-size-fits-all approach to nutrition-mediated wellness, and our dependence upon symptom relief rather than cause-relief medicine is negatively echoed throughout, in a bevy of wellness statistics.

The World Health Organization (WHO) and the Food and Agricultural Organization (FAO) have gone to great lengths to rate the average U.S. health status poorly when compared to the rest of the world. In a society where we spend over a trillion dollars per year on health care—more than any other country in the world—you'd expect the best health in the world. Unfortunately, we're not getting our money's worth and for many valid reasons (the following is based on postulations by the WHO and other agencies):

- Our dependence on crisis-relief and symptom-relief medicine rather than cause-relief medicine

- Our dependence and overuse of both legal and illegal drugs

- Our lack of regular exercise and recreation

- Our stressful lifestyles

- Our polluted environment

- Mass production methods for food production, processing, storage, and distribution which depletes nutrient density and bioactivity

- Nutrient-depleted topsoil

- Our lack of emphasis on preventive medicine including (and especially) proper eating habits

I would like to add one more reason to this list: our reliance on a one-size-fits-all approach to the preceding eight reasons given, especially as it applies to the last reason.

The inference here by the WHO and others is that, if we would remove or improve the eight (or nine) health-restricting dilemmas stated above, the average health status for Americans would improve significantly. This makes sense! Then maybe we'd finally get our money's worth from our trillion-dollar-plus-per-year healthcare budget.

As should be clear by now, this book's primary focus is on reaching the final frontier of nutrition as a people, at which point we may overcome the majority of nutrition-related wellness obstacles that plague society. Unfortunately, one-size-fits-all thinking predominates throughout the current nutritional themes distributed in our nation. Its negative repercussions and health-threatening consequences will become apparent to you in the following, highly condensed overview of statistics and research. The progressive shift of research interests toward the final frontier of nutrition, (i.e., personalization) among health authorities will become dramatically apparent. While the following research clearly demonstrates the ineffectiveness of one-size-fits-all nutritional precepts, it will comfortably bring you to the logical and inevitable wellness solution that we seek, which is to address the needs of each person on a specific, for-your-body-only basis.

Let the Research Speak

The following quotes help to illustrate the point that one-size-fits-all nutrition is totally obsolete and repeatedly confuses the issues concerning wellness. My comments and questions to these research quotes are in parentheses ( ).

Welcome to that zany madcap world of epidemiology, where you, the ambitious scientists, attempt to unequivocally prove your theory of diet and disease. But watch out for those nasty pitfalls! They're out to undermine your work at every turn.
— Bonnie Liebman, M.S., "Playing The Research Game," Nutrition Action Health Letter, Vol. 21, No. 8, October 1994.

From the Update *Mayo Clinic Health Letter*, April 14, 1994, "Beta Carotene Supplements—Do They Prevent Or Promote Lung Cancer?" (Good question! According to studies in the *New England Journal of Medicine*, it cuts both ways. No surprise in a one-size-fits-all world.)

That's when researchers from Finland and the National Cancer institute dropped a double whammy: not only did betacarotene and vitamin E supplements fail to reduce the risk of lung cancer, they might cause harm . . . . "It was totally unexpected," says Charles Henneteens, researcher from the Harvard School of Public Health. Robert McLennan from the Queensland Institute of Medical Research said quoting from his study, "People taking betacarotene developed 40% more precancerous polyps of the colon." Dr. Ziegler from the U.S. National Cancer Institute stated, "It's conceivable that certain amounts of a single form of beta carotene could interfere with the absorption, transport or utilization of other forms of betacarotene, other carotenoids, or other important compounds in fruits and vegetables."
—*Nutrition Action Health Letter*, Vol. 21, No. 5, June 1994.

The research presented in the preceding pages offers evidence (in this case regarding betacarotene) that one-size-fits-all nutrition serves only to confuse the issue of what's good for you and what's not good for you. (It's hard to be sure when even the authorities can't figure it out.)

When you take an herbal supplement, you do so at your own risk.
—*Mayo Clinic Health Letter*, Vol. 12, No. 6, June 1994.

Fish oil did not lower blood pressure—as some researchers have suggested—in one study of 18 people with mild hypertension and a second study of 38 middle-aged men with normal or elevated pressure.
—*Nutrition Action Health Letter*, Vol. 2, No. 6, July/August 1993. (You mean fish oil doesn't lower blood pressure? Earlier studies have demonstrated that it does. What gives? The studies referred to above were taken from the *American Journal of Clinical Nutrition*, Vol. 57, No. 59, 1993, and the *American Journal of Public Health*, Vol. 83., No. 267, 1993.)

". . . two European studies say that margarine trans fats don't raise the risk of heart disease . . . . The studies were fatally flawed," according to Walter Willett of the Harvard School of Public Health, "When people are fed trans fat their cholesterol levels rise."
—*Nutrition Action Health Letter*, Vol. 22, No. 4, May 1995. (The moral here is that you can't trust most research because it can change the latest news headlines from moment to moment. This only serves to confuse the one-size-fits-all state of mind.)

I also don't believe in over-the-counter supplements. They help some people, harm others, and have no effect on most. Popping vitamins doesn't do you any good . . . . We get all the vitamins we need in our diets and taking supplements just give you expensive urine . . . . Sometimes Vitamin C is a pro-oxidant—it creates free radicals and promotes disease... None of the antioxidants are pure oxidants. They are all redox agents—sometimes antioxidant—sometimes pro-oxidant.
—Dr. Victor Herbert, M.D., "What You Should Know About Vitamins—The Case Against Supplements," *Bottom Line*, Vol. 15, No. 23, December 1, 1994. (What's a one sizer to do!? Dr. Herbert, after all, is considered to be the "Godfather of the RDA's")

More is not always better.
—*From the Mayo Clinic Health Letter*, Vol. 12, No. 9, September 1994. (You can do more damage than you may think when it

comes to overdosing foods and supplements—shotgunners beware!)

A person taking high doses of niacin to lower his cholesterol developed severe life-threatening hyperglycemia (high blood sugar levels).
—*Archives of Internal Medicine*, Vol. 153, No. 2050, 1993. (You take niacin to lower your cholesterol and then risk suffering from diabetes? Be brave, one sizers!)

Question—Do I need calcium supplements? Answer—It depends on who you are and how much calcium you get from foods.
—*Nutrition Action Health Letter*, Vol. 22, No. 4, May 1995. (This answer probably doesn't make much sense to a one sizer.)

I don't want to suggest that there's no such thing as an age-related decline in immune function. But the rate of decline is much greater than it needs to be, because we can slow it down through nutritional interventions . . . . So the U.S. Recommended Daily Allowance (USRDA) of 2 mg. (vitamin B6) wasn't enough? That's right. It was inadequate to maintain optimal immune function."
—Jeffrey Blumberg (Associate Director for the U.S. Department of Agriculture's Human Nutrition Research Center on Aging at Tuft's University), *Nutrition Action Health Letter*, Vol. 20, No. 3, April 1993. (According to Dr. Blumberg, you could be making a big mistake if you practice one-size-fits-all nutrition and expect your immune system to be up to par—especially if you use the RDA's as your guide.)

Can I overdose on vitamin A? Yes, vitamin A overdose may appear if you take five to ten times the Reference Daily Intake.
—*Mayo Clinic Health Letter*, Vol. 12, No. 8, August 1994. (Shotgunners take heed!) Also from the same health letter: "No more standard diet—the new recommendations (from the ADA— American Diabetes Association) stress the need for personalizing your diet but the key is individualization." (Surprise, surprise! Even the ADA doesn't like one-size-fits-all practices!)

Natural Doesn't Mean Safe.
—*Mayo Clinic Health Letter*, Vol. 12, No. 6, June 1994. (In reference to supplements:) "Yet there's scanty proof that supplements can actually help you." (This is something we'd expect from one-size-fits-all supplementation.)

Today's physicians perform just 20–60% of the preventative health services recommended by expert groups.
—*Harvard Health Letter*, Vol. 20, No. 3, January 1995. (The WHO told us this a long time ago).

People who are allergic to latex are likely to have problems with certain fruits.
—Harvard Health Letter, Vol. 19, No. 5, March 1994., (Are you one of these people? How can you tell?)

Anesthesia with nitrous oxide (a painkiller dentists and surgeons often use) can cause severe neurological damage in people with vitamin B12 deficiency, suggesting that patients at risk should be checked before surgery.
—*Nutrition Action Health Letter*, Vol. 21, No. 3, April 1994.

"Coffee appears to reduce bone density only when calcium intake is inadequate," according to Barrett and Courer.
—Excerpted from *Journal of the American Medical Association* (JAMA), Vol. 271, No. 280, 1994. (But, one sizers, when is calcium intake adequate?)

The benefits of taking aspirin outweighs the risk in men over age 40 who have never had a heart attack as well as in women and men of any age who have already had one. Researchers don't know if the benefits outweigh the risks in women who have never had a heart attack.
—*Nutrition Action Health Letter*, Vol. 22, No. 2, March 1995. (It all sounds risky to a one sizer.)

The tamoxifen trial was halted briefly for reevaluation of the cost/benefit equation. An analysis from the National Cancer Institute predicted that the trial will prevent 133 cases of breast cancer, while causing 83 cases of uterine cancer.
—*John Hopkins Health After 50 Medical Letter*, Vol. 6, No. 8, October 1994. (One-size-fits-all drug taking can be very tricky and exceedingly dangerous to your health. In this case, I call it the "Hurt Peter to Help Paul Syndrome," because while this particular drug helps to prevent one problem, it causes another.)

High temperature meat ended up with more heterocyclic aromatic amines (HAAs). HAAs are formed when juices from meat, poultry, and seafood are broken down by heat . . . . HAAs become carcinogens only after the body activates them . . . . After a week of eating the high temperature meat, 72% of volunteers had more of the liver enzymes that activate HAAs.
—Rashmi Sinha, M.D., *Cancer Research*, Vol. 54, No. 6154, 1994. (Is this a case for or against one-size-fits-all cooking?)

Researchers studied hunter-gatherer societies whose eating habits haven't changed for 40,000 years. Heart disease, stroke, osteoporosis, diabetes, hypertension, and breast cancer are unknown in these societies despite a diet consisting on average of 35% meat.
—From the book *The Paleolithic Prescription*, as noted by Harvard University. (This is in contrast to the 30% protein and 30% fat recommended by *The Zone*: "Meat consumed is 4% fat instead of the 35% fat found in domesticated beef and 65% vegetable." This book makes a strong statement against one-size-fits-all thinking, in favor of individualizing one's diet according to your tribe or genotype. If you're a "hunter or a gatherer" by ancestry or genotype, do as a hunter or gatherer does.)

Nutrition was better before the agricultural revolution than afterwards.
—S. Boyd Eaton, radiologist at Emory University in Atlanta, Georgia. (This is why nowadays it's even more critical that your food intake and supplements be more precisely fit to your individual needs.)

The risk for developing AIDS was 3 times higher for those who consumed more than 20 mg zinc per day.
—*Nutrition Action Health Letter*, Vol. 21, No. 3, April 1993. (This information was also published in a Harvard study found in Science, Vol. 265, No. 1464, 1994: "High levels of zinc may contribute to Alzheimer's." Shotgunners take note of this and one sizers remember not to hurt Peter to help Paul.)

Megadosing vitamins cut in half the reoccurrence of superficial bladder cancer.
—According to a West Virginia University study. (The study subject intake was 40,000 iu vitamin A, 100 mg vitamin B-6, 2,000 mg vitamin C, 400 iu vitamin E, 90 mg zinc—watch out for AIDS and Alzheimer's at this dosage level. This study actually condones shotgunning supplements if you don't mind the extra risks for AIDS and Alzheimer's that taking 90 mg of zinc will create: "A lifetime of coffee drinking will weaken your bones if you consume too little calcium." This last quote brings up the phenomenon of nutrient and anti-nutrient (drug) interaction. This is yet another phenomenon that complicates one-size-fits-all. Even our drinking water is suspect in this regard. A study published in the *Journal of Toxicology*, Vol. 42, No. 109, 1994, found that "Fertility rates proportionately decrease in countries with increased levels of fluoride in water." Many of the most essential nutrients may be lost from your body because of the interactive eating and drug taking habits you have. Sometimes seemingly innocent habits can create major metabolic conflicts which only serve to undermine your health. Are you aware of the metabolic conflicts which specifically plague you? The moral of this and all the preceding narrative is that, sometimes, something we are led to think is good for us may not be, and this problem becomes very tricky when trying to achieve optimum health.)

A low fat diet reduced bad cholesterol even more in people whose genes gave them small LDL (Low Density Lipoprotein) particles than in people with large LDLs. The smaller your LDL, the greater your risk of heart disease.
—*Nutrition Action Health Letter*, Vol. 20, No. 1,   January/

February 1993. (My question to one sizers is do you have big or small LDLs in your blood?)

Question—Is it true that drinking cranberry juice can cure a urinary tract infection? Answer—For the first time, we have evidence that cranberry juice can reduce bacteria in the urinary tract.
—Dr. Jerry Avorn, Associate Professor of Medicine at Harvard Medical School, *By The Way Doctor*, Vol. 19, No. 10, August 1994. (It's about time you found this out, Doc! I've known about this for years from other previous research. Cranberry juice still doesn't work for everyone in the same therapeutic way due to individual differences.)

Tea is impressive because it inhibits such a broad spectrum of cancers.
—Chung S. Yang, Ph.D., Rutgers University. "(But according to a research survey by the *Nutrition Action Health Letter*, Vol. 21, No. 9, November 1994: "One cup of coffee can prevent your body from absorbing about 40% of the iron you've eaten up to an hour before or after—regular black tea is even worse with a 60% decreased absorption of iron." Are we to drink tea to prevent cancer but foster anemia . . . or do we look at tea consumption on a more individualized basis and in conjunction with other nutritional factors?)

The most frequently cited cause of cancer in the news was man-made chemicals followed by food additives, pollution, radiation, pesticides, hormone treatments, sunlight, diet and asbestos . . . . Diet has been linked (by research) to 30% of all cancers.
—*John Hopkins Health After 50 Medical Letter*, Vol. 6, Issue 10, December 1994. (citation of research by the American Association of Cancer Research). (Actually, this last statement is a gross understatement but still brings out the need to scrutinize one's own diet and environment even more carefully again—something that one-size-fits-all practices simply cannot accomplish.)

Can vitamin C supplements cause kidney stones? They may promote kidney stones in those who are at risk for them.
—*John Hopkins Health After 50 Medical Letter*, Vol. 6, Issue 8, October 1994. (Under one-size-fits-all premises, how do you know who's at risk and who's not unless, of course, you already have kidney stones and then again, what kind do you have? Maybe vitamin C doesn't cause your particular kind of kidney stone.)

Asthmatics should not use royal jelly to treat insomnia and liver disease.
—*John Hopkins Health After 50 Medical Letter*, Vol. 6, Issue 6, August 1994.

. . . severe asthma attacks and one death by the use of this product (royal jelly).
—*John Hopkins Health After 50 Medical Letter*, Vol. 6, Issue 6, August 1994 (citing an article from an Australian medical journal). (All I can say here is, piecemealers, shotgunners and one sizers beware. By the way, I personally have completely overcome my own asthma and just love royal jelly!)

Comment: Medical academics continue publicly to support the position that vitamin and mineral supplements are unnecessary. Privately, however, many of them are not so sure. By taking supplements they hope to prolong their lives. By refusing to talk about the benefits of supplements, they hope to prolong their careers.
—Alan R. Galsey, M.D., *Townsend Letter For Doctors,* No. 108, July 1992. (from comments based on a Harvard Medical School study where 80% of the study's respondents reported supplement use and/or dietary manipulation to increase vitamin intake). (From the same health letter, according to Jonathan Collin, M.D., "In testimony before the House Subcommittee on Health and the Environment, Claire A. Farr, President of the National Counsel For Improved Health, claimed that for several decades the FDA has been engaged in an ugly and unjustified vendetta against the foodaceutical industry. It has harassed and persecuted the

manufacturers of vitamins, minerals, and other foods for special dietary use." Politics has only served to make the one-size-fits-all dilemma more confusing, as authorities say one thing and do another to get you to think a certain way even if they don't believe in what they're saying in the first place. Doctors who don't practice what they preach are evident in the Harvard Study. FDA politicians have persecuted a whole health-oriented industry for capitalistic reasons we may never fully understand. All in all, politics and hypocrisy are very much responsible for the occurrence of the one-size-fits-all phenomenon in our society.)

Myth I: You can get all your nutrients from food.
Reality: The majority of people don't eat a healthy balanced diet.
Result: You may not be getting all you nutrients from healthy foods—even if you eat what the government says you should eat. Many trace minerals are deficient in food because of our current farming methods. The biggest problem I see is imbalance—taking a lot of one nutrient and not enough of another without understanding the relationship between the two.
Example: There's a link between magnesium and calcium and between copper and zinc (and all other nutrients). Also, a few vitamins can be taken in excess. Don't overlook red meat. An optimal diet varies from person to person due to individual metabolisms.
—Robban-Sica-Cohen, M.D., "What You Should Know About Vitamins," *Bottom Line*, Vol. 15, No. 22, November 15, 1994. (Dr. Robban-Sica-Cohen, M.D., understands the fallacies inherent in one-size-fits-all thinking and has journeyed into the final frontier of genetically correct, metabolically measured, applied nutrition.)

It is well accepted that nutritional deficiencies or imbalances can adversely affect the health of individuals and delay healing and recovery.
—Luke R. Bucci, Ph.D., CCN, CCA *Journal*, Vol. 19, No. 3, March 1994. (Here's one more reinforcement of the diet-wellness connection and the need for more nutritional individualization to

eliminate deficiencies and imbalances.)

Major health problems are diet-related; the solution to illness can be found in nutrition and the real potential from improved diet is preventative in that it may defer or modify the development of disease state.

—*An Evaluation of Research in the United States on Human Nutrition*, Report 2, Benefits from Nutrition Research,1971, prepared by a Joint Task Group of the U.S. Department of Agriculture and the State Universities and Land Grant Colleges. (This was actually considered a very secret document at one time, when the prevailing political forces wanted to keep the role of diet in disease eradication a secret from consumers for political purposes.)

After reading the preceding information, it should be easier for you to see just how confusing the field becomes when one-size-fits-all nutritional practices are evaluated by one-size-fits-all research, in order to reveal the nutritional keys to total wellness. You can begin to see how politics, common societal practices, and conflicting research just confuse the issues even more in a one-size-fits-all society that is simply not making the grade when it comes to optimizing nutrition-related wellness.

By now, you should also be able to see that the solution to this confusion lies in the direction of individualizing nutrition according to our biochemical and metabolic uniqueness. The following research excerpts will further reinforce the presence of this trend toward scientifically individualized nutrition while decimating any remaining convictions you may still have to one-size-fits-all beliefs.

When it comes to diet-related disease the literature reports that "consistent, long term nutrient deficiencies may evolve into subclinical ailments and ultimately contribute to disease processes such as arthritis, cardiovascular disease, cancer, and immunological dysfunction (to name a few)." This conclusion comes from *The Kellogg Report*: "The Impact of Nutrition, Environment, and Lifestyle on the Health of Americans" by Dr. Beasley, M.D., and Swift, M.A.

Now consider that, in addition to the more obvious nutrient deficiencies viewed as medically harmful, even marginal or "hidden" nutrient deficiencies are also medically harmful. According to the *Vitamin Nutrition Information Service*, Vol. 2, No. 2:

> Marginal vitamin (and mineral) deficiency is a middle ground between adequate nutritional status and the point at which frank deficiency disease symptoms develop. Because there are no specific symptoms, this intermediate stage of depletion is frequently not apparent. In more common terms, it may be the difference between feeling one's best or being under the weather.

One-sizers can only guess about how to avoid deficiencies both obvious and hidden. If people weren't guessing about proper nutrition in the first place, this dilemma wouldn't occur. By the way, "under the weather" is the typical answer of the majority of drug-taking Americans when asked at random how they feel.

Furthermore, according to the *Vitamin Nutrition Information Service*,

> Marginal deficiency may affect the body's ability to resist disease and infection, its ability to recover from surgery, stress or disease, the ability of the brain to function at a higher level and, in general, the optimal development and efficient functioning of the total person.

Also consider the fact that the 1988 Surgeon General's Report on Nutrition and Health concluded that fifteen out of every 24 deaths in the U.S. involve nutrition. (That figure is even higher now.) According to Dr. Wiley, in 1900, the first head of the Department of Agriculture and the FDA reported that only one in seven people died from heart disease (14%); now, statistically, 44% of people die from heart attack, which is categorized today as the number one killer of U.S. citizens and the easiest disease to treat nutritionally.

The story is much the same for cancer. In 1900, only one in 30 died from this disease. Nowadays, one out of every four deaths is attributed to this notoriously diet-related disease. Why would anyone practice one-size-fits-all nutrition, knowing the serious consequences on oneself because of nutritional mistakes? For some perspective, bear in mind that drug side effects are the number four killer of U.S. residents, according to same study—very scary!

The proof of one-size-fits-all failures—and (of course) our general inattention to individualizing diet in the first place—is manifest in the fact that the outright majority of Americans are nutrient deficient. As already mentioned, according to the HANES, studies I and II identified nutrient deficiencies in 81% of *all* persons tested, including those persons taking supplements. However, Meta Metrix Laboratories and others have reported an even greater (over 90%) incidence of nutrient deficiencies in people already taking supplements. In my own nutritional practice, I have *never* encountered a patient who didn't have deficiencies when tested. And the majority of my patients are one sizers who think they eat well and take the "correct" supplements. Are *they* ever surprised when I metabolically type/profile them!

It's no wonder there is such a widespread deficiency problem, when you consider that the RDA's for nutrition are misleading. RDA's confuse attempts to estimate the adequacy of diet and vitamin/mineral/herbal supplementation in the care and treatment of individual patients (of mine or of any other nutrition specialist.) Unfortunately, reassuring *mis*information about RDA's is presented as scientifically founded, government approved, AMA (American Medical Association) endorsed standard nutrition for "average" people. Consequently doctors, nutritionists, and their patients falsely assume that maintaining the RDA level for each nutrient will assure that each patient's requirements are met.

According to the Food and Nutrition Board (*National Academy of Sciences Recommended Dietary Allowances*, 9th Edition): "RDA's should not be confused with requirements for a *specific* individual. They are not guidelines for formulating diets nor for assessing the nutritional status of individuals." The Food and Nutrition Board designed the RDA's in the first place and now have announced their ineffectivity in gauging the needs of specific individuals. What's a one sizer to do? There goes his/her entire belief system!

Numerous studies conducted at the Clayton Biochemical Institute (University of Texas) have demonstrated the therapeutic value of individualized supplementation. They all indicate that deficiency patterns are random and uniquely individualized to different patients and disease processes. Therefore, "each patient should be tested and an individualized nutritional repletion initiated" according to this Institute. These studies have further demonstrated an overwhelming improvement in the symptoms of persons with subclinical ailments (remember that the *Kellogg Report* cited the subclinical ailment dilemma) who followed supplementation guided by nutritional and metabolic test results.

It should be plain by now that simple (generalized) vitamin and mineral supplementation is not adequate health insurance. Scientific data from the analysis of essential micronutrients shows that, of those individuals with clinically demonstrated functional nutrient deficiencies, 53% (tested in this case) were already using some form of dietary supplementation based on RDA levels. These results were found in a study performed by the University of Texas.

Obviously, indiscriminate shotgun and piecemeal vitamin and mineral supplementation do not ensure adequate functional nutrient levels and concomitant protection from advancing chronic and debilitative diseases. This dilemma is further compounded by indiscriminate diet variations because again, each person is biochemically individual with uniquely different food nutrient requirements. These nutrient requirements are not demonstrated by *conventional* medical questionnaires, examinations or laboratory tests. The appropriate "unconventional" tests and procedures, however, will provide a scientific analysis which precisely identifies each person's individual requirements and will specifically indicate those essential nutrients that require therapeutic intervention.

After reading through the previous section, is it any wonder why Harvard University, for one, has withdrawn its support from the "indiscriminate use of diet and supplements" to preserve wellness? This University knows better—that one-size-fits-all nutritional philosophy doesn't work and that individualized nutrition specific to scientific analysis does work. Either way, Harvard doesn't have much faith in the way most people currently go about developing their nutritional programs.

Summary

As a country, the United States is plagued by a growing epidemic of diet-related, degenerative disease. Obesity, heart disease, osteoporosis, cancer, diabetes, arthritis, allergy syndromes, immuno-dysfunction, and many more diseases head the list of our most pressing ailments. Their presence undermines our average health standing when compared to the rest of the world. Our symptom-relief oriented drug-mediated modern medical system is not effectively "treating" these problems.

The majority of the population in the U.S. acknowledges this disturbing health phenomenon, and it is this upsurge that is pushing our society back into a more natural and conservative approach to common illnesses, actively seeking alternative healthcare, better nutrition, and more exercise.

Theoretically, this back-to-natural-health movement should be helping us. But, when it comes to proper nutrition—the absolute foundation of overall wellness—across the board we are not achieving the fullest beneficial results we'd expect. Over time, research statistics have demonstrated little change in our diet-related disease epidemic, other than the progressive emergence of new and more diet-related problems (such as widespread nutritional deficiencies and excesses). The progressive and intensifying appearance of these diet-related problems, now better understood, is helping us to metabolically and genetically explain why we're not achieving the optimum wellness levels we're striving for so intently.

From a nutritional standpoint, our failures all boil down to what I deductively term a "shot in the dark" approach to proper nutrition, a concept we have defined as the one-size-fits-all practice. From one study to the next—whether it's the perplexing research conflicts, hard to explain nutritional interactions, or one-size-fits-all research that only piecemeals nutritional information in the most generalized sense—*one-size-fits-all is just not working!* The attainment of true wellness evades us (and confuses us at the same time), especially taking into consideration some of the conflicting research and opinions presented in this section. Remember, the comments and statistics give here represent only a tiny fragment of the overall research base, which strenuously disproves the validity of one-size-fits-all.

The body of research on nutrition—and on drugs, for that matter—is full of tentative information, conflicts, and contradictions. Today, a given substance is shown to save lives or promote wellness; tomorrow it takes lives and deteriorates health. With precise body type differentiation for research subjects fewer conflicts will occur.

There will come a day when a given study on humans lists the effects of what is being tested on a body type by body type basis. Perhaps a given nutrient works on the Thyroid Dominant body type but has no effect on the Pancreatic Dominant type but is found to be harmful on the Adrenal Dominant type. Or perhaps a given nutrient only works for those showing a particular deficiency, but not for those with other deficiencies, and so on.

The good news is that culminating research demonstrates overwhelmingly that one-size-fits-all nutrition is eventually going to be completely replaced by highly scientific individualization in accordance with our biochemical uniqueness. As this scientific individualization process permeates our society, we will experience a progressive shrinkage of diet-related disease incidence and a profound upsurge of wellness advancements on a scale never before thought possible.

Given this, I would venture to say that between the geneticists helping to correct some defective genes and the nutritionists correcting faulty nutrition by individualizing nutrition to measurable metabolic and genetic standards, both diet-related and some gene-related disease will disappear from our society! Since these types of diseases (especially diet-related disease) account for the majority of illness in society, disease will become rare in the future.

Say good-bye to one-size-fits-all thinking and nutritional practices. It is truly obsolete in every way. The final frontier of nutrition lies before your: in the following sections, you will learn how to take the guesswork out of what your body really needs to be healthy, so that your life's quantity and quality will reach its peak.

CHAPTER THREE

You Are 100% Unique
The Health Implications of
Biochemical Individuality

The natural healing force within each one of us is the greatest force in getting well.
— **Hippocrates**

That true bible . . . the human body.
—**Andrew Vesalius**

If anything is sacred, the human body is sacred.
—**Walt Whitman**

Have you ever wondered about why your best friend, who happens to be skinny, can eat three helpings of food without gaining weight, while you so much as look at what he or she is eating and you gain two pounds?

Or why one person is short and fat, another tall and thin, and yet another highly muscular? Or why you have a big nose while your sister or brother has a small one? Why one person has long, straight, silky hair and another has curly, short, coarse hair? Why we have different "slopfactors?" (a concept Dr. Sears has postulated in *The Zone*). Why do we all have different body odors, intelligence quotients (IQ's), and personalities?

The reason is because *we are all unique*—inside and out, physically and chemically, intellectually and psychologically.

Why RDA's Are Not Adequate for Most Individuals

Roger Williams, Ph.D., published *Biochemical Individuality* in 1956. In this research publication, he presented evidence provided through hundreds of research studies that each person is biochemically unique in terms of their anatomy and chemical composition. It was shown that people differ in the size of their brains, bones, muscles, glands, organs, and in the amounts of their enzymes, hormones, vitamins, minerals, and amino acids. They also differ in their clinical measurements, such as pain thresholds, blood pressure, pulse, and taste reactions. All of Dr. Williams' research extrapolations showed wide variations among healthy "normal" humans. He related these differences to genetic inheritance and labeled it the "Genotrophic Concept."

Dr. Williams further revealed numerous diet patterns and focused upon specific nutrient needs, digestion, and food allergies. He showed that we inherit unique needs for particular nutrients because we inherit unique digestive, absorptive and enzymatic patterns along with our abilities to transport nutrients and excrete by-products of metabolism. In effect, he demonstrated that RDA's were not adequate for most people because they actually need more of one nutrient or another specific to their biochemical individuality.

Interestingly enough, over 40 years after Dr. Williams' primary publications, the Food and Nutrition Board qualifies its RDA data with the statement: "RDA's should not be confused with requirements for a specific individual. They are not guidelines for formulating diets nor assessing the nutritional status of individuals." This is in direct contradiction with the purpose for which RDA's, MDR's, and even Daily Values were originally designed! We really have come full circle in the last 40 years! Even the RDA's, historically a nutritional bible to many, have been negated as being applicable to the needs of the individual. Perhaps the Food and Nutrition Board members should have read *Biochemical Individuality* and Dr. Williams' other books before placing so much emphasis on RDA's in the first place. It's truly unfortunate that so much nutritional research before and after Dr. Williams' projects has been neglected by mainstream medicine until only very recently.

Dr. Williams and others have found that each person has a distinctive and unique pattern of amino acids (protein's smallest constituents) in both their urine and blood. A chemist, Dr. William Walsh, discovered that individuals separate into one of six fundamental hair analysis categories. He relates these groupings to six body chemistry types. In 1941, Charles Stockard, published research on animals demonstrating that endocrine gland hormones shape specific body and personality patterns. He also found that these patterns were inherited. Further research on humans has shown this phenomenon among people as well.

TABLE 3
CATEGORIES OF HUMAN UNIQUENESS

External Differences	Height, weight, hair distribution on body, hair texture and color, degree of baldness, skin thickness, skin activity, skin color, skin oil content, body shape, head and face shape, muscularity, bone size, retinal image, eye color, size of eyes, size and shape of teeth, finger and toe shape and size, length and proportion of limbs and torso, fingerprints, auras, and body odor.
Internal Differences	Size and shape of all internal organs, including brains, bones, muscles, glands, stomach, intestines, etc.; quantity and composition of enzymes, hormones, vitamins, minerals, amino acids, blood type, composition and pressure, pulse rate, systemic and organic strengths and weaknesses, pain threshold, taste reactions, pH, digestive, absorptive, utilization, detoxification, and elimination patterns, anabolism and catabolism rates, number of body cells, cell division rates, cellular metabolism, composition of tissues and tissue amount, oxidation rates and efficiency, genetic structure (DNA), fertility rates,
Psychological Differences	Mental and emotional activity levels, emotions, beliefs, values, attitudes, personality, intelligence quotients (IQ), interests, likes and dislikes, behavior and energy levels, quickness of thought, intuition, dream states

NOTE: Refer to APPENDIX A: Psychological Typing Combined With Body Typing.

Why No Two Diet Patterns
Can Ever Be Quite The Same

"Each person uniquely requires
more of one nutrient than another."

Continuing research has demonstrated certain patterns among people when it comes to diet. Much of this same research has focused on nutrient needs, digestion and absorption, and food allergies. Dr. Williams demonstrated that we each inherit unique needs for specific nutrients. We inherit these needs as a genetic legacy, received in the form of unique digestion characteristics, absorption traits, enzyme patterns, and nutrient transport and excretion factors. This is the primary reason why the government's one-size-fits-all, recommended dietary allowances of vitamins, minerals, carbohydrates, fats, and proteins are inadequate for many people. It's all due to the nature of our innate "genotrophic" design. Each person uniquely requires more of one nutrient than another.

German Army research has identified a distinctive pattern of digestive fluid and amino acids from person to person which further confirms the presence of human digestive patterns. Dr. Richard T. Powers, Ph.D., has found relationships between food allergies, blood types, and immune systems in his research. The process of "human uniqueness" investigation continues in universities, laboratories, and amongst independent researchers.

Underlying these schools of research is a general consensus, which views humans as fitting into three (very) basic categories of diet: vegetarian, meat-eater, and omnivore. There are established subgroupings within these categories which are variations of the basic category. An example of one of these subgroupings can be found within the vegetarian category where you have ovo-lacto-pesca-vegan types of vegetarians. The etymological basis for these terms is as follows: *ovo* = eggs, *lacto* = milk, *pesca* = fish, *vegan* = vegetables. Within these subgroupings even further distinctions about each specific food and nutrient need can be made using the appropriate laboratory procedure. This ultimately culminates in a nutritional specificity per person never before possible.

The Achilles Heel of Popular Diet Systems

The biggest mistake lying at the heart of today's popular diet systems is their inability to allow for human uniqueness. They are predominately of a one-size-fits-all nature, and in some cases are very extreme and one-sided when it comes to nutrient recommendations and other factors. A large number of modern fad diets have been derived from untested personal experience, capitalistic manipulations, trendy "logic," and/or uninformed advertising.

Popular modern diets include:

- High protein or high carbohydrate content
- Low cholesterol diets, low fat diets
- High monounsaturated fat diets, 1983 low glycemic index diets
- Fruitarian diets
- Raw food diets
- Alkalinizing diets
- Detoxification diets
- Ethnic diets
- Zone diets
- Blood type diets
- Numerous other weight loss programs, including ketogenic diets

Because we are each unique, these diet and supplement plans are generally very limited and lead to confusion by those who undertake to use them. In fact, many of these plans can actually be dangerous for you, because they do not accommodate your nutrient needs properly.

The mismatching of diets can upset your body's metabolic balance, causing a deterioration of health and well-being. That is exactly why various research authorities—most notably Harvard University—have withdrawn support for the indiscriminate practice of diet (and supplementation) to promote health and wellness. The FTC and FDA are constantly "pulling the plug" on products and programs that are actually dangerous for your health.

Considering the widespread utilization of these common diet programs, combined with our one-size-fits-all attitudes, is it any wonder why people are not achieving the health and well-being they truly deserve? I think not. Are you designed to be a vegetarian, taking extra vitamin C, iron, copper, and B12, and eating four times a day? Maybe or maybe not. Only your personal metabolic nutritionist knows for sure . . . but he or she has to determine your metabolic "profile," "type," "pattern," or "body type" first. (These four terms are basically synonymous, although "profile" refers more to the lab testing part of typing.)

What Is Metabolic Typing?

The art and science of Metabolic Typing interconnects genetically predisposed human patterns, dividing everyone into distinct physiological categories based on similar characteristics. This process, once completed, is then used for nutritional evaluation and therapy. Metabolic analysis can be based on one's blood type, nervous system characteristics, endocrine gland balance, oxidation pattern, body shape, body composition, personality, hair and facial features, and even more.

The process of Metabolic Typing can be further reinforced and differentiated with laboratory assessments of both long- and short-term metabolic factors and up to the moment overall nutrient status. This is called Profiling, a practice that allows us to see what you've "done" to yourself chemically—remember, you are responsible for your own dietary intake, and you are what you eat! And only a certain part of the food chain (approximately 25%) is best for you.

Ultimately, Metabolic Typing and Profiling can lead to a fully customized and foolproof nutrition program for each individual with the exact foods and supplements in the proper proportions for optimum wellness.

Where Do Metabolic Types
Come From and What Are Their Implications?

Quite simply, metabolic types come from our human genetic "pools" or more accurately termed Genotypes and Phenotypes.

Genotypes reflect the entire genetic constitution of a person distinguished from his/her physical appearance.

Phenotypes reflect the entire physical, biochemical, and physiological make-up of an individual, a profile that is determined both environmentally and genetically.

In effect, we have groups of humans possessing similar genetic characteristics based on an **original** genetic "set" (or pattern), which has been modified over time due to the influences of environment. Simply speaking, we all come from identifiable **ancestral**, tribal origins. (See "Ancestral Typing" in the Glossary at the end of this book.) Due to environmental variations such as climate, diet, lifestyle, and socialization factors, our genetic set has been further differentiated from its primal origins into other races and body types with certain genetic characteristics indigenous to each race and still others found in all races.

That which has been genetically delivered to each of us—individually, here in modern times—is a body type variation based on a 40,000+ year chronology of environmentally affected evolution. Whether your ancestors were hunters, gatherers, farmers, fishermen, savage warriors, peaceful citizens; whether they lived in cold climates, warm climates, high altitudes, low altitudes, etc., all of those factors have had a pronounced effect on **what you are**, as an individual, and what you require from the environment to be your healthy best.

"There is an eternal wellness benefit
built into traditional lifestyles
that we are rapidly losing in modern times."

From an environmental standpoint, diet is the single most important factor in "feeding your genes" properly. Stay within the path of your genetic origins and their antecedent environmental patterns, and you'll thrive physically and mentally. Stray from this path as "one sizing" would have you do and you'll suffer the consequences of diet-related disease.

There is an eternal wellness benefit built into traditional lifestyles that we are rapidly losing in modern times as collectively we stray far and wide from the essence of our genetic design. Is it any wonder, then, that here in the U.S.—where extensive multi-cultural variations and anti-tradition attitudes cause us to digress from our traditional eating patterns moment by moment—diet-related disease is at an all-time high?

After all, we Americans represent the world's largest "melting pot."

Where else in the world can you find someone genetically designed for vegetarianism wolfing down a burger and beer, just to fit in with friends... only to return home and wolf antacids to counteract the severe digestive stress such behavior produces?

Where else in the world can you find a genetically programmed meat-eater adopting a straight vego-vegetarian diet, for "religious reasons," and subsequently suffering from anemia, parasites, chronic fatigue, and premature aging?

Where else in the world can you find someone designed to be an omnivore trying out the latest "grapefruit diet," thereafter suffering from chronic pathological diarrhea, all the while thinking that it's okay because he's been mistakenly told by others that this represents a "detoxification process"?

Where else in the world can you find someone with a pronounced magnesium deficiency consistently megadosing calcium, which only serves to worsen the magnesium deficiency?

Where else in the world can you find an Asian Thyroid Dominant Type (an Endocrine Type) subsisting on a "40-30-30 zoned" macronutrient proportion (carbohydrate/protein/fat), when they really require a 70-20-10 proportion for best results?

If we were all "typed" correctly, none of this distress would be suffered, and our average combined health status, as a nation, would dramatically improve.

You certainly cannot forcibly change what's been genetically built into your body over the last 40,000 years overnight, but with "Typing and Profiling" you can certainly learn to work with it and improve upon it now and for all generations to come.

Religous and Evolutionary Perspectives on Metabolic Types

It may very well be that when God put man on this earth, he placed him in the valley of the Euphrates River. This region has continued to be semi-tropical in nature for more than four millennia. Fertile with trees and plants bearing nuts, seeds, fruits, and vegetables, the lands along the banks of the Euphrates provided all the foods necessary to nourish the "type" of metabolism man was initially endowed with. At this time in history, man could reach up and pick food from the land whenever he desired it. For the purpose of discussion, let's call this first metabolic type," "Type 1," since in theory this was man's first body type. (Geneticists contend that they have found human DNA 1.8 million years old.)

When man began to migrate outside of the Euphrates region, he adopted goats' milk and some other foods into his diet. These small modifications in diet only slightly altered his Phenotype, and he slowly became a "Type 1A" metabolizer. Over time, through the generations, the "Type 1A" metabolizer was better able to fully utilize these initial diet modifications through more efficient processes of digestion, absorption, assimilation, and elimination.

Another dietary addition came when those people who settled in Greece and Northern Italy had to learn to add grains to their diet, because of the lack of other food in those regions. They could no longer reach up and pick their food year round. At first, babies born to this group could not adapt well as they grew. They often became weak, sickly, and many died. The stronger children who survived this environmental stress in turn had babies who were a little stronger and better adapted to the new grain-rich diets. Gradually, this tribal line mutated into a "Type 2" metabolizer, with the ability to efficiently utilize foods that would undermine the health of "Type 1" metabolizers thanks to newly acquired genetic capabilities not found in "Type 1's."

As people continued to spread out and populate the colder climates to the north, with their higher altitudes, the new settlers had to increase their dependency on grains and stored foods for survival. And they were forced to consume small animals to fill the gaps in food scarcity.

Further Phenotypic mutation took place over time to form another metabolic type that we'll arbitrarily call "Type 3." During these difficult periods in history, anyone born with incompatible metabolic "types" for their respective environment would die prematurely in infancy, childhood, or early adulthood. This phenomenon is called (famously, thanks to Darwin), "natural selection."

As civilization moved even further north, the people had to hunt and consume animals like deer and bear to survive. As in the case of "Type 3," children born who could not adapt to this diet change died prematurely. Those who were left were quite hardy and thrived on heavy purine (red meat) diets, giving rise to our next metabolic category: "Type 4."

This same type of mutation pattern occurred as people populated China, India, and the islands of the Pacific and Indian Oceans. Those born in these particular regions had to become "Type 1A" metabolizers, or remained as "Type 1." Numerous religious sects indigenous to these areas forbade meat and animal products, so that "Type 4's" rarely appeared in these groups. And again, those born into these societies with the wrong metabolic "type" would not survive.

At the least, there are between 8–10 basic types of metabolizers with differing nutrient needs. Interestingly, when East Indian and Asian philosophers and teachers come to America, they believe that all Americans should practice vegetarian diets, because the peoples of their Eastern homelands are predominantly vegetarians. These philosophers completely overlook the fact that we cannot change any metabolic "type" in one or even two generations, let alone in a person's own lifetime. It takes a minimum of eight or more generations to successfully effect any permanent Phenotypic changes.

Don't be frustrated about the "type" of metabolism you have inherited. You cannot help being what you are, other than by learning to work with your metabolism for optimum health results. Ignoring one's metabolic "type" can only cause harmful effects, especially when diet is modified for purposes of "fitting into" someone else's philosophy or religion. The dietary needs of one's own body as measured by Typing and Profiling are the only real protection from one-size-fits-all traps.

In ancient days, people died quickly when they were born into a rigid environment mismatched to their genetic set because they had no choice— there were no supermarkets around the corner to supply them with the right foods that their bodies could healthfully metabolize. Sadly, it's not much different nowadays, even with the supermarket around the corner, because without "typing," you really can't tell exactly what you need from that supermarket to achieve your best health. The direct result of this guesswork problem is our current epidemic of rampant diet-related disease. This nation is carelessly overfed yet seriously undernourished!

We're attempting to keep people alive, not with the proper nourishment we each require, but with nutritional stereotyping, generic drugs, pills, lotions, potions, and surgeries which have no direct connection to the root cause of our ailments. These "quick fixes" are just false substitutes for the real thing. No wonder we have an extensive degenerative disease plague crushing the quantity and quality out of life!

A Contemporary Message About Evolusiton and Genes

Recently, I came across a best-selling book stating outright that our genes haven't changed in 100,000 years! This is truly an absurd statement, which points up how widespread are one-size-fits-all fallacies and beliefs in our society.

If you already haven't deduced that this statement is incorrect out of simple logic and/or from reading this book thus far, let me help to further clarify the facts of the matter.

Two genetic scientists—Michael Crawford, Ph.D., and Michael Marsh— wrote a book in 1989: *The Driving Force—Food, Evolution, and The Future*. According to their human genetic and evolutionary research, food is the driving force that has molded the shape of the species as well as the limiting force that has fixed lines of selection. Nowadays food is of such a commonplace nature that it is taken for granted and its qualitative relationship with long term biological considerations is overlooked. The historical changes in disease patterns, the contrast in disease incidence from country to country, and importantly, the socioeconomic contrasts within a country suggest that we are witnessing a signal of the potential power of food as a dominant factor in evolution.

Crawford and Marsh's research findings "pose serious questions as to the impact of present day food and agricultural policies on immediate and future generations," according to Beatrice Trum Hunter from the *Townsend Letter* in reference to this book. Crawford and Marsh believe that "among other follies, agricultural practices have emphasized yields stressing quantity rather than quality." Nutrition has not been a prime goal. For example, in animal feeding practices, both the protein and nutrient values of animal food products have been diluted by fat. In her analysis of their work, Hunter states that the authors find that food has always been a crucial factor in shaping life's evolutionary process on this planet— from the earliest time when life first emerged, up to the present, and that it will continue into the future.

If only Darwin had been a "nutritional" geneticist! The role of nutrition would have been fully empowered by his support, shaping our conception of phenotypes and perhaps giving metabolic "typing" science a boost to the forefront of our health concerns to this day—rather than the "back seat" it currently occupies.

A good example of how our genes have changed in the last 10,000 years was brought out in an article "Unkind Milk," appearing in the *Harvard Health Letter* (Vol. 18, No. 12, October 1993). Stephen E. Goldfinger, M.D., et alia, state that "about 10,000 years ago, according to scientists' best guess, a genetic mutation occurred among the populations of northern and central Europe that had learned to herd dairy animals and consume milk products." This historically new genetic development, which leads to the occurrence of blood type B, allowed 80% of these people and their descendants to produce ample lactose into adulthood, making them an exception to the human rule for drinking milk.

TABLE 4
LACTOSE INTOLERANCE IN "HEALTHY" ADULTS

Group	Number Studied	Lactose Intolerant By:		
		Symptoms	Blood Sugar	Lactose Assay
Caucasians, (U.S., Great Britain, Australia) (several studies combined)	217	17	19	15
Black, U.S.A. (several studies c ombined)	107	63	74	73
Black, Central Africa, various Countries)	16	50	88	–
Black, Bantu, various tribes	66	40	59	70
Black, Hamitic tribes	10	–	0	–
Oriental, U.S.A.	31	70	95	100
Oriental, Australia	20	95	85	–
Oriental, India	18	22	22	11
Oriental Thailand	215	88	97	95
Australian, aborigine	19	–	79	–
North American Indian	3	–	67	–
South American Indian (Colombia)	24	58	100	–
South American Mestizo and "many" Antioqueno	"high"	"high"	–	–
Greek Cypriot	17	–	88	–
North American Arab	3	67	100	–

Source: L. Lutwak, 1970 "The Significance of Lactose Intolerance in Nutritional Problems– Eastern Experiment Station Collaborators' Conference on Human Nutrition," ARS 73-67, U.S. Dept. of Agriculture, October 28, 1969.

Lactose intolerance is very common among other ethnic groups. For example, milk disagreed with about 50% of all adult Hispanics and with at least 75% of people of African, Asian, or Native American descent in one government study. (Refer to Table 4: Lactose Intolerance In "Healthy" Adults and also to Appendix B, #1: Omnivore Diet For Blood Type B and AB.)

Our genes have changed many times over the last 100,000 years and will continue to do so until the very end of time. This is why we have differing body types and our own unique biochemical individuality in the first place!

Truth About Alergies

Where do you think most food allergies come from? You've probably surmised by now that straying from your path of genetically predetermined eating patterns will increase the likelihood of incidental food allergies and sensitivities. Your body is simply not used to certain foods (and some new manmade additives, mutations, and residues in those foods), because their metabolic compatibility has not been genetically programmed into you. Chapter IV addresses this subject in more depth, dealing with the implications of allergies and sensitivities and their relationship to metabolic types and biochemical individuality. For now, suffice it to say that a properly "Typed and Profiled" person will know what foods to avoid completely for optimum wellness. The good news about food allergies is that many food sensitivities can be overcome with the right nutritional approach.

Do We *Really* Need Metabolic Typing?

After what you've just read, this may seem like a silly question; but it warrants further explanation. In the first place, very, very few people really know what their proper diet should be. This holds true especially for Americans. With the constant interbreeding of genetically different populations, combined with the increasing rejection of traditional ethnic diets, new "modern" diets have emerged. These "modern" diets no longer correspond to our individual genetic digestive, absorptive, assimilation, and excretory capabilities.

The problem really starts with digestion. Not everyone's body can digest every kind of food. Undigested or partially digested food can lead to a multitude of problems, including gas, cramps, bloating, constipation, diarrhea, ulcers, fat and weight gain or loss, "cellulite," rashes, liver, kidney and other organic stress . . . and **allergies**. The proportions of proteins, fats, and carbohydrates each person needs is highly specific to them. Equally important are their vitamin and mineral requirements.

Diet-related disease and its symptoms are now at an all-time high— literally epidemic in our society—because most of us do not know exactly what our choices are and how much, and in which combination, to eat our foods. If you follow the correct nutritional plan for your specific metabolism, diet-related disease will vanish from your life and at the same time your life span and functional energy span will lengthen considerably. Metabolic Typing is our only hope when it comes to putting our bodies back in balance—and this is no secret, nor was it to the ancients of humanity's antiquity.

The Historic Origins of Metabolic Typing

Metabolic Typing, as a science, really began with Hippocrates, "the father of medicine," and his followers in ancient Greece. Hippocrates held that different sorts of people have different maladies. He diagnosed his patients on the basis of what he termed "the four humors" (or fluids), developing a typing system consisting of four temperaments and two body types. His nutrition and lifestyle treatments were specific to each of these patient categories, and he adopted a favorite motto as the essence of his philosophy: "thy food shall be thy remedy." Were he alive, I think Hippocrates would be well received in modern times, thanks to what he believed and practiced.

The ancient Chinese, Egyptians, Buddhists, and Hindus were also "body typers," as represented in the chart below:

Ancient Metabolic Typing	Constitutional Types
Ancient Chinese Medicine and Acupuncture	5 Elemental Types
Ancient Egyptian Medicine	7 Organ Systems
Ancient Greek Medicine and Hippocrates	4 Humors, the Liver-Bile Type
Ancient Buddhist and Hindu Traditions	7 Energy Center Types and Vata, Pitta, Kapha (5 elements)

Some Ancient Metabolic Typing Systems

Chinese Typing

The ancient Chinese philosophy of medicine focuses on the balance of life in relation to each person, and requires the use of diet, hands on therapies, exercise, proper rest, and herbs to restore balance. The Chinese concept of basing therapeutic treatments on the nature of each person rather, than on the nature of the diseases they suffer from, is an embodiment of the overall purpose of Metabolic Typing. Many people in the West who have experienced therapeutic success through the Chinese medicine system can attest to its efficacy, despite some of its inherent limitations.

The ancient Chinese referred to their body typing system as "Constitutional Types." Practitioners divide each person to be treated into their specific Constitutional Type before any therapeutic intervention commences. The fundamental principles of constitutional therapy originated in approximately 3000 BC, and its use has spread throughout Asia, the Middle East, Europe, and the West to this day.

In order to properly "type" an individual, the Chinese healer closely examines the patterns of responsiveness and creativity that develop during childhood and which persist throughout life. The constitutional characteristics of each individual are not perfectly fixed and can therefore be slightly modified by environmental factors and internal development. However, in the majority of cases, constitutional types rarely change significantly and never become another type entirely. This is due to a history of behavioral and physical tendencies, which began early in life and centered around physical, spiritual, and mental development. In effect, a person's constitution is determined on the basis of present conditions and long-term patterns. Is it any wonder an ancient Chinese proverb states that "nature, time, and patience are the three great physicians"?

In the West, by comparison, our personality types can be categorized as Type A's and Type B's, or as those individuals "at risk" or "not at risk." Type A's are categorically ambitious, very motivated, always productive, highly goal-oriented, constantly pushing the upper limits of their abilities, and very considerate of working associates; they eat too quickly, drink in excess, and don't get enough rest. In contrast, Type B's are generally relaxed, taking things in stride, allowing for pleasure and leisure; they let others worry about deadlines and satisfying work demands, and they tend to eat slowly and sleep a lot.

Of course, not everyone fits cleanly into either one of these categories, but this type of categorization does help to better clarify and classify differences we Westerners see in each other. Western health practitioners classify persons into two further categories, based on tendencies that they exhibit during illness:

At Risk—people who may be severely debilitated after contracting common influenza. After contracting the flu, these individuals may suffer a secondary infection or a worsening of symptoms due to a chronic degenerative disease state that they already have. This compromised health status may undermine their resistance to the flu to the point of death or prolonged hospitalization. Examples of "At Risk" individuals include elderly and very young children, people with transplanted organs,, ongoing or recent cancer therapies, those with chronic respiratory diseases, and morbidly obese people.

Not At Risk—people who, after coming down with the flu, suffer only minor symptoms of discomfort. Maybe they miss a day or two of work or school, and ultimately recover in about a week or less. These people are considered constitutionally healthy and uncompromised, with a characteristically normal, healthy response to viral infiltration.

Conventional Western health practitioners look at these four "rough" body types (Type A, Type B, At Risk, Not At Risk) in relation to their treatment recommendations. The doctor tells the Type A person to slow down a little and let the body heal. He or she then makes special therapeutic allowances for At Risk individuals by very closely monitoring their progress.

CHINESE TYPING SYSTEMS: FIVE ELEMENTS

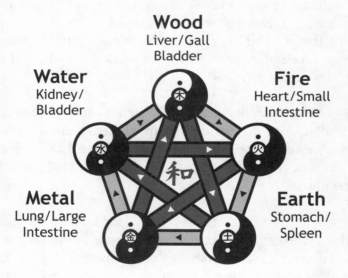

Wood
Liver/Gall
Bladder

Water
Kidney/
Bladder

Fire
Heart/Small
Intestine

Metal
Lung/Large
Intestine

Earth
Stomach/
Spleen

Contrast this method with the Chinese system, where medicine specialists utilize their Five Constitutional, "Elemental" Types and the law of Yin and Yang (based on opposing forces and their interrelation) when calculating the nature of disharmonies. Individuals are most likely to suffer from specific maladies based on their "type," and the symptomatic progress of any disease can be mapped for that "type." On top of a balanced diet, Chinese practitioners use special foods (i.e., herbs) to resolve underlying constitutional imbalances that, when present, increase a person's initial susceptibility to disease; if the patient has already contracted the disease, the practitioner can determine a response to it for the long term.

The so-called constitutional imbalances that Chinese practitioners focus upon are really metabolic imbalances, which when properly aligned maximize immune functions. The Chinese Elemental Types are wood, fire, metal, earth, water, heat/dryness, and energy. (Heat/dryness and energy are more modern-day additions to the five traditional, primal elements.)

Each fundamental "type" is further divided by the Chinese into two subgroups, very similar to "At Risk" and "Not At Risk" Western types. Each "type" is more differentiated beyond the Western Type A's and B's in terms of behavior patterns. Each of the "At Risk" and "Not At Risk" subgroups in Chinese medicine are referred to as weak and stressed constitution. Those with weak constitutions tend to become sick more easily, have more nutrient deficiencies or basic energy deficiencies, take longer to recover from ailments, are easily upset or damaged by environmental influences, and require interventional therapies to strengthen and nourish their bodies. Stressed constitutional (or metabolic) "types" are less susceptible to illness and when they do become ill, they recover faster with less disruption. Stressed types tend to be more resistant to environmental irritations as well.

In essence, the Chinese system of metabolic types consists of 7 behavioral types and 14 constitutional types: 2 subgroups (weak and stressed) for each of the 7 elemental types (wood, fire, metal, earth, water, heat/dryness, and energy).

The law of Yin and Yang divides up the universe's opposing forces within each of us and throughout the entirety of existence. Yin and Yang distinctions include:

- Cosmic bodies
- Temperament
- Time of day
- Season
- Magnetic pull
- Temperature
- Physical density
- Speed
- Relative moisture
- Heavenly body location
- Organs
- Height
- Distance
- Sides
- Light
- Sexual characteristics
- Constitution

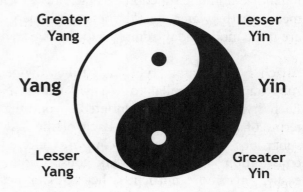

CHINESE TYPING SYSTEMS: YIN AND YANG

Greater Yang

Lesser Yin

Yang

Yin

Lesser Yang

Greater Yin

These distinctions help to reveal the characteristics of movement and energy within us and around us due to the natural attraction between Yin and Yang.

The ancient Chinese system of medicine helps to clarify laws of nature for each of us. It is quite an achievement, given these ancients' lack of understanding about the human body, most particularly about the nervous system.

Ayurvedic Typing

Ayurvedic science was derived from the religious belief that the god Indra conveyed "the knowledge of long life" to one of the Hindu *rishis* or seers. It originated in the fifth century BC and is based on the Vedas, which represent the world's oldest philosophical writings.

Ayurvedic philosophy sees health within a universal context, where human life is thought to be an extension of the life of the creator, also known as the "Cosmic Consciousness." An individual's health is based upon their relationship with the Cosmic Consciousness. Ayurvedic healers attempt to reestablish harmony between an individual and the life of the universe by balancing the universal forces indigenous to each person.

The lifeforce as expression of the Cosmic Consciousness is called *prana*. Prana is the animate power of life that provides vitality and endurance to each human being and is the basis for healing. This lifeforce or energy is expressed in terms of five "Great Elements": earth, water, fire, air, and ether. These are seen as both functions and aspects of the human body, holding it together in vital synchrony.

The three forces that balance the form and substance of the body are known as the *Doshas: Vata, Pitta,* and *Kapha*; these act on the Five Great Elements as their motive forces. Vata and Kapha types are opposites, while Pitta is the mediating force between the two extremes. When all the Doshas are in balance, the body functions in optimum harmony; when such balance diminishes, disease takes over.

AYURVEDIC TYPING:

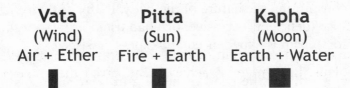

Vata	Pitta	Kapha
(Wind)	(Sun)	(Moon)
Air + Ether	Fire + Earth	Earth + Water

The Doshas combine uniquely in each person, giving to rise to body types that lean towards one Dosha or another. These Doshas create tendencies in each person but one or two Doshas are dominant in the shaping of one's personality and constitution. Dosha dominance and resultant imbalances provide unique strengths and weaknesses which create tendencies toward certain illnesses and disorders. Kapha types may be prone to lung, heart, stomach, and immune disorders, while Pitta types are prone to liver, gallbladder, blood, small intestine, stomach and spleen disorders and are prone to strokes and cancer.

The three Doshas affect how Prana flows through the body, in an either balanced or unbalanced fashion. This ancient philosophy also contends that the Prana flows through the body in a specific pattern of meridians, or "rivers of energy." These rivers of energy correspond roughly to points in Chinese acupuncture. Similar to the Chinese, the Ayurvedic practitioner uses pulse and physiognomy for patient diagnosis and treats each individual with foods, herbs, and special treatments related to each Dosha, the Five Great Elements, and the body's meridian pattern.

Greek Typing

Hippocrates was born on the Greek island of Cos in 460 BC. He created the first school of medicine dedicated to the scientific understanding of health and the body. He did not consider good health and bad health as gifts or punishments from the gods, as did his contemporaries. Instead, he believed that states of good and bad health were consequences of natural and orderly processes, which could in turn be understood and treated by man. For his beliefs, Hippocrates was considered a towering and revolutionary figure in his time, and is still revered for his insights by modern practitioners to this day.

Hippocrates postulated from his text, *The Nature of Man*, that the human body contains blood, phlegm, yellow bile, and black bile (the Four Humors), constituting the nature of the body. If any of these elements falls out of balance (deficient, excessive, or unadjusted in relationship with the other Humors), pain is experienced and illness persists.

Hippocrates utilized the triad of healing in relation to his patients by approaching each patient with specific roles with himself as physician, the patient him or herself, and the controllable aspects of the patient's environment. Treating each patient differently, according to their uniqueness, Hippocrates used proper and specific foods and drink, suitable exercise, and calmness of mind and body during his healing interventions. He further believed in opportune moments during the healing process, aside from prevention, where a crisis could be averted if acted upon soon enough. He called these moments "kairos," the root word for crises where life or death could hang in the balance. "*Pepsis*," or "the forces of healing," could be accelerated or left alone, depending on the physician's discretion and factors of the disease's timing.

GREEK TYPING:
FOUR HUMORS

Blood	**Yellow Bile**	**Black Bile**	**Phlegm**
(Air)	(Fire)	(Earth)	(Water)
Sanguine	Choleric	Melancholic	Phlegmatic
△	△	▽	▽

Hippocrates felt that, when properly treated, illness could have beneficial effects by helping to create a new order among the Four Humors. With this new order, each individual could eliminate poisons and impurities from their specific system.

The ancient Hippocratic methodologies are no longer strictly practiced, but their influences have followed man throughout history, from Galen and Paracelsus to Avicenna and many traditional healers in practicing down to our present time. Medical doctors continue to take the "Hippocratic Oath." The sciences of Naturopathy, Chiropractics, and Osteopathy embody many of the Hippocratic principles. Nutritional cleansing or detoxification is still an important part of nutritional sciences, millennia after Hippocrates' life ended.

The three ancient Metabolic Typing systems discussed in this chapter provide many insights into human differentiations of type, well beyond one-size-fits-all thinking. Unfortunately, these systems are very limited, from a scientific standpoint, when it comes to putting the body under the microscope. Due to their primitive nature and "artistic approach" to individuality, they pass over the atomic and molecular level distinctions we now comprehend in regards to the human body as discernible through the modern sciences of anthropology, genetics, physiology, anatomy, neurology, psychology, embryology, biochemistry, biology, clinical nutrition sciences, barietrics, psychiatry, genealogy, and physics. Using these modernized sciences, to update the ancient natural medicine philosophies with new metabolic medicine insights, has given us more information about ones biochemical uniqueness and how to balance it than ever before.

Modern Metabolic Typing and Profiling

Numerous researchers and research studies have appeared that created the body of knowledge we now classify as Metabolic Typing, Metabolic Patterning, Metabolic Profiling, Body Typing, or simply "typing" (my preferred term).

To stay within the scope of this book—and because of space considerations—I have purposely condensed the history of "modern typing" to contain what I subjectively ascertain to be the most important research and noteworthy researchers from 1900 to the present. I sincerely apologize for leaving out certain other significant researchers who have so conscientiously contributed their efforts to improve our awareness of the human condition. Those I do mention, and those I haven't mentioned, are owed our undying gratitude for their role in helping us to reach the final frontier of nutrition.

Historical Overview

1900   Carl Landsteiner, M.D. discovers the ABO blood types.

1919   Dr. M. Kretschmer Publishes *Symptoms of Visceral Disease*.

1925   Dr. Kretschmer investigates and categorizes body types based on the proportion of derm most developed in the embryo (endomorphs, ectomorphs, mesomorphs).

1931   Dr. Cary A. Reams, a student of Albert Einstein, begins developing "The Theory of Biological Ionization" and the ability to differentiate thousands of metabolic types..

1940   ABO blood types linked to diet by German Army doctors.

1941   Charles Stockard, Ph.D. demonstrates through animal research that endocrine gland hormones form specific body and personality patterns. Human research later confirms his observations.

1950 William H. Sheldon, Ph.D. develops Kretschmer's research further.

1952 A state-sponsored German research group shows that each healthy person has a distinctive pattern of amino acids in their intestinal digestive juices, proving human digestive patterns.

1954 Dr. Sheldon publishes the *Atlas of Men*.

1956 Roger Williams, Ph.D., writes *Biochemical Individuality and Nutrition Against Disease*, which demonstrates the true uniqueness of each of our bodies from a physiological and biochemical standpoint.

1965 Henry G. Bieler, M.D., develops the first endocrine typing system based on European research. Also develops the first modern system to match body type to diet. Writes *Food is Your Best Medicine*.

1970 Thomas M. Riddick, M.S., develops the principles of "Zeta Potential" in relation to the human body, with findings published in *Heart Disease, A New Approach To Prevention And Control*.

1970's James D'Adamo, N.D., researches and develops the first blood typing system for diet (based on 20 years of research.)

George Watson, Ph.D.—Developed the first oxidation typing system. Wrote *Personality, Strength, and Psychochemical Energy*, 1979, which utilized a five "type" psychological system based on oxidation rates, pH, psychochemical odor analysis, and a personality self-rating. Involves diet and supplements matched to each "type."

William Kelley, D.D.S., develops the first nerve typing system as an extrapolation of Watson's work and Francis Pottenger's Ph.D. research on the autonomic nervous system. This involves three nerve types with four variable levels of oxidation efficiency each and subsequent individualized nutrition therapy.

1980   Dr. D'Adamo writes *One Man's Food*.

1982   Dr. Reams Publishes *Choose Life or Death*.

1989   M. Abravanci, Ph.D., publishes Bodytype Diet and Lifetime Nutrition Plan, an updated weight-loss version of Bieler's project.

1980's James Braly, M.D., pioneers the development of food allergy testing and methodologies, relating this information to the biochemical uniqueness of each individual. (Writes *Food Allergy and Nutrition Revolution*, 1985.)

D.L. Watts, Ph.D., links tissue mineral assays to metabolic type and nutritional needs.

Gerald Berkowitz, M.D., writes *The Berkowitz Diet Switch* and attempts to match diet to Sheldon's original body types.

Richard T. Power, Ph.D., and Laura Power, B.A., expand, combine, and refine preceding Metabolic Typing systems relying heavily on endocrine typing and blood typing methodologies. The team writes many articles over a series of years.

1990's Deepak Chopra, M.D., writes *Perfect Health*, popularizing the ancient system of Mahareshi Ayurveda, featuring Vata, Pitta, and Kapha.

Gregory H. Tefft, D.C., N.D., further expands upon and updates previous Metabolic Typing systems, incorporating the use of herbs in the rebalancing process.

Dr. Elliot Abravanel, Dr. Jeffrey Bland, Dr. Donald Donsbach, and Dr. Michael Colgan have also contributed a great deal to typing research and information along with Drs. Linus Pauling and Francis Pottenger.

There are numerous researchers and laboratory projects worldwide in the process of investigating further the biochemical uniqueness of each individual and the relationship of diet to that uniqueness. New technologies and information breakthroughs appear on an ongoing basis, and this scientific pursuit can well be thought of as the "last frontier of wellness medicine."

The Landmark Systems

Next, we will explore the art and science of body typing in the process of identifying biochemical uniqueness. A brief overview follows, describing the seven primary systems of Metabolic Typing.

The Sheldon System

The *Atlas Of Men* (1954) by the psychologist Dr. Sheldon popularized this body typing system based on European research by Dr. Kretschmer. This system was the first "coherent" modern body typing system. It contained only three body types each based on that portion of the derm (the three primal tissue types) developed the most in the embryonic stage of life.

The three derm types are the Mesoderm, Endoderm, and Ectoderm. Sheldon's body types were named accordingly.

- The *Mesoderm* forms the connective tissue and muscles and is therefore associated with the typically muscular Mesomorph Type.

- The *Endoderm* forms the skin, body linings, and fat storage tissues of the body, hence the round, soft, and usually overweight Endomorph Type.

- The *Ectoderm* forms the nervous system which relates to the high strung, highly intelligent, usually underweight or thin Ectomorph Type.

Overall, this system has validity in relation to body shape but demonstrates very little direct relationship to metabolism, diet, or nutritional needs. In 1981, Gerald Berkowitz, M.D., attempted to link diet to Sheldon's three types in his book, *The Berkowitz Diet Switch*. Many texts about exercise physiology features Sheldon's work in the classification of body types.

The Bieler System

This was the first endocrine typing system, developed by Henry G. Bieler, M.D., and based on European research. His body types (the Thyroid Type, Pituitary Type, Adrenal Type) were based on an individual's dominant gland. Bieler further developed the first modern process to directly match body type to diet pattern. Bieler's diet therapies were partly based on the works of Hippocrates and Sir William Osler. *The Bodytype Diet and Lifetime Nutrition Plan* by Dr. Abravanci is what most would term a "trendy" weight-loss version of Bieler's work.

Endocrine glands have been shown to control many aspects of body shape and personality. Examples of this include the pituitary and thymus that control growth hormone which in turn effects many factors of immunity, size, shape, fat deposition, etc. The adrenals control muscle development and energy and oxidation levels. The thyroid gland exerts an influence on mental function and controls the metabolic rate overall helping to inhibit fat accumulation. Various nutrient needs are connected to the production of hormones exemplified by the thyroid's need for iodine, tyrosine, and B6, and in the pancreas' special need for zinc and protein. Glandular function is also connected to digestion through digestive enzyme production and intestinal motility.

Shortcomings in Bieler's work were apparent only due to the fact that, at the time of his research, the functions of all the endocrine glands were not known.

The D'Adamo System

James D' Adamo, N.D., is credited with developing the first blood typing system for diet. He utilized the works of Dr. Carl Landsteiner, who discovered the ABO blood types, and German Army research that linked them to diet in the 1940s.

Blood typing is partially effective for basic distinguishing of diet and potential food allergies. Blood types are directly related to the immune system, based on the presence of antigens (allergic substances, in this case) on the surface of red blood cells that react with specific antibodies on white cells. For example, many foods (and especially seeds) contain antigens called lectins, which are responsible for food allergies in some people such as allergenicity to milk. (More on this in Chapter IV.)

The Watson System

George Watson, Ph.D., created the first oxidation typing system based on five psychological types. These psychological types are categorized by the oxidation rates of blood sugar, blood pH levels, psychochemical odor tests, and personality self-ratings. Blood chemistry and personality disorders are correlated by this system. Interestingly, this system is not based on genetic inheritance but on one that is conditional. Its therapeutic objective is to change its characteristic four abnormal types into one normal type through diet and supplements.

The Kelley System

William D. Kelley, D.D.S., developed the first nerve typing system, based primarily on Watson's work and the work of Dr. Frances Potenger, who closely researched the autonomic nervous system. This program involves three basic nerve types with three to four variable levels of oxidation efficiency, each adding up to ten subtypes altogether.

The autonomic nervous system is directly responsive to stress, giving rise to our "fight or flight" mechanisms. When stress is perceived, the sympathetic nerves automatically respond by constricting muscles and elevating pulse. When stress is reduced, the parasympathetic nerves compensate by relaxing muscles and lowering the pulse rate. These autonomic responses make certain demands on our body's oxidation process, therefore sapping nutrients such as electrolytes, oxidants, and antioxidants from the body. These same nerves affect hunger and digestion as well.

This typing system is conditional and not based on genetics. It is much like Watson's system and defines one's response to stress, as opposed to examining one's inherited individualities, in order to decipher long-term nutritional needs, precise diet patterns, and body shape factors.

The Power System

Designed by Richard Power, Ph.D., and Laura Power, B.A., this system provides a logical combination of the other systems, with further knowledge expansion and correlation, and a functional resolution of observable discrepancies between them. It relies heavily on endocrine typing and blood typing, genetically inherited features that help to accurately define body shape, personality, metabolism, digestion, diet, supplements, and allergies. The Power System utilizes over eight body types.

The Tefft System

Further expanding on the Power and other systems, this system relies heavily on endocrine and blood typing. It brings into play the role of herbs in metabolic rebalancing, most directly in connection to observed endocrine patterns. The Tefft system also utilizes expanded laboratory assessments (i.e., Profiling) on a highly specific level and in conjunction with body type criteria. Blood, urine, feces, hair, saliva, and cell scrapings are incorporated into the Metabolic Typing process to further identify biochemical uniqueness, genetic design, up-to-the-moment metabolic and nutrient status, and resultant nutritional specificities. This system's therapeutic intervention is fully customized to each person's needs, on the most sophisticated levels.

Metabolic Typing—The Process

The process of Metabolic Typing is a systematic, constitutional analysis of an individual's physiology to determine a long-term nutritional pattern. It is assisted by designated laboratory research on body specimens to further clarify and refine both long and short-term nutritional needs. The Metabolic Typing process, in combination with appropriate laboratory protocol (Profiling), is essential in order to:

- Determine the most efficient and long term protein pattern for an individual

- Anticipate and measure unusual individual nutrient needs regarding all foods, special forms of foods or supplements, and very high or low amounts of certain nutrient factors

- Determine the best long or short term diet and supplement pattern for an individual

- Detect hidden or suppressed inherent genetic strengths and develop them nutritionally

- Better elucidate any metabolic ramifications reflected from long and short-term nutritional patterns as measured by nutritional or metabolic deficiency/dysfunction analysis

- Design the appropriate macro/micronutrient food, water and supplement ratios within the diet pattern and monitor results with retests

As you can see, the science and art of Metabolic Typing is designed to go to great lengths to "dig out" the facts of the matter when it comes to our own biochemical uniqueness, and what is precisely called for when it comes to diet and supplementation strategies for the attainment of optimum wellness results.

The Metabolic Typing process entails categorizing an individual on the basis of factors such as:

- Blood type
- Height
- Weight range
- Pulse rate
- Blood pressure
- Hair characteristics
- Skin traits
- Muscle size

- Shape and tone
- Bone factors
- Overall shape
- Head and face shape
- Personality
- Ethnicity
- Intelligence factors
- Dream states

It is further refined by using laboratory tests that reveal even more specific information about every metabolic and nutrient function we can scientifically measure and understand. This process entails extensive information gathering on the subject: detecting all allergies, toxins, nutrient deficiencies and excesses, breakdowns in digestion, absorption, utilization and excretion, pre- and post-disease states. A properly "typed" individual will know exactly what his or her metabolic and wellness status is up-to-the-moment, what foods and supplements he or she will thrive on, what foods and supplements to completely avoid, and ultimately will have a fully customized diet and supplement program for his or her body type only.

In essence, a properly "typed" individual need never haphazardly guess about what foods and supplements he or she needs to be in accordance with how he or she was genetically designed to live. Since our bodies were designed from the start to be healthy (the process is termed "homeostasis"), the precise nutritional program that "typing" yields will insure wellness in direct accordance with nature.

No magical pill, no one-size-fits-all supplement or food, no one-meditation technique, and no one special exercise can foster the metabolic balance of true health. Only the Metabolic Typing process can identify, assemble, and organize all of the many constituents of what it takes to be your healthy best.

In Retrospect

There are 76 minerals, 17 vitamins, 38 fatty acids, 12 essential amino acids, 28 non-essential amino acids, hundreds—perhaps thousands—of phytonutrients and vitamin-like compounds found in nature—all of which the individual chemistry of our body (and mind) is designed to utilize. These vital nutrients were in existence long before man made an appearance on earth. Much of our genetic setup is based on the amounts and types of these nutrients found in the specific regions that saw the beginning of our ancestors' development as humans (see above, "Where Do Metabolic Types Come From . . . ?" etc.).

These various nutrient groupings have shaped our bodies, mind, and lives for centuries and this process continues. It is only in the last century or so that we have stepped out of the pre-determined nutritional boundaries in our "melting pot society" and, as a result, created fundamental problems of incomplete wellness. These are the problems that are cumulatively plaguing us as a current and ever-intensifying epidemic of diet-related disease. The epidemic is further compounded by our synthetic and mass production agricultural methodologies, nutrient-depleted and disappearing topsoils, extensive food processing, improper food storage, poisonous food additives, pesticides, herbicides and other environmental pollutants, preparation of "enzyme dead foods," and so on. Combined, these poor practices only serve to further undermine the foods that we consume and add extra toxins to our bodies, toxins we have not evolved to handle efficiently over the last 40,000 years of our development as a species.

Is it any wonder, then, that Metabolic Typing should be considered the most important process to retrieve our "lost" health once and for all? Metabolic Typing uncovers our individual biochemical identities, and is the only way to precisely measure what it is that we are doing wrong nutritionally. With typing, we will finally be able to get back on the healthy track, and without Metabolic Typing you are only at best "guessing in the dark" about nutrition and therefore risking your health. It should be clear by now that our quest for the medical magic bullet has overlooked body typing and kept us in the dark about the true healing powers of nature. One-size-fits-all thinking, lodged as it is in our culture's attitudes toward health and nutrition, is hampering our wellness progress. To combat its bad influence, typing is our only hope to right the wrongs of ineffective modern-day nutritional practices. If you agree with these statements, then you are seriously committed to entering the final frontier of nutrition.

A Word About Tribes

In modern times, it's very difficult to find "pure" societies that have changed little or not at all in the last 40,000 years, and still possess much of their given environment intact. In Chapter II, I mentioned a book called *The Paleolithic Prescription*, in which scientists were able to find a group of "untainted" hunter-gatherer societies and study them extensively. Add to that the wealth of information scientists have compiled about the Hunzas, Georgians, Tibetan tribes, Titikakas, Armenians, Abcasians, Azerbaijanis, Gauchos, Vilcabombe Indians, and others—from these tribal exemplars we gain a genuine look at how it used to be for all of us, when we were settled in our most appropriate environments.

These "pure" hunter-gatherer, fisherman, and agrarian societies are exactly matched to their environments, whose characteristics spawned their inhabitants' genetic makeup. These tribes still practice the same eating, exercise, and lifestyle habits that their ancestors practiced thousands of years ago. Each of our ancestors was in a similar setting at one time, practicing the same habits and rites of life, generation after generation. Nowadays, in our "anything goes" society, we are living completely outside of our primal nourishing elements and the natural patterns of life and wellness.

What do you think the scientific research on these unchanged ancient tribes demonstrates? An *absolute lack of diet-related disease and results of longevity well over 100 years old for most individuals*. Based on his studies of these tribes and his own clinical experience, Joel Wallach, D.V.M, N.D., believes our proper lifespan to be 130 to 140 years; such longevity can be achieved, if the diets ingested are appropriate. I agree with Wallach's findings. Even the researchers living in the Arizona Biosphere, under ideal conditions, were projected to have over 160 years of life expectancy, if they maintained their place in the controlled environment (based on UCLA computer predictions).

When examining long-lived primal tribes up close, researchers have found that their people simply don't suffer from osteoporosis, heart disease, diabetes, obesity, allergy syndromes, arthritis, cancer, and many more across-the-board diet-related diseases. In fact, the vast majority of these tribal people are energetic, active, productive, and disease-free . . . up until the day they die, which is nearly always from natural causes (such as old age). (By the way, the diets and behaviors of the tribal people studied did not fit squarely into the "40-30-30 zone" classification.) Most of these tribal people pass away due to ever so slight nutrient deficiencies that finally "catch-up" with them, after they are well into their 100's. An example of this phenomenon is typified by the bone tuberculosis that has taken the lives of some Hunzas (who are most often centenarians when they die); this disease is linked to an ever so slight protein deficiency, manifesting itself over hundreds of years.

Wow! To think the average American only lives to be 75.4 years old. The majority of that 75 years of life is plagued by a host of varying diseases, obesity, low energy, and all kinds of routine symptoms, from headaches to constipation to fatigue to indigestion to joint pains, and so on. While your average Hunzan is out in the fields, able to work ten to twelve hours a day consistently, well into his/her hundreds, and is naturally thin, optimistic and energetic, the average "old" American can barely get out of their chair to go to the restroom. While Georgians are reaching their sexual peak well into their 40's, 50's, and beyond, the average "middle-aged" American regards complete sexual fulfillment as a pleasant memory at best, or obtains virility and libido through drugs.

At this point, you may be thinking to yourself, "In order to be healthy I'll have to move to Lake Titikaka and do as the Titikakas do." The disease-free status and longevity success of these tribes confirms completely the need to do as our ancestral roots dictate.

But if you do move to Lake Titikaka, it might not help your wellness status, thanks to one problem you may not have thought of: your Metabolic Type does not match that of the Titikakas. Your tribal ancestry follows a line of people who lived in an entirely different environment, under entirely different circumstances, which have genetically formed your constitution accordingly. Your primal tribe may have been carni-vegans who subsisted on completely different foods than the Titikakas do. However, if you were a genuine Titikakan who left the tribe to become a lawyer in New York City over the past fifteen years, and then moved back home due to your brand new set of society-imposed diet-related illnesses, you would be happily rewarded with optimum health again in a very short period of time. You'd be back in your primal element doing what your genes were designed to do.

Because we can't all return to our tribes or countries of origin, we must utilize Metabolic Typing to reveal the essence of how our bodies function and what they specifically require to operate at peak efficiency, no matter where we are in the world. When we know our "type" we can efficiently organize our diets (and lives) very closely to the way it used to be for our ancestors, who rarely strayed from their tribes or countries and who typically practiced life in harmony with their environment.

Outside of the U.S., many countries fare much better when it comes to overall health status. Japan, for instance, is one of the top seven healthiest countries in the world, and for good reason: even with all of the health-inhibiting factors of modern civilization (such as stress, pollution, drug dependence, etc.), the Japanese adhere closely to the ritualistic life patterns of their ancestors. This is true for many Asian countries where tradition reinforces the diet and lifestyle practices of their country's past. In essence, these peoples are doing more of what their specific body type was designed to do and enjoy the absence of most diet-related diseases.

The Eskimo Versus the Indian

A dramatic metabolic contrast is evident when you consider the differences between an Eskimo's and an East Indian's dietary patterns.

Traditional Eskimos eat as much as ten pounds of very fatty meat per day, thrive physically, and are able to successfully survive the harshest climate on earth. Historically, their overall incidence of diet-related disease has been minuscule, with no traces of cardio-vascular disease or cancer until only recently, with their adoption of "advanced" civilization. (Progressive dental decay and diabetes is something that modern man has lately given the Eskimos, with the introduction of refined sugars into their diets.)

During countless generations, the Eskimo's physiological constitution became perfectly suited to their environment through natural adaptation and mutation (Phenotyping). Their bodies became progressively more efficient at metabolizing the "types" of food naturally occurring within their harsh living environments. In essence, the Eskimos have developed a genetic need for high protein and high fat in their diets in order to healthfully survive. Without fatty meats, their health and survival would rapidly deteriorate.

The East Indian vegetarian diet offers the most vivid contrast on earth to the Eskimo's carni-vegan diet adaptation (bear in mind that Eskimos are almost pure carnivores, as are the Masai Tribes in Africa and the South American Gauchos). East Indians have an opposite food need, based mostly on vegetables, grains, and fruits with no animal meats or fat.

If either Indians or Eskimos completely switched to the other's typical diet, they would suffer an overwhelming dietary-disease plague that could potentially end the existence of both races very rapidly. Interestingly, many paleontologists blame changes in the food chain many millions of years ago for both dinosaur mutations and their eventual extinction. It isn't inconceivable, when you think about it, that man may suffer the same fate as the dinosaurs from changing his dietary patterns too quickly for the necessary Phenotypic adaptation to keep pace. Man could potentially bring on his own extinction by altering his nutrition too drastically in too short a period of time.

The nutritional principles of VATTA, PITTA, KAPHA and others spawned in India aren't going to healthfully sustain a carnivore (like Eskimos) or red meat – carni-vegan (like most Americans). In fact, these misapplied principles may actually doom him or her instead to poor health. Our only protection from accidental food-related extinction is to pay closer attention to our body-specific nutritional requirements and not take any drastic leaps into incompatible nutrition plans.

The Death of Soil Quality

The last 50 years or so have seen extreme change in the farming industry. Prior to this time, most farms in the U.S. were small and managed by the families who lived on them. These agrarian families tended their own gardens and lived off the land. They grew potatoes, corn and other assorted vegetables and grains. Typically, they had a flock of chickens, some dairy cows, some hogs, a horse or two, and perhaps some apple, pear, or plum trees, and some blueberry or raspberry bushes. What they did not consume themselves they sent to local markets for sale. These farmers ate fish occasionally and other wild foods that they fished, picked or hunted, like trout, berries, wild turkeys or deer. They took shavings, peelings, leftovers, and other natural organic garbage and used it as compost plowing it back into the soil as fertilizer. They collected their cow, horse, chicken, and pig manure and plowed it back into the soil as well. Through this ecological process, the soil was constantly being recycled so that all of the nutrients originally found in the soil remained there. Crops were also rotated for this expressed purpose owing to the fact that some crops deplete certain elements of soil more so than others while still others help to synergistically recharge certain elements found in soil.

In this way, the soil was kept in a state of nutrient balance and yielded healthy crops from within its own natural ecosystem with few outside influences. During winter, the soil rested and all of the micro-organisms, worms, and bugs in soil would continue to break nutrients down into forms usable by plants. This winter "rest and recycling" period made more nutrients available for next years crop. The lowland fields near streams and rivers were naturally flooded during winter's thaw and rainy seasons and experienced large scale flooding every one to three years, which served to bring in new layers of silt. These layers of silt leached from the surrounding mountains and highlands brought in even more minerals and nutrients to the farming soils.

This was a period in farming history when chickens were free to roam around, eating whatever bugs and seeds appealed to them; the typically "small udder" dairy cows were likewise free to roam the fields and sample whatever elements of nature they chose. Collectively, this natural feeding process resulted in food that looked, felt, smelled, and tasted much different than our mass-produced foods of today. Eggshells and egg yolks defied breaking and milk was thick and tangy—versus today's brittle eggshells, pale yolks, and watery milk (from hybridized "big udder" cows). This was a time when vegetables had deep, tangy flavors and whole-grain breads were dark and heavy. to satisfy our appetites versus the waxy tasteless vegetables and crumbly, air-filled breads we currently find in the supermarket.

It is obvious to anyone who is old enough to remember the farms of yesteryear, or who was fortunate enough to be able to tend his or her own private gardens through the years, that typical food was totally different fifty years ago.

The changes to our modern farming system began with the emergence of gigantic, high-profit farms which progressively replaced the status quo of small farms in America. These large farms were measured in square miles instead of acres, as their small farm predecessors had been. This shift into large farming operations was widespread throughout the U.S. and Canada. The new gigantic farms were extremely productive turning out huge surpluses of grains, dairy products, vegetables, and livestock on a magnitude never seen before. This potent agricultural force became the backbone of U.S. supremacy in the world as a superpower. In a land of such great abundance, we go so far as to pay our farmers not to produce product (subsidies), and either give away or practically give away food for the political manipulation of other countries in the world—charity?

In this mass-production world of super-productive farming, the soils are pushed well beyond their limits of natural balance. Many of these same soils—where previously one crop per year was grown—are now subjected to two, three, or even more crops per year, with no rest in between. This holds true especially for the warmer climates in the U.S., where there is an eternal, year-round harvest.

The typical large-scale modern farm uses powerful insecticides to kill bugs and deadly herbicides to destroy unwanted plants. These poisons are dropped from the air by planes, from the undersides of tractors, and in some cases by hand, in order to contain agricultural pests. Unfortunately, these poisons also tend to destroy beneficial bugs, worms, and micro-organisms needed in the soil to keep it nutrient-rich.

Rivers that used to follow their natural courses are now dyked and dammed to prevent flooding. The minerals they used to carry in from the surrounding highlands and distant mountains to deposit as silt over agricultural topsoils are now whisked directly out to sea and lost forever.

The growing soils of today are pushed to the limit, "toxed up" with deadly poisons, and typically miss out on the majority of nutrient-recycling phenomena common just fifty years ago. Our modern soils are no longer replenished within the fundamental ecology of nature. Instead, man has brought in billions of tons of artificial chemical fertilizers to help enrich the soil for productivity purposes, not ecological purposes. By this, I mean that these specific fertilizers are put into the soil only to keep crop yields up and not to restore the natural ecological balance of the soil and what grows on it and feeds on it. Crops produced nowadays can look good (even without artificial colors, which are often used to optimize food's appearance). Corn still looks like corn, and may even grow to be twelve feet tall; strawberries and melons look good; lettuce, tomatoes, carrots, and potatoes all look colorful, and full and well shaped. But looks aren't everything, and when you get down to the finer science of what's in that food—something major is missing.

Plants build themselves out of about seventy to eighty different elements provided that they are available in the soil as the plants grow. Commercial growing fields are continuously overused and the chemical fertilizers added to maintain productivity inadequately replace nutrients that the plants have been extracting from the soil. Typically, the most common synthetic fertilizers are composed of only three to five different elements such as nitrogen, potassium, phosphorus, and calcium. These few elements are used because they are the only ones that are needed to make the plants grow big and appear healthy.

Unfortunately, these elements are not all a plant should have. Plants by nature want about seventy or so different elements as sustenance for life if available. But these natural elements just aren't in the soil anymore. All that is left in the soil in dense amounts are potassium, phosphorus, nitrogen, and calcium. The other necessary plant nutrients are found few and far between if at all in "modern soils." This nutrient-deficient soil crisis has affected our food in many ways, but in particular has undermined the nutrient qualities of food drastically.

According to the *Firman E. Bear Report,* published by Rutgers University, variations in the mineral content in foods vary by hundreds to even thousands of percent in some cases. Please see the Appendix: I ("Variations of Mineral Content In Vegetables") for more details.

On his audio tape, "Who Stole America's Health?" Dr. Erwin L. Gemmer comments that, at the turn of the century, "wheat was 40% protein . . . now it's 9%. If two slices of bread were to give you a certain amount of food value in 1900, now you may have to eat ten slices to get the same nutrition." Also according to Dr. Gemmer, "In 1948, spinach had 150 mg of iron per 100 grams . . . . In 1965, spinach had 27 mg of iron per 100 grams . . . . In 1973, spinach had 2.2 mg of iron per 100 grams . . . ."

Another expert weighs in on this issue: Dr. Joel Wallach, D.V.M., N.D., 1991 Nobel Prize Nominee in Medicine, echoes these serious concerns about the state of soil depletion in his tape, "Dead Doctors Don't Lie." The lack of nutrients in the soil is undermining the mineral content of our growing soils, which in turn is compromising the mineral density of our foods. Dr. Wallach grew up on a farm and worked with plants and livestock for many years. Further commenting on this crisis, Senate Documents 264 and 268 demonstrate over 90% average mineral depletion from farming soils.

From my personal experience—having had access to my grandparent's vegetable garden covering about half an acre—I was always delightfully spoiled by the rich flavors, crisp freshness, and complete appetite satisfaction I experienced with our home-grown foods, as compared to the supermarket produce that didn't look, taste, smell, or satisfy my appetite as well.

So far, in my professional research, I haven't been able to isolate the source of Dr. Gemmer's wheat and spinach statistics, but I have seen many similar statistics in relation to other foods, as assayed by consumer groups, government agencies, and from other professional publications, including research work done by Dr. Michael Colgan, Ph.D. These statistics demonstrate a wide array of varying nutrient densities in foods, usually far below the values you'd expect. Imagine oranges with only a trace of vitamin C left, and other produce completely devoid of selenium and other vital minerals we count on for our good health.

That isn't all, unfortunately: we have a new host of toxic residues in food from pesticides, herbicides, and other mass production, storage, and refinement aftereffects. Meats are full of fat, antibiotics, and steroids; milk is pasteurized and homogenized to compensate for dirty cows; and our meats are deficient in nutrients not apparent in livestock feeds or supplements. (Yes, even farm animals need many of the supplements humans do, because their foods are not up to par, either.) Scientists have developed new genetic food hybrids (plants and animals) aimed at increasing the quantity of yields but not necessarily the quality of nutrient density. It all tastes different and affects us differently than food grown in the "good old days."

This disturbing "hit or miss" phenomenon, where we come into contact with varying nutrient and toxin density in our foods, is only one more reason why we all need to be properly "typed." We should not leave our foundation of good health to chance.

"Good" Foods, "Bad" Foods, And "Compatible" Foods— How to Know What is What For You

After considering the existence of our biochemical individuality, is it fair to think of any food as good or bad? The answer is simple: any food in and of itself cannot be considered either good or bad. A given food is good or bad relative only to its effect on a specific metabolic "type." Is whale blubber compatible to an East Indian's metabolism? I doubt it, just as much as a whole-grain rice dish is not compatible to an Eskimo's metabolism. I choose the word "compatible" over good or bad in my reference to foods, in order to avoid falsely judging one's food. Is a food compatible with you? Only "typing" can tell for sure.

There is a category of generically bad food in existence, and no matter what body type you possess, this bad food simply is not compatible with human beings. I'm referring to highly processed, heat-treated, chemical-laden, nutrient- and enzyme-dead, overcooked foods. By nature, these foods undermine the health of all "types," because of their toxin-laden and nutrient-scarce nature. Organically grown, fresh and simple foods are more "nutrient-alive," and are generally preferred over synthetically altered, highly processed, mass-produced foods in every case.

There is a whole new breed of food that should be taken into account as well. Known as "super-nutritious food," it contains an even greater nutrient density and less toxic accumulation than our best standard organically grown foods. (More about this in Chapter 5).

Within the hierarchy of healthy foods, fresh is always best; frozen is the next best; canned, freeze-dried, and boxed are last in line. In the hierarchy of healthy food preparation, fresh and raw is best (except for meats and some dense starches like potatoes); low temperature, long-term cooking or high temperature "flash" cooking (like broiling and stir fry) is next best; baking, stewing, and microwaving follows the others as a healthy technique for cooking; boiling, long-term sautéing, and pressure cooking is considered worst on the list, since they have the potential to undermine the nutrient values of food. No matter what type of food preparation, over-cooking should be avoided at all costs. Fried foods are generally undesirable for all "types" due to trans-fat accumulation (more on trans fat in Chapter 4), excessive calories, free radical buildup, and nutrient deprivation.

Forced Feeding Incompatibility Syndrome (FFIS)

"FFIS" is a phenomenon where one-size-fits-all symptom relief marketers encourage unsuspecting consumers to risk their health by eating foods that are either generally unhealthy or specifically incompatible with any individual's metabolism, while they promise to relieve the symptomatic consequences that one will suffer from eating these foods with their special wonder drug. This type of drug is specifically designed to allow you to survive the discomfort of eating the wrong foods, which would normally (without the drug) cause a great deal of discomfort to eat and digest.

A good example of FFIS can be seen in a current TV commercial for antacids that encourages the viewer to eat the foods that we already know will typically cause acid indigestion, heartburn, digestive distress (and worse); as the advertisement promises, taking this antacid drug in advance will protect us from experiencing painful symptoms. "Go right ahead and eat that 'bad' (i.e., incompatible) food," the commercial seems to be blatantly telling us. "After all, if you take this drug you won't feel the food hurting you—so, based on this commercial, why worry?"

This incredibly irresponsible suggestion encourages us to indulge in an unhealthy practice, where one can use artificial pain-relief drugs to block the body's messages that certain foods we are eating are damaging us! Don't buy into this unbelievable insanity if you value yourself in the least! In this particular commercial, the kids are about to put away a serving of greasy fast foods, while one parent questions the other for ordering the same fast foods as their kids. Both parents openly acknowledge that these foods are exceedingly unhealthy (and will cause stomach upset and other problems once eaten). They obviously don't value their own kids' health by endorsing the intake of indigestible fast foods! What's worse, the parent explains to her friend that it's okay for her to eat this junk food, since she's got a drug that will block the pain it causes!

In another prime example of FFIS, an advertisement encourages the consumption of certain milk products, which many people cannot digest due to lactase deficiencies. Promoters push a so-called "drug"— actually an enzyme complex—to "help" one eliminate digestive stress from these products.

The apparent analogy present in this mentality is that, again, it's okay to indulge in foods that are completely incompatible with your Phenotype (body type) and biochemical individuality, and which are ultimately harmful to your health. Chemical incompatibility causes uncomfortable symptoms and physical damage, all of which does not seem important anymore, when you can cover up the problem by popping pills.

In effect, the promoters' drug products in the above examples (and many others commonplace in our society) artificially "cover up" your body's natural defensive responses (that is, pain that you experience consciously) to incompatible foods. This natural defensive pain response to incompatible foods is termed "symptoms" or "dis-ease." If you willingly go along with the logic behind such advertisements as those described above, then with drugs in hand you can literally "force feed" your body with food that it would normally reject...and you will (seemingly) get away with it—at least from a symptomatic standpoint.

But you really don't get away with anything when you consider the metabolic damage these foods cause to your system; such damage will still occur, whether or not you experience painful symptoms. When your body hurts, it's trying to let you know that something is wrong. In the case of all pain relief medications, conscious symptoms are artificially reduced while the root physical cause of the pain goes uncorrected and is allowed to progress. At least with food-induced pain the cure is most obvious: simply avoid incompatible (or symptom-provoking) foods and/or food combinations! Prevention is the key.

Metabolic Typing and Profiling science systematically sorts out food incompatibilities for each individual, revealing whether food-related symptoms are due to genetic factors or actually due to other measurable metabolic and nutritional inconsistencies which can be overcome **naturally**. Typing and Profiling will answer the question "is this food right for my body or is my body not right for this food?" It also answers the question, "can my body be made right for this food?" In all cases, understanding your biochemical individuality can ensure optimal health. Avoiding foods or food combinations, which require pain-relief medication, is a quantum leap in the right direction for eternal wellness.

CHAPTER FOUR

Personalized Nutrition . . .
The Next Megatrend

Let thy food be thy medicine.
—**Hippocrates**

To a significant degree, our body, face, and voice reflect our habits, emotions, thoughts, and lifestyle. Our innermost thoughts, neuromuscular tensions, and habits form, in large part, the shape of our bodies and the topography of our faces.
—**Dan Millman**

Never trust a weight loss expert that has never been there.
—**Bob Schwartz, Ph.D.**

For each essential factor there is a "too little" deficiency, a minimum, a maximum, a "too much" (excess) and a Goldilocks's "just right" (optimum) daily amount.
—**Udo Erasmus, Ph.D.**

One man's meat is another man's poison.
—**Lucretius**

The therapeutic expression of Typing and Profiling—including all of its healthful implications—lies within the creation of a fully individualized and customized diet and supplement program. Just knowing that you're a

Thyroid Dominant Type with an underactive digestive system and B12 deficiency, for example, isn't going to help you, without a precise nutritional plan to go along with it.

In this chapter, I will treat you as if you were my nutritional client and take you conceptually through the five steps of typing, in order to help you better understand how this process actually works. The end result is the creation of a fully customized nutritional program scientifically matched to **your** own biochemical uniqueness.

Before I get started typing you, I would like to present a brief overview of some half-hearted attempts in common practice to personalize or individualize nutrition for you. These attempts at personalization are only slightly better than one-size-fits-all nutrition and are extremely limited in scope. They do, however, represent the beginning of the mainstream societal acknowledgment of, demand for, and the acceptance of nutritional personalization. Furthermore, these programs and their ancillary products have historical value, because they have sequentially opened up the door to the next (and final) megatrend in nutrition—the final frontier: personalized nutrition—our only alternative!

The Limitations of Pseudo-Individualized Supplements

You go to your favorite health food store, pharmacy, or supermarket to buy a multivitamin and mineral supplement . . . are immediately bombarded by shelf after shelf of multivitamins! You ask yourself, "which brand should I choose?" Then you notice the female formula (you happen to be female). "Ah ha!" you say to yourself, "this makes sense because I don't want to take **manly** vitamins, now do I? Of course not! Maybe they're dangerous for me . . . they might even turn me into a man!"

Fears aside, you then step up to the shelf and notice the "over-40" formula next to the female formula. You say to yourself "you'd think they'd have the over-40 **and** female formulas all rolled into one." Maybe they do, maybe they don't. The point is that you are naturally drawn to a more body-specific formula. You instinctively want this personalization factor built in—it makes sense.

"Or maybe you are that average person —roughly 1–2% of the population— and this formula (by luck) actually helps you."

The problem is, these generic supplements are merely take-offs based on RDA levels, and therefore have no direct connection to your specific needs. At best, your average gender-specific, age-related multivitamin is a slightly improved generic guess at what is predicted for your body needs. But without typing or testing your metabolism, it is still a "shot in the dark" in terms of fulfilling your actual nutrient needs.

You may still buy the female, over-40 multivitamin, but you really don't know if it's going to work or not. Perhaps it's so mismatched to your biochemically unique profile that it will actually create deficiencies or megadosing overload syndromes, or else liver, heart, or kidney stress. Or maybe so many other components of your diet are out of balance that this formula couldn't possibly make up for other dietary mistakes. Or perhaps the supplement is "dead" (i.e., lost its bioactivity) because it's been sitting on the shelf for so long. Or maybe you are that average person—roughly 1–2% of the population—and this formula (by luck) actually helps you.

Without typing you really haven't a clue, unless of course you literally "gag" on this pill because you are so allergic to it and have to dump it immediately. Or maybe you continue forcing yourself to take it because it doesn't have to taste (or feel) good to be good for you, right? Or maybe your body just isn't ready yet for this pill . . . or the pill is not synergized— but how can you really know without typing?

The Fatal Flaw of the "Body Type" Diet

I have observed a number of body type diets, including the aptly named "Body Type Diet." I applaud the efforts of the inventors of these plans for attempting to further differentiate us as individuals using certain person-specific criteria. It represents a step in the right direction. These plans are certainly a lot closer to providing a healthier nutrient balance than some of the other extremist plans I've seen in use.

The inherent weaknesses in these types of diets is their requirement for respective personalization strategies. This undermines their effectiveness and validity. These weaknesses all fall under one category: speculation.

The criteria required for entry into any one of these body type programs are usually based on questionnaires or charts. Aside from the scientific controversies about the inconsistencies, discrepancies, and limitations of some of these programs (like Sheldon's or Kelley's Systems) they all make the fundamental mistake of speculating about—rather than actually measuring—your nutritional needs directly.

To better understand this "speculation factor," let me ask the following question: Would you expect your family doctor to diagnose and treat your health condition from a mere phone call, without the benefit of a physical exam, blood and urine tests, x-rays, or other evaluative modalities, and without a follow-up? Of course not! It works the same in these chart-driven or questionnaire-mediated "Body Type Diet Programs." Without directly measuring and classifying your body's metabolic functions and nutrient status, you can't possibly tell what's right for you. Questionnaire and chart programs simply make too many unprovable assumptions without true body specific criteria. Human error further compounds this issue rendering even more inconsistencies into the assumptive criteria. Most people fill out questionnaires inaccurately in the first place.

With true typing, there are very little speculative and assumptive criteria because there are so many body-specific measurements taken directly from the person in question. In typing speculation is at an all time minimum. A typer would know if his urine was too acidic and that he had a full-blown folic acid deficiency, based on actual lab tests. He would know what to do about it and then be able to double-check his/her progress with a retest to validate improvement. The process of typing goes well beyond what questionnaire and chart mediated body typing can do.

If You Were My Patient...

Let's pretend that you've sought my help and you are now in my office, ready to be typed and profiled. You have already been to a fair number of doctors, nutritionists, trainers, and the like, all of whom have not fully addressed your symptoms, objectives, and lifestyle needs. (This is the typical case for many of my patients.)

Nobody has fully "connected the dots" of wellness for you and you're still suffering! Perhaps the last medical doctor you visited couldn't find any **overt** problems or disease present, and therefore told you "it's all in your head." Maybe you believed him or her, or maybe you really didn't and that's why you sought my help! After all, you still have a lot of nagging symptoms plaguing you like fatigue, intermittent digestive stress, nagging headaches, weakness, weight problems, recurring rashes, joint pain, high blood pressure, and many more symptoms. You may have already been to an Herbologist, Acupuncturist, Iridologist, Kinesiologist, and other assorted healthcare practitioners. You may even have brought your diet plan and a host of other supplements and drugs with you for me to examine along with all of your medical records. Maybe you've gotten to the point of pure desperation and that's why you're giving the "guy down the street" (me) a chance. After all, what have you got to lose that you already haven't lost!

Maybe you found me likable when you saw me on a TV program. Or maybe you liked it when Dr. Bob Torman on "CBS This Morning" called me "quintessential," because it appealed to your rebellious instincts to "break out of the mold" and look for alternatives. Maybe you simply felt that I knew something that no one else seemed to know and could actually help you (for a change)!

None of this really matters now, because here you are in my office ready to be typed and profiled. You are committed to seeing this process through We start off by having you fill out an extensive medical, nutrition, and exercise history. This allows me to better understand your personal wellness experiences.

"The greater the 'gray area' the greater the success potential."

Next, we have an initial consultation. We discuss your health history and what has and has not been done for you in the way of fully analyzing and fulfilling your wellness needs. I accomplish all of this by taking a very close look at your diet, supplements, exercise (or non-exercise) patterns, and your lifestyle at large—I look for imbalances. I do this in the hope of identifying "gray areas" in your health history. These "gray areas" represent the need for investigative procedures that have not been performed on you to date such as typing or profiling analysis. The more of these "gray areas" that become apparent, the greater the chance that we can fully restore you to optimal health.

Most people have huge "gray areas" with regard to clinical nutrition intervention. The larger these clinical nutrition "gray areas," the greater the success potential. My goal is to nutritionally rebuild you from the ground up and create a foundation of wellness that will never deteriorate again. Because nutrition is the absolute cornerstone of wellness and in your case you've historically had little, if any **proper** intervention (which is typical of patients), we have a lot to work with and can expect many dramatic improvements. I've already noted your ethnicity, family disease patterns, personal disease pattern, you and your family's ages, your weight (on **my** scale, of course), gender, and other background information.

After I give you a brief overview of what one-size-fits-all thinking is, stressing its ineffectiveness in promoting optimal health on an individual basis, we next get down to business.

Step 1: Quantification and Qualification (Computing Calories and Food Patterns)

We begin the first step by discussing your health and fitness objectives. You tell me that you're hoping to eliminate the various and variable symptoms that you've included on your health and history forms, but first and foremost you simply want to feel younger. Some of the nagging symptoms you've noted include:

- Headaches
- Depression
- Rebounding constipation and diarrhea
- Overt sugar cravings (you're a confirmed "chocoholic")

- Fatigue
- Indigestion
- Joint pain
- Poor sleep patterns
- Constant scarring
- Intermittent skin rashes

- Hair loss
- Gum sensitivity
- Heart palpitations on occasion
- wrinkly skin
- Inability to concentrate
- Intermittent blurred vision
- Flabby untoned musculature
- Excessive fat that just won't come off
- Extreme mood swings
- Chronic sinus congestion and post nasal drip
- Chronically dry and bad tasting mouth
- Very dry or oily skin (depending on the body area)
- Craving for stimulants (like coffee)
- Cold feeling extremities
- Occasional dizziness
- Poor memory
- Slow-healing wounds
- Halitosis (bad breath)
- Muscle cramps (especially in your legs)
- Multiple "age spots"
- Premature graying hair
- Pale complexion
- Redness in the eyes
- Cellulite
- Heavy PMS
- Constant gas
- Anxiety attacks
- Foul-smelling stools and urine
- Stomach pain
- Excessive sweating
- Bad body odor
- Constant burping
- Blood in the stool
- Stiffness
- Excessive temper
- Inconsistent appetite

. . . and others still.

You may find, to your surprise, that many of these symptoms are of extreme importance to me as your typing doctor. Prior to our meeting you were told by other health professionals that "it's all in your head," that "it's not that important" or "learn to live with it because there's nothing that can be done anyway." Then, when you think about the quality of your life, you realize that these "dis-eases" are making you absolutely miserable even though the previous doctor said you weren't really sick.

Our first objective through typing is to naturally eliminate any and all of these symptoms (if possible) so you can feel better. And, of course, you want to live a longer life under improved conditions with. the youthful vitality of earlier days.

Your second objective, according to your statements, is to drop body fat and tone up: get fit again. Maybe you're a person who doesn't exercise at all; or maybe your exercise program is just not cutting it; or maybe you have an even more pressing need to get into shape again. Maybe you're a world-class athlete looking to peak for the next Olympics; or are preparing for a future bodybuilding competition; or you're a movie star who needs to show some muscle for your next movie which is being filmed in eight weeks. Perhaps you are truly obese and need to drop the fat and get into shape as a matter of an immediate life or death scenario. Maybe you need to rehabilitate a nagging injury that just won't go away or perhaps you are an average person simply searching for the answers to simply feel and look better.

Now that we know your desired objectives of fat loss and health gain, we can begin a general physical examination, including testing blood pressure, heart rate, listening to your heart and lungs, palpation for abdominal masses; examining your body structure and range of movement, measuring limb and trunk size, doing a body fat analysis; looking at your eyes, ears, nose skin, hair and throat under magnification, and perhaps taking a standard blood and urine sample for conventional analysis (if not performed very recently); maybe we will even take an x-ray of an injury site or have an x-ray performed. if warranted for some other reason. Once we accomplish the standard examination phase of Step 1, we can move on to the next phase which is quantifying (or assessing) your actual macronutrient caloric need given your lifestyle and objectives. How many calories does it take to run your body most efficiently? We'll find out directly.

By the way, the majority of nutrition patients I've worked with have been to other so-called nutritionists (mostly novices) who have never quantified their diet for them. Instead of assessing caloric need scientifically for each client, these novice nutritionists simply guess about this procedure or in some cases are not even aware that it exists in the first place, due to their lack of training and expertise in its application. Many of my patients have walked into the office with what I term "standard form diets" taken from a generic source with no real direct connection to them as the patient.

In one instance, a patient of mine handed me a Pritikin Diet plan. Apparently, this patient had walked into a nutritionist's office, plopped down $150, talked to the novice nutritionist for about fifteen minutes (with no formal exam or medical history taken), and was then handed this generic Pritikin Diet. It had been taken from a notebook. The patient had been told to follow through on it, though no quantification or qualification process to determine exact calorie needs was performed, no typing, no metabolic analysis, and no diet analysis of any kind was given. To add insult to injury, my new patient plopped down an additional $150 for a group of one-size-fits-all supplements, which of course had no connection to the actual measurable needs of this patient. And, there was that same pile of partly used supplements placed on my desk, pills that my patient had barely taken because they made her feel even worse after she ingested them.

What a joke! My disgust with this treatment of my new patient intensified further when I found out that the particular novice nutritionist in question is a (somewhat) famous nutritionist "to the stars." In reality, this person has no discernible or accredited academic qualifications at all. Truly a case of the "blind leading the blind." What's worse is that this is not an isolated case—this kind of fraud occurs every day to thousands of unsuspecting consumers. Don't be one of them!

The Quantifying Process

Our first task is to assess your Basal Metabolic Rate (BMR). The BMR, expressed as calories, is the daily rate at which your body consumes calories in a resting state, in order to sustain life. This rate represents an amount of calories that your body needs if you were to lay in bed all day (24 hours). If you were to match this exact rate (BMR) to the exact amount of calories from foods you take in (properly proportioned), your body would not gain or lose any weight whatsoever. You would not gain so much as an ounce of fat, muscle, bone, organ, tissue or water. The total BMR represents a culmination of the differing rates at which each cell, tissue, and organ uses energy It is an ideal calorie amount and it is unique to you only.

Your BMR is a sustained calorie level that changes throughout your life as you grow and mature. It is a level of calorie consumption which can be altered by disease onset, stress, dietary, and exercise modifications in your life. Direct and indirect *calorimetric* studies have measured these levels in humans and there are some mathematically derived norms I can employ to decipher your particular BMR.

Your BMR is then computed based on age, gender, height, weight, and other factors (all of which are mathematically corrected for). In effect, I am estimating your BMR levels without having to utilize expensive, sophisticated, complex in-lab calorimetric assessment, although a lab can be contacted to do this if you wish (as my patient).

The Energy Usage of Physical Activity

Once we have computed a mathematically derived BMR for you (or tested you on a BMR tester), we then add in the caloric energy needs of your body as a result of "getting out of bed," moving around, and exercising. We call this the "Energy Level of Physical Activity"—also known as Daily Physical Activity Need (DPAN)—it requires an individualized computation of calories. Whether you sit in an office all day, are a blue collar laborer, a professional athlete, exercise intermittently or consistently—all modes of life have a direct effect on how many calories your body requires daily, over and above your BMR levels.

As my patient, we will look at what physical activities you are performing, covering literally every hour of your day (and night). When you exercise, I will assess both the "type" of your exercises and the intensity at which you perform them. Whether you are a heavy, medium, or light laborer, this too has a bearing on the process of determining the exact amount of calories your body requires. I will assess the rate at which you burn calories throughout the day during different activities using mathematical norms based upon calorimetry studies conducted on exercising and sedentary humans. When you sit down you'll burn so many calories, when you lift heavy objects, you'll burn so many calories and so on.

If you'd like to have this more directly assessed, there is new lab technology that allows us to more precisely monitor your caloric consumption during your daily routine. As part of your treatment, I can arrange for this procedure.

Once we've determined the specific calorie needs for your individual pattern of activity, then we can add this amount to your BMR. In our hypothetical case, as my patient we determined your BMR to be 1,500 calories per day. Your Daily Physical Activity Need was found to be another 600 calories per day, so the combined figure is 2,100 calories per day. In other words, your body requires 2,100 calories per day to sustain itself without any net weight gain or loss in and out of bed. But we're not finished with the quantification process yet.

Specific Dynamic Activity

The Specific Dynamic Activity (SDA) represents the caloric energy required for the processes of digestion and reflexive **brown fat thermogenesis** after eating. Thermogenesis is a term referring to heat production by the body.

Our body is actually a "heat factory" with about 75% of the caloric energy that we consume as food going into heat production. About a quarter of what's left goes into energy production for muscular movement, thinking, and all other bodily processes—except for the 6 to 10% that consumed by the SDA. A certain amount of energy usually—expressed as a percentage of overall body energy—is consumed by digestion and brown fat metabolism automatically.

After eating, that "warm feeling" you experience is a reflexive response to the increased calorie consumption of brown adipose tissue which gives off extra heat for better digestion. This brown adipose tissue is a primary **thermoregulator** (i.e., a heat regulator) of the body, and is specifically designed to create heat to stabilize body temperatures. (By the way, white (or yellow) adipose is designed strictly for fat storage and body part insulation.) There are many thermogenic supplements designed to stimulate brown fat metabolism to increase calorie usage by the body. MaHuang is one of those herbal supplements used for this purpose—but is it right for you? Only typing will tell!

So far, we've been able to compute your SDA as a fixed 6% of your BMR and DPAN combined.

Next, we add all three figures together:

BMR	1,500 calories	(Laying in bed all day.)
DPAN.	+ 600 calories	(Exercise, job, lifestyle.)
SDA	+ 126 calories	(6% of 2,100) (Digestion)
TCND	2,226 calories	

This adds up to 2,226 calories, which equals your Total Calorie Need Per Day (TCND). Your body requires this amount to maintain itself at its constant weight, based on all your lifestyle factors.

Dangerous Territory

"Dangerous territory" can be found above the Total Caloric Need Per Day figure or below it. If you're consuming more calories than the 2,226 TCND level (remember, this is a hypothetical figure—your own number outside of this example may be quite different), you will gain weight, primarily as fat. (Most people in our country, over time, tend to exceed their TCND's. This has lead the U.S. to become the most overweight country in the world.)

Over time, our metabolisms slow down as we age and exercise less and less. During the aging process we tend to eat more and more of the wrong foods due to stress, less free time, and inattention to our precise nutritional needs. This problem is compounded further by the fact that most of the foods we consume typically have low nutrient densities with a greater proportion of empty calories, which satisfy our appetites less while serving to increase our appetites more. In response to this situation, our bodies reflexively seek more nourishment. Subsequently, we eat more to make up the difference for low nutrient densities and end up accumulating more body fat from empty calories.

Aging in combination with a lack of exercise allows our valuable calorie-burning muscles to shrink away, while non-calorie consuming storage fat (white or yellow fat) greedily accumulates in its place. It has been postulated by physiologists that between the ages of thirty and sixty, the average American woman and man loses 30% of their strength and the muscle that creates it as they gain approximately 30% more fat on their bodies.

In our hypothetical treatment of you (as my client), your stated objective is to lose ten pounds in the next ten weeks and thereafter keep fat accumulation controlled for the rest of your life for both health and cosmetic reasons. Excess fat accumulation is a generic health risk and also considered by most to be unsightly. Once you are fully typed, your worries about fat gain will dissipate once and for all.

If your actual daily calorie consumption level is below the TCND level of 2,226—say, at 1,600—you are still in dangerous territory if you are chronically underweight. At this level, you would be consuming 626 fewer calories than your body actually requires to maintain itself, which in turn would force it to burn whatever fat or muscle is available to it, in order to make up the calorie difference. Being chronically underweight carries its own set of health risks ranging from deficiency states to immunodeprivation, growth and maturation impairments.

In the above example of chronic underweight, you would need to actually gain "good weight" to be optimally healthy. By "good weight" I mean muscle, bone, and teeth density, better hydration (water weight), and maybe even a little "reserve fat." In order to accomplish steady weight increases, you would have to consume more than your TCND level and then back your calories down to the TCND level once your ideal weight has been achieved; this would allow you to maintain yourself at the ideal level.

As a typical American nutrition patient, you've already expressed the need to lose some body fat (ten pounds in ten weeks). Let's say that my evaluation of your eating habits reveals that your Actual Daily Calorie Consumption (ADCC) is in reality 2,700 calories per day, 474 calories over your calculated theoretical need per day of 2,226 calories (TCND). It is quite clear that you are consuming more food than your body actually requires. No wonder you've accumulated some fat and are overweight!

Put graphically:

ADCC	2,700 calories
TCND	-.2,226 calories

= 474 calories

So you're "in the red" by 474 calories. This means that you are taking in almost 500 calories per day more than your body actually requires to sustain itself, given your daily average lifestyle.

What happens to this extra 474 calories? You answer, "I'm not exactly sure, maybe this extra fat layer on my body?" Exactly: what calories your body can't use for energy and heat it stores as fat.

The only way to **subtract** this fat from your body is to **subtract** some calories from your current daily intake, but this cannot be done in a haphazard fashion! There is a method to our madness (you've probably heard about this before): given that one pound of fat equals 3,500 calories, we will quantify your customized diet so that fat will progressively and naturally come off of your body at a rate that's healthy and safe, until you reach your ideal weight and fat percentage. This is accomplished by subtracting calories from your TCND and ADCC. Under these terms your body will be slightly starved for calories and have to burn fat in order to compensate. In the future, once your ideal weight is reached, your diet will again be adjusted so that calories are added in to bring you up to your TCND caloric level; then you will be able to maintain that ideal fat percentage and weight level. Otherwise, you would continue to lose too much weight.

This new TCND level may have to be adjusted higher than your current 2,226 TCND level because your metabolism and caloric consumption rate has favorably increased since we first typed you. Of course, a faster metabolism is highly desirable because, thanks to the process set in motion through typing," your body uses more calories in less time, producing more energy than ever before! This means that you can eat more without gaining fat.

For now, we'll subtract 750 calories from you current ADCC level of 2,700 calories, or approximately 250 from your TCND 2,226 calorie level for a New Target Level of 2,000 calories per day.

Organizing your nutritional plan at 2,000 calories per day as your caloric target will force your body to take 250 calories per day out of fat storage from under the skin, between your muscles, and from around your internal organs, in order to make up the difference. We call this a "Calorie Deficit" or "Negative Calorie Balance."

250 calories of fat melting off your body every day over a seven-day period equals 1,750 (7 x 250) calories of fat per week lost from your body, or about half a pound of fat (half of 3,500 calories) lost each week you stay on the 2,000-calorie-per-day target level. So, in ten weeks, you'll lose five pounds, at least theoretically.

Because I'm going to redesign your daily exercise program so that you will burn off an extra 250 calories per day with physical activity that your body isn't replacing with diet, the calorie deficit will grow to 500 calories per day less than what your body needs to sustain your current weight (250 calories from diet + 250 calories from exercise = 500). In effect, you'll be in a 500-calorie-per-day Negative Calorie Balance (or deficit).

Now you'll be losing fat at a rate of approximately one pound per week (3,500 caloric deficit per week), for a total loss of ten pounds in ten weeks: exactly what your stated objective was. (See Workbook Step 1: How To Quantify and Qualify Your Diet, for more details and your own self-application of this process.)

This all sounds simple, but when strategizing diet, most people and novice nutritionists "blow it" from the start because they don't quantify caloric needs properly. This happens either due to ignorance or imprecision, but however this occurs, the result always undermines effectiveness.

Now, with your new 2,000-calorie-per-day Target Calorie Level, you may think that you're all set to go—but you're not even close! Now I'm going to take you to the next phase of Step 1—qualification.

The Qualifying Process

Now that we know (theoretically) how many daily calories your body needs to healthfully lose ten pounds in the next ten weeks, we need to divide this number up into the proper proportion of macronutrients and their correct caloric amount to fulfill our 2,000 calorie-per-day target. Macronutrients are the basic nutrients we need to consume on a daily basis in "larger than gram" amounts for survival (I classify air as a macronutrient although most scientific texts do not because it is not considered a weight measure. The fact is that the atmosphere weighs 14.7 pounds per square inch so air does in fact have weight). These macronutrients are protein, fats, carbohydrates, air, and water. They each have their own calorie value and metabolic value.

According to the Atwater Coefficients:

1 gram of protein = 4.35 Kcal = Calorie   1 gram of carbohydrates
    = 4.1   Kcal = Calorie
1 gram of fat = 9 Kcal = Calorie
1 gram of water = 0 Kcal = Calorie
1 gram of ethanol = 7 Kcal = Calorie (alcohol is not a true
(alcohol)   macronutrient because
                          we do not require it
                          for survival).

Simply stated, the metabolic value of macronutrients (besides as calories) is:

PROTEIN: Provides the building blocks of the body (amino acids) for all cells, tissues, organs, hormones, neuropeptides, etc. Protein tends to speed up metabolism and stimulate the Central Nervous System (CNS). It has diuretic qualities. It cannot be stored significantly as usable protein and therefore must be replenished daily. It can be turned into fat when taken in excess.

CARBOHYDRATES: Provides the primary "high intensity, short term energy source" all body cells and tissues require, especially nerve and muscle cells. Excess carbohydrates tend to slow metabolism down and hold water in the body in larger than ideal amounts. Carbs can be easily stored as glycogen and then fat if not used for energy purposes.

FATS: Provides the primary "low intensity, long term energy" source most body cells and tissues require and are involved in a multitude of metabolic processes ranging from immune function to fat digestion, forming body linings and nerve insulation, for prostaglandin formation and more. Fat tends to slow metabolism down but not to the same degree as carbohydrates in excess. In excess, fat is easily stored as fat.

The improper proportion of one macronutrient to the next has a profound effect on body metabolism leading to increased or decreased metabolic rates with subsequent fatigue, serious nutrient and metabolic imbalances and disease states, and premature aging. The proper apportionment of proteins, carbohydrates, and fats within the nutritional plan is very important in terms of overall health impact.

At this stage, within the five steps of typing, we are still only at the initial theoretical levels that have not been fully adjusted to "typing/profiling" specifications yet—this comes later. For the moment (in your case as a hypothetical patient), we are only mathematically estimating your macronutrient needs. Before we apportion the macronutrients into your 2,000-calorie-per-day formula, we need to take a closer look at these macronutrients.

The Protein-Carb-Fat Connection

PROTEIN: Of the types of proteins found in nature, all have different properties within our body's metabolism. Foods rich in proteins consist of eggs, milk, fish, poultry, beef, pork, soy, lamb, legumes, nuts, seeds, grains, etc. (See Appendix D, Common Food Families Used Through The Centuries). They each have different body and tissue building characteristics, various digestive implications, and allergy factor potentials specific to your biochemical uniqueness. Proteins require the presence of fats and carbohydrates for efficient metabolism. Their carbon skeletons can be denitrogenized and transformed into sugar (deaminization) which in turn can convert into adipose tissue (fat) but all at a very expensive metabolic and health denigrating cost.

To rely on protein as a substitute for carbohydrate and fat needs is completely erroneous and risky to your health. Excessively high protein diets can kill, as demonstrated by the recorded deaths of some people who were on high-protein diets. Proteins need to be in proper balance with carbs and fats specific to your "type," in order to be maximized properly.

CARBOHYDRATES: There are 4 basic categories of carbohydrates:

Complex—Calorie Dense (starches with high caloric-to-fiber ratio)
Complex—Calorie Dilute (vegetables with high fiber
                    and low calories)
Natural Simple Sugars (fruits, high sugar vegetables, and honey)
Manmade Refined Simple Sugars

Each of these carbohydrate types has different effects on the body, some good and some not so good in terms of digestion, hormonal and neuropeptide responses, blood sugar levels, acidity and alkalinity, short and long term energy production, and overall health. The vegetables and fruits, which contain concentrated carbohydrates, have a variety of properties including different acidity and alkalinity levels before and after entering the body, varying glycemic index factors, and differing phytonutrient contents.

For optimum metabolism, these different types of carbohydrates should be properly proportioned to each other and in relation to protein and fat within the diet, as well as the amounts taken in being determined by the specifics of your "type." Excessive carbohydrate intake, especially in regard to refined carbohydrates, will slow the metabolism. Excess carbs also hold body water, strain organs and body systems, damage teeth and the digestive system, and most definitely cause fat accumulation, since carbohydrate readily converts to fat.

FAT: There are three basic types of fat from varying food sources:

MUFA—(Monounsaturated Fatty Acids)—Found in a variety of foods from all macronutrient categories.

PUFA—(Polyunsaturated Fatty Acids)—Mostly from plant sources, particularly grains, seeds, and vegetables. Also from fish and poultry.

SAFA—(Saturated Fatty Acids)—Predominantly from animal sources. The dietary apportionment of each of these types of fat—in relation to one another and in relation to proteins and carbohydrates—is critical to a balanced healthy metabolism and is very individual to your "type." When people indiscriminately cut fat from their diets, they tend to remove "good" fats as well as "bad" fats, which in turn creates health problems and metabolic dysfunction.

The PUFA's are categorized by three primary essential "good" fatty acids: *"alpha"* linolenic, "cis" linoleic, and *"gamma"* linolenic acid, which are absolutely critical to the immune system and metabolism at large. Many people are deficient or unbalanced in these essential fats and their derivatives due to indiscriminate diet practices, enzyme inhibition (delta 6 desaturase for one), and cofactor deficiencies. (Cofactors are vitamins, minerals, and hormones.)

Probably the most significant consequence of this fat dilemma is immune system dysfunction. All in all, these fat factors need to be balanced in relation to each other and to carbs and proteins, and in relation to your typing specifications for healthiest results. And, as you probably know by now, excesses of saturated fats (most particularly) increase fat accumulation in the body, cause higher blood cholesterol and triglyceride levels, and also put a pronounced unhealthy strain on your body's frame and metabolism in general.

We next need to proportion protein, carb, and fat origin foods into a theoretical, "inter-proportion" category. I call this "Zone I," of perhaps 40/30/30,or some other "rough" ratio to build from as we move through metabolic typing Steps 2, 3, and 4. Within each category of nutrient, I will build a list of food selections with the proper "intra-proportion category." For example, your theoretical "rough" diet will consist of:

Theoretical Zone I

> 50% of its calories from carbohydrates
> 30% of its calories from protein
> 20% of its calories from fat

50/30/20 = INTER PROPORTION of the 3 food categories

Theoretical Zone II

> 25% of its total protein calories from fish sources
> 25% of its protein calories from vegetable sources
> 25% of its protein calories from eggs and dairy sources
> 25% of its protein calories from red meat sources

25/25/25/25 = INTRA-PROPORTION of each Protein Type

Theoretical Zone III

40% of its total carbohydrate calories from complex calorie dilute high fiber vegetables

25% of its total complex carbohydrate from dense starchy vegetables

25% of total carb calories from natural simple sugars in fruit

10% of total carb calories from the manmade natural simple sugar category of sweets

4 0/25/25/10 = INTRA PROPORTION of each Carbohydrate Type

Theoretical Zone IV

40% of its total fat calories from PUFA'S

35% of its total fat calories from MUFA'S

25% of its total fat calories from SAFA'S

40/35/25 = INTRA PROPORTION of each Fat Type

Steps 2, 3, and 4 of the typing process will enable us to understand exactly what specific foods will be eliminated or retained based on your "type," allergy factors, mineral ratios, and pH (acidity/alkalinity ratios). The last component of the qualification process is to check the proportion of micronutrients to one another. This process and the final refinements made upon the qualification process is reserved for Step 4 when all of the other criteria for your biochemical identity is compiled. At that time, you will have a completely customized nutrition program meal-by-meal, food-by-food, zone-by-zone, essential nutrient-by-nutrient that's for your body only.

Step 2: Pure Metabolic Typing

As my hypothetical patient, you've already visited me twice—once for the initial evaluation and once to go over the quantification/qualification process. Now its your third visit and we are going to metabolically "type" you using non specimen related laboratory data except for noting your specific blood type. This is the part of your typing process that's going to allow me to place you into your basic tribal ancestral line or Phenotype and to deduce other categorizable conclusions about how your body functions so that I can place you into the proper diet category for your "type" of body.

It is in this step that we will determine if you are an omnivore, carni-vegan (a type of meat-eater), or a vegetarian blend. We will develop a working idea of what exact foods are best for you, what foods are the worst for you, and what substances are likely to cause an allergic reaction. We will be able to better understand what the best "inter" and "intra" proportions of macronutrient and individual foods are right for you (Zones I—IV). Do you need a 55/35/15 (inter) and 40/30/20/10, 25/25/25/25, 30/30/30 (intra) or some other "inter" and "intra" combination of proportions to be in the so-called "zone" for you, without a "slopfactor"? Of course: Only typing can tell! (The "slopfactor" is what Dr. Sears calls the inherent imprecision 40-30-30 has in regards to individual differences, as mentioned previously.)

Your proper micronutrient ratios will also become more evident as will the proportion of raw to cooked food you'll require. The majority of the food we match to your biochemical uniqueness in the proper proportions will automatically yield the right vitamin/mineral/ phytonutrient/amino acid composition but, thanks to the nutrient depletion of food in modern times, we will have to precisely customize and synergize your supplements "just to make sure" your diet plan doesn't fail you in the slightest. I'll take no chances with your health and well being—neither should you.

Metabolic Typing Procedures

I will now take you through a series of typing worksheets which will allow me to "score" your body type characteristics and group them into discernible categories of metabolism.

I begin to type you by scoring you on the basis of the following:

- Your blood type (ABO)
- Height, weight range
- Body fat percentage
- Pulse rate
- Hair characteristics curly, profuse, balding pattern
- Skin factors smooth, soft, rashy, thick, bumpy, eruptive, sensitive
- Bone and muscle descriptions small, thick, highly toned, soft, medium, long, large
- Overall shape long, thin, compact, symmetrical, curvaceous, broad shouldered, angular, round,
- Forehead size
- Skin color black, white, brown, yellow, red, albino
- Dream states PSI transmitter, PSI receiver
- Personality factors nervous, high-strung, meticulous, aware, sensitive, receiver, physically oriented, flirtatious, sensual, food oriented, jolly, charismatic, love-oriented
- Intelligence characteristics creative, leadership, survival, social, flexible, practical, intuitive, technical

The net result of this process is to fit you into an endocrine gland category based on glandular dominance and to identify the recessive glands and their proportions of balance in relation to one another.

Blood type and endocrine type are closely correlated. Blood typing will help in categorizing foods as theoretically right and wrong for you while endocrine typing helps delineate micronutrient needs and proportions.

Let's say that in your case you have a "B" type blood and your height is medium (5'5" female). Your weight range is usually pretty stable and medium (except for the ten pounds you just put on), your pulse rate is 66 beats per minute, your blood pressure is 120/80 mmHg, your hair is curly, your skin is thick, your muscles are toned and thick, your bones are pretty thick and dense, your overall shape is compact, your head and face shape is rather square, you dream a lot, and you're very practical when it comes to the physical, and you're mildly athletic. In this case, skin can be any color.

After rating you from the above criteria, it becomes clear, based on typing science, that you are a characteristically pure "Adrenal Type." Your adrenal gland is most dominant and the remainder of your other glands are proportionately recessive, though your thyroid is probably one of the weakest glands in your body.

I have charted the Physical Functions of the Endocrine Glands in Table 5. For the purposes of this book a full explanation of all the known metabolic types is outside its scope, but will appear in a following text. Typing is a very complex science. It is too expansive for a complete discussion in *For Your Body Only*. For now, for best results, refer to Table 5: Physical Functions of the Endocrine Glands, Table 5A: Overview of Endocrine Glands, Hormones, and Functions, Table 6: Nervous System, Endocrine Glands, and Oxidation Patterns, and Table 7: Metabolic Typing Systems Overview. Then continue following through the five typing steps (Quantification/Qualification, Pure Metabolic Typing, Laboratory Assessment, Diet and Supplement Customization, and the Final Step: Re-Evaluation); a hypothetical Adrenal Type would go through as my client and *grasp the concepts* of what we are doing for the moment.

I chose the "Adrenal Type" to bring you through the metabolic typing steps as my hypothetical patient, because it is a common body type mentioned in most typing systems. The Quick Check Workbook Chapter at the end of this book provides a simplified self-help workbook for typing yourself (pure typing), once you've gone through and understood the "body of" *For Your Body Only*.

In Table 5, each of the target glands, numbers 3–7, put out hormones that affect the organs listed next to them. The Pituitary or Master

TABLE 5
PHYSICAL FUNCTIONS OF THE ENDOCRINE GLANDS

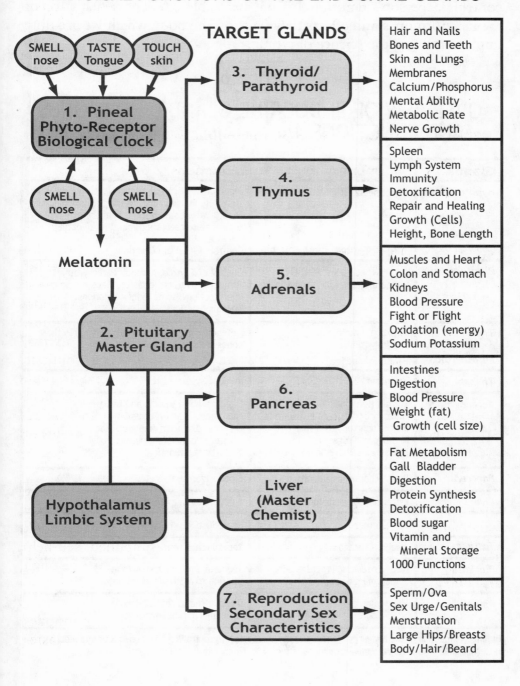

TARGET GLANDS

SMELL nose | TASTE Tongue | TOUCH skin

1. Pineal Phyto-Receptor Biological Clock

SMELL nose | SMELL nose

Melatonin

2. Pituitary Master Gland

Hypothalamus Limbic System

3. Thyroid/ Parathyroid
- Hair and Nails
- Bones and Teeth
- Skin and Lungs
- Membranes
- Calcium/Phosphorus
- Mental Ability
- Metabolic Rate
- Nerve Growth

4. Thymus
- Spleen
- Lymph System
- Immunity
- Detoxification
- Repair and Healing
- Growth (Cells)
- Height, Bone Length

5. Adrenals
- Muscles and Heart
- Colon and Stomach
- Kidneys
- Blood Pressure
- Fight or Flight
- Oxidation (energy)
- Sodium Potassium

6. Pancreas
- Intestines
- Digestion
- Blood Pressure
- Weight (fat)
- Growth (cell size)

Liver (Master Chemist)
- Fat Metabolism
- Gall Bladder
- Digestion
- Protein Synthesis
- Detoxification
- Blood sugar
- Vitamin and Mineral Storage
- 1000 Functions

7. Reproduction Secondary Sex Characteristics
- Sperm/Ova
- Sex Urge/Genitals
- Menstruation
- Large Hips/Breasts
- Body/Hair/Beard

Gland (2), is controlled by the Hypothalamus which in turn is impacted on by the Limbic System which is connected to all other parts of the Basal System of the Brain. The Basal System primarily controls a person's emotional behavior. Table 5A represents a list of the key hormones and effects they have on the body which we are now implementing in the science of typing.

TABLE 6

OVERVIEW OF ENDOCRINE GLANDS, HORMONES, AND FUNCTIONS *(Use in conjunction with TABLE 5)*

Glands	Hormones	Functions
Hypothalamus	Direct neural stimulation	Blood pressure, pupil dilation, satiety, shivering, hunger, rage, feeding reflexes, thirst, water conservation, heart rate, temperature regulation, panting, sweating
	TRH, CRH, GHRH, GHIH, LRH, PIH	Control of Pituitary Gland
Pituitary	GH, TSH, ACT, TSH, FSH, LH, Prolactin, MSH, ADH, Oxytocin	Control of Thyroid, Adrenal, Parathyroid, Pancreas, Ovaries, Testicles, Placenta, some liverfunctions, some kidney functions, Thymus functions
Thyroid	Thyroxin, Calcitonin, Triodothyronine	Metabolic rate, mental state, nerve growth, bones and teeth, mental ability, etc.
Parathyroid	Parathormone	
Thymus	Thymosin	Immune system , etc.
Adrenal	Steroid Hormones: Glucocorticoids, 17-Ketosteroids, Mineralocortocoids, Estrogens, Androgens, Progestins, Epinephrine, Norepinephrine	Fight or flight, muscle and heart functions, Sodium/Potassium balance, oxidation amounts, blood pressure, kidney functions, colon and stomach functions, etc.
Pancreas	Direct chemical stimulation	Blood sugar levels , etc.
Liver	Estrogens, Progesterone	1,000 metabolic functions, etc.
	Testosterone	Reproduction, etc.
Testicles	Insulin, Glucagon	Reproduction, etc.
Placenta	HCG, Estrogens, Progesterone, Somatomammotropin	Regulate embryonic growth in relation to mother's metabolism
Pineal	Melatonin	Direct effect on gonadatropic hormones in time/light cycle

The interconnection of the Endocrine system and Nervous System in controlling human behavior and metabolism is better clarified when using the modern science of typing in the application of nutritional elements.

TABLE 7

NERVOUS SYSTEM, ENDOCRINE GLANDS, AND OXIDATION

All the endocrine glands are composed of 2 parts or "types" of cells: acid and alkaline. Each of these cells produce distinctly different hormones that balance each other's effects within the body. The nervous system controls the Yin/Yang balance or the calming and stimulating balance of these hormones. The acid cells known as acidophils are controlled by the **Sympathetic Nervous System** which is that part of the nervous system which prepares our bodies for "fight or flight." The alkaline cells or basophils are controlled by the **Parasympathetic Nervous System**, which is that part of the nervous system that has a calming affect on the body. Your overall response to is a function of the **Autonomic Nervous System's** balance. Dr. Kelley's research demonstrated three types of stress response patterns.

SYMPATHETIC TYPE—Usually blood type A. Response to stress includes:
1. Effect on the adrenal glands which contracts muscles and constricts blood vessels which raises blood pressure.
2. Input to the thyroid which speeds up metabolism, heart and pulse rates.
3. Stimulating the pancreas to elevate blood sugar, constrict digestive juices, and suppress hunger.
4. Effect on the thymus which mobilizes the immune system for defense and repair also known as the "fight or flight" response."

(A Sympathetic Dominant "type" of person has a weak Parasympathetic response. Continuous stress resultantly causes: migraine headaches, nausea, chest pains, diarrhea, rapid pulse, low blood pressure, physical weakness, an adrenal crisis, and ultimately suffocation, cardiac arrest and death.)

PARASYMPATHETIC TYPE—Usually blood type O. Response to stress includes:
1. Initially weak Sympathetic response.
2. Followed quickly by an exaggerated Parasympathetic response.
3. Muscles and blood vessels relax.
4. Blood pressure and pulse lower.
5. Heart rate and metabolism slow down.
6. Hunger increases and digestive juices flow.

(A Parasympathetic Dominant "type" when exposed to prolonged stress suffers from obesity, fluid retention, sexual tension, mental fogginess, ulcers, heart

BALANCED TYPE - Usually blood type B or AB. Response to stress includes:
1. A Balanced Sympathetic response initially followed by a gentle Parasympathetic response.

OXIDATION PATTERNS
The **Parasympathetic** Nervous System **conserves** oxygen while the **Sympathetic** Nervous System **burns** oxygen.

SYMPATHETIC TYPES—Must conserve oxygen by taking greater amounts of antioxidant nutrients including sulfur proteins such as chicken, eggs and shellfish and vitamins A, E, F, C, B5, selenium, and manganese.

PARASYMPATHETIC TYPES—Must burn more oxygen by taking oxidants such as iron, phosphorus, copper, B6, iodine, and B12.

Generally speaking, oxidants are red in color and antioxidants are yellow. The following table (Table 7) represents a highly simplified representation of 6 Primary typing Systems.

TABLE 8
METABOLIC TYPING SYSTEMS OVERVIEW

I. Sheldon/Berkowitz   II. D'Adamo   III. Bieler   IV. Watson   V. Kelley   VI. Power   VII. Diet Categories

Omnivore(+)	Vegetarians (+)	Meat-Eaters (+)
I. **Mesomorph**—muscular, great strength and endurance, enjoys physical activity, noisy, callous, competitive	I. **Ectomorph**—tall, thin, small bones and muscles, restrained, self conscious, fond of solitude	I. **Endomorph**—short, round and soft, relaxed, sociable, even tempered lethargic
II. **Blood Type** Medium build	B II. **Blood Type A & AB** Trim/lean build	II. **Blood Type O** Large bones/large build
III. **Adrenal Type** Strong,, muscular, curly hair, large features, energetic, very physical, good digestion, easy-going disposition	III. **Thyroid Type** Small bones, thin, easily fatigued, Insomnia, delicate features, high pulse, rashes, sensitive, high strung	III. **Pituitary Type** Lanky and tall, wide mouth, large forehead, arms and legs, artistic, creative, flirtatious, sexually oriented
IV **Medium Oxidizer*** Balanced blood (pH 7.41-7.46) Warm, cooperative, optimistic	IV. **Fast Oxidizer*** Alkaline blood (pH 7.47 +) Irritable and impatient	IV. **Slow Oxidizer*** Acid blood (pH 7.3-7.4) Sullen and depressed
V. **Balanced Nervous System** During stress: sympathetic response first followed by parasympathetic response then balance, medium blood pressure	V. **Sympathetic Dominant** During stress: high pulse, no hunger, migraines, nausea, muscles constrict, chest pains, low blood pressure	V. **Parasympathetic Dominant** During stress: slow pulse, hunger, relaxed muscles, lethargy, fluid retention, high blood pressure
VI. **Adrenal Type B** Muscular, large features, medium bones and build, athletic, high blood pressure, heart strain **Balanced Type AB** Medium bones and muscles, balanced mental and physical orientation, affable, and adaptable	VI. **Thyroid Type A** Thin, quick, small bones, delicate features, high strung, creative, very mentally oriented **Pineal Type A** Domed head in back (occiput), aware, sensitive, dreamer, receiver **Thymus Type (any ABO)** Tall and lanky, long limbs, knobby Joints, wide chest	VI. **Pituitary Type O** Large, wide forehead, obsessive, charismatic, "transmitter" **Pancreas Type O** Fat, round, soft, jolly, food-oriented, diabetic tendency **Gonad Type O** Male: baldness, heavy body
VII. **3 large meals** High protein, cultured dairy products, eggs, butter, whole grains, nuts, seeds, almost any vegetables, fruits, all red and white meats, potatoes, yams, bananas, high fiber,(roughage/beans)	VII. **5 small meals.** High starch, medium fat, raw milk, eggs, cheese, yogurt, kefir, whole grains, bananas, vegetables, fish, Poultry, shellfish, acidic fruits, tomato, roughage, *no* beans, low purine meats, unsaturated fats **Thymus Type** High intake of raw foods, few animal products, rotation diet	VII. **4 small meals** High protein, no milk, no cheese, no wheat, some grains in limited amounts, alkaline vegetables and Fruits, *all* red and white meats, potatoes, yams, squash, medium roughage, high purine meats, saturated fats

+ SUPPLEMENTS—Some basic supplements do match typing categories. But each persons needs are so unique to their biochemistry—age, disease, genetics, gender, food patterns and sources, lifestyle, etc.—that further differentiation is ed for the sake of accuracy. Eating patterns are corrected with appropriate specimen evaluation to precisely differentiate individual needs.

* Not completely accurate due to indigenous discrepancies and limitations.

NOTE: VATA, PITTA, and KAPHA types (Mahareshi Ayurveda) do not properly fit into the above categories due to inherent limitations this very ancient system possesses. This system works best with those of Indian ancestry, but is not complete without other typing procedures. The Chinese constitutional system has some similarities but doesn't fit well into these categories and is more usable after contemporary typing has first been performed. It also has its own set of limitations in regards to modern metabolic typing." There is a loose connection between the Water and Fire Types and the Thyroid Type, the Wood and Heat Types and the Adrenal Type, between the Metal Type and the Pituitary Type, and between the Earth and Energy Types and the Gonadal Type.

Metabolic Typing in Practice

The Adrenal Type

We have now determined that you are a Blood Type B negative, "Adrenal Dominant Type." We'll end this visit by explaining more about the implications of being an "Adrenal Type" in terms of the way your body functions metabolically and in what nutrients it specifically requires. (Refer to Table 8: Metabolic Typing Systems Overview).

Physicality

"Adrenal Types" generally have muscles that are strong and prominent, with large and/or dense bones and large features. Hair is usually curly and coarse, the skin dry, warm and thick, neck and fingers are usually short and thicker than average with generally large and round jaws and teeth. Males tend to be more adrenal than females, although there are many exceptions to this. Animal examples would include the bulldog, tiger, and draft horse. (Think of the greyhound, cheetah, and the thoroughbred racehorse in sharp contrast.)

Personality

"Adrenals" tend to be fairly easy-going and possess great energy and endurance levels. They are strong and physically oriented, like and in most cases "love" exercise and prefer "physically" oriented careers. Professional sports, the police force, the military, business (very competitive), and skilled trades are attractive to "Adrenals." They tend not to live in fear or suffer much anxiety but do tend to be less sensitive and creative than some of the other types preferring concrete things over abstract things. Anger is slow to build but can lead to violence when aroused. Generally, "Adrenals" are more competitive and aggressive than "average."

Metabolic and Dietary Factors

"Adrenals" have a large amount of oxidation at a medium rate which has much to do with their great energy and endurance properties. Along with these properties, they have excellent muscle control and are dependent on vigorous exercise for optimum metabolic function. They have good digestion and are rarely ill. "Adrenals" have a full range of digestive enzymes which makes for a good digestive function in the consumption of foods and are therefore classified as "omnivores." However, they are one type that thrives on a high protein diet to maintain their musculature and require a high protein to carbohydrate proportion with medium fat amounts within their personal "zone."

Their autonomic nervous system is Sympathetic-Parasympathetic balanced which is a very healthy characteristic. They typically don't suffer from confusion much, nor are they overtly lazy and mentally "out of it." Milk digestibility is a function of other dependent variables like race and upbringing. The intake of dense starches are limited to exercise output. The thyroid gland tends to be weak in "adrenals" while toxin elimination is primarily handled by the bowels and kidneys. The greatest lifestyle problem "Adrenal Types" tend to have is that they abuse their bodies sometimes through improper food choices, inconsistent exercise, and inadequate rest all due to an inherent attitude of invincibility. They think of themselves as physically tough and almost able to withstand anything. Because of this "invincibility" attitude, they tend to suffer from heart and circulatory problems, if this personality trait is left unchecked.

The Diet Connection

By now, as a patient you may be thinking of me as some sort of "pseudo-psychic," because of my close and highly accurate description of your way of being. You've already agreed with the majority of my typing descriptions and have found them very revealing. Now, it's time to discuss what basic foods should be good for your body and mind. As a "B" blood type, "Adrenal Dominant" categorically, your best overall **protein sources** should include:

Red Meats	Yeast	Fish
Sea Plants	Chinese Cabbage	Cucumbers
Poultry	Sprouts	Parsley
Beans	Eggs	Milk (conditional)

Your best overall **fat sources** should include:

Avocado	Egg Yolk	Butter
Raw Nuts/Seeds	Olive Oil	Cream

Your best overall **carbohydrate sources** should include:

Whole Grains (limited)	Bananas	Yams
Peaches	Plums	Potatoes
Grapes	Cherries	Melon
Citrus Fruits	Leafy Greens	Squashes
Broccoli	Celery	Cruciferous Vegetables

TABLE 9
OMNIVORE TYPE DIET
ADJUSTED FOR ADRENAL PATTERNS

Food Types	Healthy Foods	Least Healthy Foods
Dairy Products	European Descent: butter, yogurt, cottage, cheese, kefir, *no* milk	Oriental and other descent: *no* milk products at all
Eggs, Fats	Lightly cooked eggs, unprocessed seed oils, avocado	Margarine, sesame
Meats, Poultry, Fish	Meats, Poultry, Most meats: beef, lamb, liver, organ meats, all fowl, some fish (light-colored, deep cold-water fish)	Certain fish: trout, tuna (dark), Opaleye fish, salmon, salmon caviar, all caviar, turtle, snake, some shellfish
Vegetables	Leafy green vegetables: lettuce, spinach, Swiss chard, cabbage, corn, seaweeds, kelp, spirulina, snow peas, celery, bamboo shoots, water chestnuts, alkaline vegetables: squash, cucumber, starchy vegetables: potatoes, sweet potatoes, yams, beets, carrots, cruciferous vegetables: broccoli, cauliflower, Brussels sprouts, asparagus, other: tomato, pepper, eggplant	Unusual mushrooms, artichokes, pumpkin, corn, radishes
Grains	All grains: wheat, oats, rye, rice, rye, millet, barley	All bleached and highly processed grains
Nuts, Seeds	Most seeds and nuts: almonds, brazil, filberts, pecans, sunflower	Peanuts, sesame seeds, cashews, Pumpkin seeds, pignolas
Fruit	All fruits: apple, apricot, citrus, dates, papaya, grapes, plums, figs, melon, pear, berries, pineapple, nectarine	Pomegranates, persimmons, rhubarb, coconuts
Beverages	Herb tea, vegetable and fruit juices, pure water, vegetable broth	Carbonated soft drinks, coffee, black tea, hard liquor, cocoa
Miscellaneous	Carob, raw honey, maple syrup, malt, onions, herbs, spices	Chocolate, sugar, salt, junk foods, hot spices, pepper, corn syrup

(For best results the above foods should be fresh, whole, natural, and organic if possible, without preservatives, additives, or toxic residues.)

Adrenal Type

Now that we've got the basic categories for the Adrenal Type of best foods and worst foods outlined, we need to note the "best" supplements and their relative daily intake requirements. The "best" and "worst" food groups and supplements are baseline categories, to be further refined through Steps 3 and 4 as we approach total nutritional customization.

Best VITAMINS and their relative daily intake range:

Rough daily intake range most "Adrenal Types" will fit into optimally. Typing Steps 3 and 4 will narrow these levels to individual specific amounts. Amounts vary per measured individual need.

A:	10—50,000 iu as both fish oil and beta carotene
D3:	400—800 iu
E:	100—200 iu (d'alpha tocopherol)
F:	500—1000 mg (alpha linolenic, cis linoleic, gamma linolenic acids)
B Complex:	50—75 mg
C Complex:	750—1,000 mg

Best MINERALS and their total intake range:

Calcium:	400—600 mg
Magnesium:	75—100 mg
Phosphorus:	10—24 grains from lecithin origin
Chromium:	15—20 mcg
Vanadium:	5—10 mcg
Selenium:	15—20 mcg
Copper:	1—2 mg
Zinc:	15—25 mg
Manganese:	5—10 mg
Iodine:	15—20 mcg

Best Other Vitamin-Like Substances:

Presence in diet is of primary necessity but ranges have not as yet been determined by research. Intake ranges are dependent on body size, weight, and other variables.

Thyroid Extracts	Adrenal Glandular Extracts
Bee Pollen	Melatonin
Spirulina	Yohimbe Bark
Alfalfa	Shiitaki and Reishi Mushrooms
L-tyrosine	Proanthocyanadins
CoQ10	Chlorophyll
Lecithin	Capsicum
Bromelain	Aloe Vera

Best Herbs:

For nourishment and tonification of less dominant and recessive glands.

Yerba Mate	Licorice Root
Gingko Biloba	Watercress
Saw Palmetto	Yucca
Siberian Ginseng	Iceland Moss
Schizandra	Irish Moss
Smilax	Mustard
Chia Seed	Saw Palmetto
Seawrack	Parsley
Gymnema Sylvestre	Pineal Extract
Calamus	Chickweed
Dill	Marigold
Grape Seed Extract	Rhubarb Sorel
Kola Nut	

Putting It Together

We have developed a database of information about you (my hypothetical patient) in terms of your body's metabolic strengths and weaknesses, and have created an outline of what foods and supplements in their respective proportions should work optimally for you. Because you are not a "pure" tribal Phenotype descendant, like a Hunzan or Georgian, there has been some genetic interaction between other tribal lines which has modified you in some ways. If you were a "pure" Titikakan, I would put you on this society's average tribal diet but with some other typing specifications unique to your profiled biochemistry that is different from other tribal members. I would determine those differences in Step 3 (Laboratory Assessment aka Profiling). In your case of "impure" tribal descendance, I still have the majority of categorizable and correlational metabolic and nutrient data needed in order to have a thorough understanding of what is generally right for you (in theory) allowing for small race-specific and ethnicity adjustments. "Adrenal Types" are found in all races but with some recognizable race specific differences I have already noted in your special case.

The information I have collected about you so far in this step is still in a "rough" form. This Metabolic Typing data affords clearer insights into exactly how to plan the Step 3 laboratory portion of your overall typing procedures so that I only use the most appropriate specimen test analysis in the proper sequence. By the completion of Step 3, I will have a very thorough understanding of your current metabolic status—in extreme detail! With that information in hand, I will then be able to fully customize your eating and supplement program specific to your needs and desired objectives.

Step 3: Laboratory Assessment, AKA Profiling

Up to this point, we should consider all the typing that we have accomplished so far as a "fact finding research project on you" as my hypothetical patient. The process of typing works much like a Ph.D.

thesis when it's completed. We begin with the hypothesis that we can determine your biochemical uniqueness, using the art and science of typing as a given. It's then up to us to prove that we can do this beginning with assumptions about quantification and qualification and then proceeding through more stringent typing procedures to progressively narrow down the variables regarding your biochemical nature to a minimum.

By the time we employ Step 3, which represents the most revealing and scientific step of all five steps, we are able to "prove" or "disprove" the data we have been collecting and other assumptions we may be making. As an example of this, consider that as an "Adrenal Type" sesame seeds are one of your "worst foods." In Step 3, we can take a blood specimen and test the IgG4 immunoglobulin allergic response to sesame seeds, either "proving" or "disproving" our "worst food" assumption. Chances are, from an experienced clinical standpoint, your test will be positive: you are unequivocally allergic to sesame. Or your test may come up negative, which shows that our pure typing is imprecise in relation to this particular criterion.

Step 3 allows me to further separate fact from fiction as the specifics of your uniqueness are further revealed up to the moment and to the last accountable denominator. This is where the true value of laboratory assessment lies. Ultimately, your customized diet and supplements will reflect everything we've learned about your body and if you're allergic to sesame you can bet it won't be part of your customized nutrition program! If you need more magnesium in proportion to calcium, it's in there. If your urine is too acid, you can bet that you'll find alkalinizing foods and supplements in your program. In comparison to typing doesn't one-size-fits-all seem like a waste of time?

The Four Factors of Metabolism

In this step, our special laboratory tests are directed towards evaluating the four components or factors of metabolism. The designated laboratory tests will reveal your uniqueness in each of these **Digestion, Absorption, Assimilation,** and **Elimination** sub-metabolic processes. This information provides some important pieces in the overall metabolic puzzle that we could only guess about prior to recent advancements in laboratory technology. Metabolic typing procedures from previous years have allowed us many insights into these components, but some new technologies really put the "icing on the cake" in this regard, and are comprehensively increasing the precision of non-lab mediated typing as well as "lab typing."

The Four Metabolic Factors Under the Microscope

Factor One—Digestion

How can we determine just how well you are digesting your foods? Up to this point, you've probably deduced that upsets in regularity, symptoms of heartburn, nausea, gas, stomach and abdominal pain, diarrhea and constipation are all signs of poor and/or incomplete digestion. You're right, but we still need to take a closer look at this process to fully "type" you and customize nutrition accordingly. Is protein, fat, carbohydrate individually or all together difficult for you body to digest? Is it one type of protein or fat that's the problem? Is your digestion being affected by low stomach acid or some digestive enzyme deficiencies, or due to intestinal damage or from some disease or parasite infiltration?

These and other questions can be easily answered with the appropriate lab test. The laboratory tests (used for all four metabolic factors) are not typically considered conventional although at some time in the future (probably within the next ten years or so) they will become standard practice to some degree, inside and outside of the doctor's office. Cornell University's study on medical doctors, for example, equated M.D. with "mediocre diet" due to the blatant lack of concern or knowledge about nutrition demonstrated by the vast majority of the 38,000 physicians surveyed. You will find that chiropractic doctors, osteopathic doctors, and naturopathic doctors are usually "one up" in this regard. They generally have much more clinical nutrition training and may be well aware of some lab typing procedures and their role in wellness.

The key factors of digestion can be found in saliva, stool, urine, and blood specimens using the appropriate specialized lab procedures.

In your hypothetical case as an omnivorous Adrenal Type, digestion theoretically should be generally good across-the-board. However, we really can't be sure about this without the proper laboratory evaluation in this step. This specialized assessment enhances our understanding of your digestive uniqueness up to the moment and in relation to any processes of digestive deterioration we need to know about. Any part of your digestive process not functioning properly, for whatever reason, that we don't detect in your typing program can upset metabolism and health long after we've *incompletely* "typed and tested" you, no matter how good your diet and supplements may appear. So it's critical that we get it right from the start and don't miss any details.

Without going into great detail about all of the possible test procedures that we can apply to your case, I will simplify the key procedures like so:

1. We are examining digestive markers or the digestive efficiency of food components such as triglycerides (fat) proteins, chymotrypsin (an enzyme), pH (acidity/alkalinity), and immunoglobulin presence.
2. We are looking at so-called metabolic markers such as your specific short-chain fatty acid fingerprint.
3. We are examining for the presence of bacteria both harmful and beneficial to the digestive process such as salmonella (harmful), lactobacillus (beneficial), and the balance of your intestinal "microbial flora" overall. With this procedure we're looking for yeast and other parasitic infiltration.
4. Evaluation of stool color, mass, and blood content provides other data.

5. After further laboratory examination, a dysbiosis index is given representing the relative functional efficiency of the gut lining in terms of bringing the good stuff into the body and keeping the bad stuff out of the general circulation to be solubilized and/or excreted directly. The presence of a "leaky gut syndrome" is something that shows up even more clearly in the toxin profile of Metabolic Factor Four—Elimination.

When it comes to digestion (aside from poor nutrient absorption and glandular insufficiencies, which lead to deficiencies), one of our biggest health enemies is the body's absorption of incomplete or partially digested foods; this leads to allergic reactions—some of which are easily detectable, others remain hidden. Hidden allergic reactions can be difficult for self-detection because your body's response is very subdued at this point in the digestive/absorptive process. This type of subdued reaction is called a "Delayed Food Sensitivity Response" and is an allergic phenomenon that is directly responsible for much of the symptomology and degenerative disease people suffer from since conventional medicine usually doesn't detect nor focus upon this problem. When this sensitivity is properly detected and corrected symptoms disappear.

Proper digestion is very critical so I want you (as my hypothetical patient) to maximize the efficiency of this process in every way possible. Slow down when you eat, chew your food well, eat according to your "type," take the digestive enhancement supplements I'll have customized for you, and don't drink excessive fluids, especially coffee, with your meals. (More about this later.)

Factor Two—Absorption

When proper and efficient digestion takes place, nutrient absorption should proceed smoothly. Leaving nothing to chance in our quest for your true biochemical identity, we need to closely check on this process. Blood, urine, saliva, hair, and stool, evaluation all comes into play here as we look for:

1. Normal and/or abnormal amounts of long chain fats, cholesterol, all other fats, and metabolites such as indican (a by-product of tryptophan, the amino acid, from its own metabolism within the gut).
2. The presence of most vitamins, minerals, and other vitamin-like substances in blood, hair and urine which indicates that at least they are present (or not). This is known as "static status." We can't be sure of their functional status within the body until metabolic Factor Three—Assimilation, with its differential comparisons is examined.
3. The occurrence of toxic factors such as heavy metals, free radicals, and enzyme inhibitors (alcohol, tobacco, barbiturates, sulfonamides, isonazid, xenobiotics, formaldehyde, benzene rings, trimellitic anhydride, etc.).

Factor Three—Assimilation

This physiological process needs to be carefully checked in order to insure that the nutrients you consume are actually being properly utilized by the body and not just simply passing through, creating systemic stress and unnecessarily expensive urine. All laboratory specimens are utilized here as we reveal:

1. The presence of vitamin/mineral, fatty acid, and protein (amino acid) deficiencies.
2. The in proportion of macro and micronutrient ratios.
3. The presence of vitamin, mineral, and toxin overload. (Megadosers beware!)
4. Certain enzyme activity in the processing of nutrients.
5. The status of some of our body's detoxification pathways (chemical reaction pathways which convert harmful substances into harmless substances ready to excrete).
6. Pertinent hormone and immunological activities.

Factor Four—Elimination (excretion)

This metabolic end-process is just as critical as the first three metabolic factors and warrants close examination. My dear mother used to tell me (and still does), "You are what you eat" and "what goes in must come out." (This is very true, although what comes out bears little resemblance to what goes in.) Your eliminative efficiency is the "sticking point" or the "stop-gap" for the three previous metabolic factors. If it backs up or slows down, a reverse metabolic overload is a result. Your body then becomes a dumping ground for waste materials, the toxicity of which slowly consumes your health, undermining the previous three metabolic factor functions, creating high stresses and resultant energy starvation. You quickly begin to deteriorate. Improper elimination creates resistance to the very energy of life and is therefore exceedingly dangerous. **The majority of body specimens are utilized to reveal:**

1. Both hidden and detected allergic reactions you may be having to foods. The presence of food sensitivities is really a component of all four metabolic factors but I categorize them here at the end of the metabolic chain because the key to removing their presence is by eliminating them from the diet. The good news, as mentioned previously, is that many of these food sensitivities can be overcome with the right approach.
2. Your individual detoxification pathways and their efficiency is apparent since biochemical uniqueness includes your own characteristic detoxification pattern.
3. The presence or non-presence of certain key "detox" elements or precursors made by the body or lacking in the diet.

You can probably see by now that there's a lot more to being an "Adrenal Type" (or any type), than you may have originally thought. Through the appropriate assessment of your unique-to-you metabolic factors of Digestion, Absorption, Assimilation, and Elimination in combination with your previous typing procedures, we can have a very clear picture of what your metabolic/ biochemical individuality really is replete with disease tendencies. We now have all the data necessary to proceed to Step 4 of the typing process which entails fully customizing your diet and supplementation specific to what we've already learned about your human uniqueness from the preceding steps.

Step 4: Diet and Supplement Customization

Part 1

I must go back to Step 1 and adjust the Quantification and Qualification of your diet to your particular criteria, as revealed by Step 2: Pure Metabolic Typing and Step 3: Laboratory Assessment. In effect, I will correct and refine your custom diet to the necessary specifications called for by Steps 1, 2, and 3, and according to your specific personal objectives, which in this hypothetical case are a ten-pound weight loss and optimum health and fitness gain.

To accomplish this, I go through a multi-step "ruling in and ruling out" procedure. The "ruling in" procedure consists of retaining the foods best suited to your metabolic and biochemical uniqueness according to the sum total of all of our previous typing Steps 1 through 3. The "ruling out" process consists of deleting foods that you are proven to be directly allergic to or that we reveal are not right for you due to other typing factors such as pH and glycemic index. At this point in the program all other generically obvious land mines are removed as well. These land mines consist of all the known manmade food irritants and carcinogens; these include bleached flour and sugar, nitrates, nitrites and erythrobates (additives found in cured meats like bacon), as well as other food preservatives that are unnatural, and all unnatural additives, binders, fillers, extenders, etc.

Suffice it to say, your customized diet plan will recommend only the healthiest, most wholesome, properly synergized organic food selections, with options for variety and calculated rotations for favorable metabolic stimulation. The "intra" and "inter" macronutrient proportions will be adjusted to your "type" and equal the Daily Target Calorie Level (2,000 calories) when added together mathematically.

The "inter" micronutrient proportions are present in the diet but we still need to supplement precisely to compensate for nutrient density variations (beyond our control) in whole foods.

Part 2

We then proceed to the customization of your supplements through laboratories that specialize in customizing pharmaceutical grade supplements. This will be done in accordance with your specific needs as we've measured them in deficiency, excess, or in ratio to one another. Supplements are designed to account for nutrient synergy and antagonism, in order to insure that they'll work.

To go along with Steps 1 and 2 of our customization process, we may further need to build in certain short-term detoxification procedures of diet and supplements, in order to help your body to "clean out" certain elimination systems and any toxins present. Detoxification procedures should never be taken lightly. According to Dr. Udo Erasmus, "Most healers agree that degeneration can only have two causes: malnutrition and/or internal pollution (poisoning, toxicity)." Typing addresses the problems of "internal pollution and malnutrition" with equal vigor.

By now, as my make-believe patient, you've probably been overwhelmed by the complexity of what we've done so far to "correct" your nutritional program so that it's precisely matched to your actual needs. Down deep you know that this is what really needed to be done to get you back on the right track for life. In fact, by now you've learned so much about yourself that you're really becoming your own self-directed nutritionist replete with a scientifically designed plan of action at your fingertips. There's only one thing left to do in about three to five months down the line.

Step 5: The Final Step—Re-Evaluation

The final step in the typing process consists of double-checking your body's response to the nutrition program customized for you. After all, we must make sure it's working on the biochemical level—above and beyond the fact that you've lost the ten pounds you wanted to lose, and you already feel so much better overall that you can hardly believe it! We must analyze the effectiveness of the program and your personal compliance level. Your test results should demonstrate across-the-board improvements in everything we've evaluated, from your former vitamin/mineral deficiencies to your toxic accumulation factors to the overall metabolic stress indicators regarding digestion, absorption, assimilation, and elimination.

If testing demonstrates that there are more program adjustments necessary, we will make them in order to achieve more concise and/or faster results. Future tests can be used to double check progress again. At this time we'll also work with any compliance issues which have possibly inhibited optimum benefits or have not been discussed previously. We will adjust the program as needed. Now you are fully "typed" and your results are magnificent. Congratulations!

Typing Process Overview

Step 1—Quantification and Qualification

Create a calorie and food adjusted, hypothetical "rough" diet. This step is based on standard generic scientific assumptions and predictions utilizing the science of calorimetry and conventional nutritional philosophies. The information from this step is fully refined in accordance with biochemical individuality as revealed from the following steps.

Step 2—Pure Metabolic Typing

Categorize body type by measuring and grouping physical and psychological characteristics with no specimen evaluation performed (other than blood type). Identify metabolic strengths and weaknesses to strategize the appropriate procedures for Step 3.

Step 3—Laboratory Assessment, aka Laboratory Typing or Profiling

Further refine the body type categorization process into its smallest denominator of biochemical uniqueness and up-to-the-moment metabolic status through laboratory mediated specimen evaluation. Nutrient deficiencies and overloads are revealed, along with toxic infiltration.

Step 4—Diet and Supplement Customization

Correct the "rough" diet from Step 1 and customize this diet specific to the information revealed from Steps 2 and 3. This process will fully individualize diet and supplementation in direct accordance with biochemical identity and therefore manifest as a precise nutrition program replete with short and long term detoxification procedures.

Step 5—Re-Evaluation

Measure all previous data once again, in order to analyze the effectiveness of the program. This step focuses primarily upon the outcome of all the laboratory retests given in order to pinpoint exactly what metabolic improvements such as, less nutrient deficiencies/ excesses have or have not been made to help us further refine the program if necessary. In this step any compliance issues still remaining are remediated.

Typing: The Eicosanoid Connection

Achieving a balanced state of metabolism from typing automatically includes optimizing the occurrence of health-promoting eicosanoids. The following is an overview of information found in *The Zone* by Barry Sears, Ph.D., select books and articles by David Horrobin, Ph.D. (the godfather of essential fatty acids), Udo Erasmus' *Fats That Heal—Fats That Kill* by, and the Nobel Prize-winning research of Sune Karl Bergstrom, Ph.D., Berg, Ingeman Samuel, Ph.D. and Robert John Vane, Ph.D.

Eicosanoids are considered to be "super hormones," manufactured by every living cell in the human body. These compounds arise, effect a physiological response, and then breakdown all in mere seconds. There are hundreds known, and perhaps thousands yet to be discovered. They impact on all of the body's hormonal systems and also exert control on just about every vital physiological function which sustains life. Eicosanoids are known primarily to help sustain and control the immune system, cardiovascular system, nervous system, respiratory system, and reproductive system. These compounds are involved in the control and function of every system of the body to some extent. Their total effects are not fully understood at this time but ongoing research is revealing the hidden secrets of these essential-to-life molecular body constituents.

Eicosanoids form a family of biological chemical compounds, which include prostaglandins, prostacyclins, leukotrienes, lipoxins, hydroxylated fatty acids, and thromboxannes. They are derived from two dietary unsaturated fatty acids (omega 6 and 3) which are considered as essential fatty acids and one non-essential activated fatty acid known as gamma-linolenic acid which can be made by the body or found in diet. The omega 6 essential fat is called cis-linoleic acid and the omega 3 essential fat is called alpha linolenic. The omega 6 is found mostly in vegetable oils and the omega 3 is found primarily in fish oil. A related "non-dietary essential fat" is called arachidonic acid and is found in red meats or manufactured by the body. It is essential only in its ability to convert into certain classes of eicosanoids but isn't necessary in the diet.

Eicosanoid production proceeds through a series of enzyme-mediated **desaturation** and **elongation** biochemical steps from the initial dietary forms of omega 6 and omega 3 fats. Eicosanooid production depends on the initial presence of the dietary 3's and 6's (called **substrates**), the concentration and availability of all involved enzymes and their **coenzymes** (aka cofactors, or vitamin/minerals), the proportion of glucagon and insulin to each other, and the concentration of products (eicosanoids and related products) created by this metabolic sub-system. These previous factors all affect the efficiency and the outcomes of the eicosanoid's enzymatic building process.

As with any enzyme system, it has a check-and-balance feature, which can either work for you or against you depending upon your diet and exposure to the inhibitors of efficient eicosanoid metabolism. When this system is working efficiently within itself and within its connection to the overall process of metabolism, more of the so-called "good" eicosanoids will be present, with all of their health promoting benefits. If this system is inhibited or out of balance for any reason, it forms a greater concentration of "bad" eicosanoids, which adversely affect the overall metabolic balance, and consequently the health status of the body. Many diseases and dis-eases have already been linked to an abnormal balance of bad eicosanoids to good eicosanoids within the body. The good eicosanoids and bad eicosanoids have completely opposite effects to one another. If one "good" eicosanoid opens up blood vessels to decrease blood pressure, its corresponding "bad" eicosanoid does the exact opposite by closing the same blood vessels to increase blood pressure.

TABLE 10
EICOSANOIDS: THE GOOD, THE BAD (AND THE UGLY)

Good Eicosanoids (Positive Effects)	Bad Eicosanoids (Negative Effects)
Resists inflammatory processes	Promotes inflammatory processes
Inhibits blood platelet aggregation	Promotes platelet aggregation (clots)
Promotes vasodilation	Promotes vasoconstriction
Inhibits cellular proliferation	Promotes cellular proliferation
Decreases pain transmission	Increases pain transmission
Stimulates immune response	Depresses immune response

The eicosanoidal sub-metabolic system, just like the overall metabolism at large throughout the body, is in a state of balance between opposing forces—one force being construed as "good" or health-promoting, while the other as its opposite is "bad" or non-health promoting. Proper balance is achieved when the good forces significantly outweigh the bad forces. A perfect balance of good vs. bad is highly specific to each individual's biochemical identity and metabolic type. This person-specific, overall metabolic balance is no different for eicosanoid metabolism. The check and balance effect of metabolism is exceedingly easy to see when you understand the nature of eicosanoid production—and its dietary controlling forces.

Given that our goal is the promotion of well being, then our immediate objective in typing is to increase the concentration of "good" eicosanoids over "bad" in the body. Table 9: Eicosanoids: The Good, The Bad, (and The Ugly), above, lists a few of the "good" and "bad" things that eicosanoids do.

First, we have to eat enough of the two primary essential fats in nature (cis-linoleic or omega 6 fat and alpha-linoleic or omega 3 fat. These are front-line dietary fats that provide the raw product (or substrate) to make good eicosanoids. They must be present within the diet in high enough amounts in and of themselves and in relation to non-essential fats such as saturated fats to provide optimal "good" eicosanoid benefits. Unfortunately, most people don't get this right! They are so busy blindly cutting fats from their diets for the sake of weight loss and cholesterol reduction that they unintentionally create their own dietary deficiency of essential fats.

In fact, more than 70% of deaths in the U.S. are related to fat deficiencies, imbalances, and excesses. Therefore, the first step is to properly balance all fats in the diet by proportioning PUFA's, MUFA's, and SAFA's into the person-specific intra-macronutrient fat zone. According to typing procedures, we also have to properly "type" the inter-macronutrient Zone I (carb-protein-fat connection) to individual specifications. Too many of the wrong carbohydrates (high glycemic index and/or high acid-forming carbs—depending on metabolic type) in relation to essential and non-essential fats can increase insulin production, which hastens the development of bad eicosanoids. Also, too many carbohydrates in total and in relation to inter-proportional fats inhibit good prostaglandin production.

Additionally, imbalances of intra-proportional (Zone V) carbohydrates (natural simple, processed simple, calorie-dense complex, etc.) enhance bad eicosanoid production through elevated insulin activity. Then there's the proper level and type of each protein you must take for proper eicosanoid balance. Because protein in general inhibits insulin production, enough protein must be in the diet in relation to carbohydrates specific to an individual's type. This occurs when the properly typed inter macronutrient proportion (Zone I) between protein and carbs, and protein and fat is in balance. Protein and fat inter-macronutrient proportions are also critical because many fats are present in protein sources and must be proportioned properly within intra-macronutrient zones as well. The intra- and inter-macronutrient proportions of protein, carbs, and fat all have a balancing effect on one another in relation to eicosanoid metabolism and all metabolism for that matter. Again, typing determines this for each individual metabolic type (especially discernible from fatty acid chemical fingerprints). From the dietary side, proper typing ensures optimal eicosanoid balance.

Since specific diet balance controls eicosanoid balance, let me give you one non-specific or generic bit of information on fats. Superheated fats (such as those from frying) are in a form called "trans" fats versus "cis" fats. Cis fats are in their natural state and are utilized by the body efficiently. Trans fats, however, are not considered nourishment by the body and, in fact, inhibit the production of good eicosanoids. This means you should stay away from fried fat foods whenever possible, no matter what "type" you ought to minimize for your personal intake of trans fat.

When it comes to the optimum production of eicosanoids, our second concern is in our balanced intake of all micronutrients (aka coenzymes or cofactors), and especially those controlling the enzymes that catalyze the formation of good eicosanoids. Take any or all of these coenzymes away and the whole eicosanoidal system of metabolism is completely undermined. These cofactors include the antioxidants beta carotene, vitamin C complex, vitamin E (d'alpha tocopherol), and the enzyme catalysts vitamin B3, B6, zinc, magnesium, and indirectly iron, copper, manganese, melatonin, essential amino acids, cadmium, calcium, phosphorus, and other B vitamins, due to their metabolic relationships with the enzyme catalysts that make them available to the enzymes in the first place.

It should be obvious, therefore, that the overall balance of vitamins, minerals, and other vitamin-like substances is critical to "good" eicosanoid production because of their need to be available at the right time and in the right amounts. Cofactor availability in turn is dependent on dietary presence (within the foods you eat), digestion, and assimilation. These factors in turn are dependent on proper typing procedures to ensure their bioavailability for good eicosanoid production in the first place. One-size-fits-all practices can only undermine this sub-metabolic system's function, whereas typing will optimize its success in producing good eicosanoids and in balancing the super-hormones more precisely in the process, all as a matter of **cause and effect**. This cause and effect process is accomplished through the accurate inter and intra-proportioning of all macro and micronutrients, which serves to set the eicosanoid metabolism off in the right enzymatic direction and preserves its reactive expediency.

Thirdly, in this eicosanoid-producing system—as in all enzyme systems—there's always that one sluggish enzyme (known as the "rate-limiting enzyme") that all other chemical reactions have to wait for before they can happen. In this system, delta 6 desaturase is our "bottleneck" or stop-gap. Its ability to function at peak efficiency allowing the rest of the system to function efficiently is very susceptible to a number of factors. These factors when present most assuredly hasten the production of bad eicosanoids over good ones because delta 6 desaturase is unable to contribute its share in promoting good eicosanoids.

The inhibitors of delta 6 desaturase activity include all dietary imbalances and especially improper macro and micronutrient proportions (inter and intra) including of course, essential fat imbalances and the presence of **too much** trans fat and red meat containing arachidonic acid. Other delta 6 desaturase inhibitors include aging (which has to do with free energy production—more in Chapter 5), disease presence (especially viral infections), stress-related hormones such as **endogenous** cortisol and adrenaline, and **exogenous** drugs which depress immune function such as corticosteroids found in prescription and non-prescription drugs. Other overall "good" eicosanoid inhibitors are tobacco, caffeine, alcohol, all toxins, aspirin, hydrogenated fats (source of trans fat), excess saturated fats, tartrazine, obesity, and high cholesterol levels. Proper typing, specific to biochemical and metabolic specifications, ensures proper eicosanoid balance, which is one of Typing's calculated effects for the prevention and reversal of disease.

There are some good eicosanoid-forming tricks typing allows for. These tricks include the use of activated essential fatty acids both through diet and supplementation procedures. Activated essential fatty acids such as gammolinoleic acid (GLA) and eicosopentanoic acid (EPA) are those which are produced by enzymes in the body through normal eicosanoid synthesis. They can also be found in certain foods and supplements that we eat. The gammaolinoleic acid found in mother's milk, evening of primrose, and borage seed oil are good examples of such foods. Another good example is that of EPA found mostly in fatty fish like mackerel, sardines, and salmon.

Taking EPA and GLA directly from diet and supplements bypasses any faulty enzyme metabolism in the body which converts omega 6 fat to GLA and omega 3 fat to EPA. In this way, a greater concentration of GLA and EPA is attained directly without interference from enzymatic efficiency breakdowns. Using this "trick" method, a typer can exert a more direct influence on good eicosanoid balance by "forcing" another eicosanoidal enzyme delta 5 desaturase to inhibit the formation of arachidonic acid which when present immediately converts to only bad eicosanoids. More GLA and EPA in combination with lower insulin levels and higher glucagon levels greatly suppresses delta 5 desaturase activity which chokes off the production or arachidonic acid which notoriously converts into bad eicosanoids. Keeping red meat intake in balance by proportioning intra and inter-macro and micronutrient proportions according to metabolic type also complements this process. "Typing and Profiling" does so by accounting for meats' presence in the diet and within the body and balancing it accordingly.

A typer's custom diet and supplement plan automatically takes the process of eicosanoid metabolism into full account in combination with a full accounting of the other components of metabolism both directly related or indirectly related to eicosanoids on a highly individualized and specific level. Metabolically this ensures a perfect balance with optimal levels of eicosanoids and all other metabolites. Typing is designed to take you into the eicosanoid zone that's "good" for your body only, not as a generic zone.

Typing: The Fat Solution

"Out of 200 people who go on any diet, only ten lose all the weight they set out to lose. Out of those ten dieters, only one keeps it off for any reasonable length of time." This is a failure rate of 99.5%, reported the *Washington Post* (as reprinted in the *Houston Chronicle* by Arthur Frank). I believe this to be one of the saddest commentaries on the futility of one-size-fits-all weight loss. What's even worse is that this statistic is typical.

Probably the most common physical and psychological annoyance among humans is the unwanted deposition of body fat. Most people consider excess body fat unsightly and attempt to deal with it on the basis of its negative cosmetic effect. Literally hundreds of billions of dollars are spent on its "cosmetic control." The negative effects of excess body fat, however, goes much further than what is merely observed on the outside. People with excess fat accumulation usually experience certain states of disease and subclinical symptomatic syndromes that automatically accompany its unsightly appearance. A lower effective energy level, feeling less than "one's best" overall, and experiencing more strain on the feet, legs, and spine are common experiences of carrying excessive fat. But being "overfat" in combination with the predisposing causative metabolic state that typically accompanies it and preserves its excesses has much further reaching implications.

From both a metabolic standpoint and common knowledge, we understand that being over fat is a major risk factor in all disease and for all subclinical dis-ease (discomfort). It provides a primary resistance factor which inhibits full metabolic balance. Its excessive presence mirrors the fact that there is metabolic imbalance in the first place. Excess body fat deposition is easily one of the most observable signs of metabolic imbalance. Excessive body fat accumulation is a potential imbalance which can plague any body type. Even the very lean blood Type A Thyroid and Pineal Dominant Ectotonic Types can gain unwanted fat and inches when out of balance. Of course, some types typically gain weight more readily than others but in some types this unwanted tendency can actually be an advantage for greater longevity and superior athletic achievement.

The accumulation of excess body fat has different ramifications and consequences for each body type that professional typists are well aware of. Each body type has a different health and fitness tolerance for fat. Five excess pounds to a Balanced Endocrine Type with a Type B blood pattern (like a Robert Redford or Jane Fonda body type) has the health-compromising effect that an extra 15 pounds would have on a Pancreatic Dominant blood type O Endotonic Type (like Ella Fitzgerald or Jackie Gleason). In other words, a Balanced Type blood Type B, has a lower resistance to fat's ill effects than a Pancreatic Dominant blood Type O Endotonic Type, whose innate body chemistry by nature is designed to carry more fat with less health risks. In effect, some body types are genetically designed to carry more fat than others even when in a state of total metabolic balance. So when someone says they weren't designed to be "that thin" there may be some truth to this statement (whether they know it or not).

Clinically speaking, it is my aim to reduce body fat levels into an acceptable range specific to each type, and to the patient's individually specified body design objectives (like getting ready for an athletic contest, a movie role, etc.). But five extra pounds on a Thyroid

Ectotonic Asian blood Type A has a different meaning to me than five extra pounds on a Pancreatic Endotonic European or on an Adrenal Mesotonic blood Type B African-American. On a naturally slim body type, fat's health-reducing effects are much greater than on a naturally round type of body. In other words, on a naturally thinner body type, excess fat accumulation, pound for pound, has a more degenerative effect than pound for pound gains on rounder types. Ultimately, working within the phenotypic framework of each type is the all-encompassing key to restore low fat metabolic balance.

From a generic standpoint, the most common causes of excess fat accumulation (which in reality are **only** caused by metabolic imbalances) are:

1. Eating too much for the type of body and lifestyle one has have.
2. Consuming the wrong balance of macro and micronutrients for one's specific type and especially **too much** calcium and not enough iron.
3. Eating at non-fixed and variable times in the daily routine.
4. A lack of regular exercise in combination with the three points above.
5. Aging without proper dietary and lifestyle modifications to synchronize with this process.
6. Certain disease states, which slow metabolism and foster fat accumulation.
7. Certain glandular imbalances, which inhibit the efficient metabolism of food.
8. Toxin accumulation which provides resistance to metabolic efficiency and balance. (This includes drug- induced metabolic inconsistencies that lead to fat accumulation.)
9. The combination of any and all factors mentioned in factors 1 through 8 above, together or individually.

It should be obvious that all of the previous "fat growing" factors can only result from one not fully knowing his or her given type and what lifestyle modifications are specifically called for to rebalance metabolism.

Any fat loss program designed without utilizing the typing process first is exceedingly dangerous to one's health and statistically doomed to failure. The health authority-consensual statistical success figure for those who lose weight but fail to keep it off for long is less than 2%. That means that at least 98% of those who lose weight at first fail to reach their target weight level and also fail to keep the fat off because they eventually rebound into an often fatter state than ever before (i.e., the "yoyo diet" effect). What's even worse, most weight loss programs have little or no emphasis on building health while weight loss proceeds. This oversight results in people who perhaps weigh less but who are actually less healthy than when they started losing weight. This is due to the extreme imbalance that their one-size-fits-all fat loss approach utilized with absolutely no scientific regard for human biophysiological uniqueness.

So the net effect here is temporary weight loss **and** some health loss to go with it! Just losing weight doesn't guarantee better health. Eating less food on a one-size-fits-all fat loss mode further worsens existing deficiencies and metabolic inconsistencies severely undermining one's health—with no accountability whatsoever (other than an overly generalized quantitative measure of weight loss). I've seen patients who've undergone one-size-fits-all weight loss and who have lost all if not a good portion of their hair in the process. Hair loss during weight loss is an extreme sign of health loss—you'd think people would figure that out sooner! (Probably some weight loss counselor untruthfully told them that the hair loss was from detoxing or some other lie to keep them on the program).

Lying about nutrition for any reason such as ignorance, manipulation, egotism, and other reasons, is what I refer to as "nutritional terrorism." If your hair is quickly graying and/or disappearing on a fat-loss program, this is a sure sign that your health is fading fast. You're losing a lot of muscle, bone, electrolytes, vitamins and minerals, water, and other body essentials. In fact, fat may account for the least of what you've lost! I don't think that losing your hair or health from an inappropriate weight loss scheme was ever in your particular plan of life or anybody's for that matter. So don't be fooled into thinking that weight loss is automatic health gain! One-size-fits-all weight loss doesn't work this way!

Even Richard Simmons, during an appearance on Maury Povich's talk show, admitted to losing all of his hair when he first dieted. Why do you think this happened? Probably because Mr. Simmons practices one-size-fits-all diet habits, and has consequently damaged his health: an initial sacrifice for quick weight loss. And then you think to yourself, "why should I take weight loss advice from a guy who lost all of his hair when he dieted?" That's like going to a cardiologist for health advice who ends up dying from a heart attack before his fortieth birthday. This kind of ridiculous contradiction is very commonplace and happens all the time—we take advice from people who don't fully practice or understand what they preach! We tend to make the same one-size-fits-all mistakes that they're making and duplicate their failures.

So, when Maury asked Mr. Simmons why he lost all of his hair from dieting, he replied, "That was before I knew how to diet properly." The obvious implication here is that he knows how to diet properly now. But when Maury opened up Mr. Simmons' refrigerator and spied all of the partially eaten "sweet treats" he was startled again. Mr. Simmons quickly assured Maury that "nobody's perfect" and that if you exercise and eat right most of the time you can sneak treats without fatty consequences. I agree somewhat. But maybe Mr. Simmons' need for "sweet treats" (like chocolate ice cream) was due to metabolic imbalances; if these could be corrected, these cravings would probably be partly or completely eliminated.

To remain briefly on the subject of this popular weight loss "guru," I have a special question for Mr. Simmons—"where're your abs, guy?!" I've never seen any clearly defined abdominal muscles—or much tone overall, for that matter—on Mr. Simmons, or many of our so-called health and fitness gurus of today. Do you think that you could ever find your abs after listening to them and following their advice? Guess again! To help illustrate a major fat loss point, please indulge me momentarily in a fantasy of mine. I'd like to have a best-ab bodybuilding contest between some of our current health and fitness celebrities. Let's line up Dr. Deepak Chopra, Dr. Barry Sears, Dr. Julian Whitaker, Covert Baily, Tony Little, Richard Simmons, Jake Steinfeld, and Jack LaLane (and anyone else you'd like) in their swimsuits on stage, in front of a panel of judges in a "guys only" contest. Then let's ask them to flex their abs and bodies. Actually, this would turn out to be a contest for best "beer belly" or "fat stomach." The only place you'd see some real hard abdominal muscles actually showing (not hidden under layers of fat) would be on Mr. LaLane and Mr. Steinfeld. (Yes, I know Mr. Little used to have good abs when he unsuccessfully competed as a bodybuilder—but I haven't seen any on him during his media appearances for many years, and old pictures don't mean much in the here and now.)

Now, Mr. LaLane and Mr. Steinfeld obviously must practice more of what they preach to have their good state of tone, and in doing so, are perhaps closer to their typing needs either by accident or chance unless they've been professionally "typed." Unfortunately, to the best of my knowledge, these two are one sizers, but apparently they are doing more of what's right for them . . . and that's good. My initial impression of Mr. LaLane is as a very Adrenal Dominant Type, whereas Mr. Steinfeld is a Pituitary-Thymic body blend with some strong Adrenal Type characteristics. Both of these celebrities also have less to do in general with commercially pushing special diets than their other on-stage competitors. Oddly enough, they are in better shape, when you'd think the opposite would be true because of their lack of nutritional commercialization.

The superior physiques of LaLane and Steinfeld are due to a better exercise and eating patterns overall, habits much more closely matched to their individual "types" than the others. Only typing them can accurately reveal what's really going in their particular cases. All things said, I want to congratulate each of the celebrity individuals I've mentioned for their huge contributions to society, helping to inspire people to get off the couch and do something about their fitness and health. And Tony, I know you'll get your abs back with a little more effort.

The point I would really like to make from all of this jabberwocky is an observation of one-size-fits-all fat loss ineffectiveness, easily seen in the case of many of our inspirational celebrities. (Oprah Winfrey comes to mind most poignantly here.) I'm talking about—despite all of the discomforts of dieting—that last bit of fat that just never seems to come off no matter how hard you try. That lumpy fat that just seems to hang on no matter how hard you struggle, no matter how much your skin sags, no matter how much good health you lose, and no matter how many unnecessary wrinkles you've collected in your one-size-fits-all quest for rapid weight loss. Precisely typing yourself will completely eliminate that last stubborn fat deposit and protect you from the health loss which predisposes you to sags and wrinkles typical of improper weight loss techniques.

A freshly achieved and maintained optimal metabolic balance will prevent yoyo fatness rebounds, maximize energy levels, completely eradicate food cravings, restore appetite balance, ensure optimal health and fitness, and provide a long satisfying low fat life span. To attempt permanent and healthy fat loss without typing and profiling is suicidal at best, because it robs you of vitality, "killing you softly" on a most subtle physiological basis, and will simultaneously doom you to fat loss failure, replete with all of the psychological suffering and aggravations typically associated with that yoyo experience. To me, attempting fat loss without typing is like taking a shower in a raincoat! Yes, it looks like you are going through the motions of taking a shower, but without taking off the raincoat and getting the soap out, you'll never fully accomplish what a shower is really supposed to do for you. Typing will always balance your unique biochemistry so that you can once and for all rid the body naturally of something it was never designed to have in excess in the first place— fat.

Typing and the Athelete

The fundamental goal of all athletics is to specifically feed and train the body into a state of **hyper-functional** metabolic balance. This is a metabolic state wherein all body and mind adaptations to a given sport stimulus have efficiently taken place maximizing the development of continuous free energy to push the body beyond its previous limitations of performance. It is obvious that typing is just what the athlete ordered because it provides them the opportunity to individually strategize nutrition, training, and their synergistic combination in order to achieve a complete state of metabolic balance. This typing advantage effectively brings one closer to his or her biological potential for fitness than by any other means.

A metabolically unbalanced athlete is truly a physically handicapped one and will not go far in his or her achievements. An athlete's metabolism in a state of disarray only provides unchecked resistances to free energy production which in turn limits performance potentials drastically. Even athletes with the best genetic predisposition to their given sport still cannot fully liberate their biological potential without typing. These genetically gifted athletes may pass by those who possess fewer genetic advantages, but they still won't individually achieve all that is physically and mentally possible in their given sport without being typed.

A fully typed athlete has a profound advantage over non-typed athletes in all of the parameters of physical and mental challenge their sport provides, from injury protection to endurance and strength development, to a concentrated performance focus and positive attitude, and to the duplication of peak performance. As a specialized sport's medicine health practitioner, I have always utilized typing and profiling on my athletic patients whether world class or weekend warrior.

I agree with Dr. Joel Wallach, D.V.M., N.D., when he says "exercise without supplementation is suicide." But I would like to qualify his statement further by saying that any exercise or sports related physical undertaking, without typing and profiling, is foolhardy and, while it may not cost your life on the spot, it may cost you the thrill of victory in favor of the agony of defeat.

Many world-class and pro-level sports teams currently use elements of typing and profiling science to maximize their athletes' performance levels with much success. It is due to typing science that world records continue and will continue to be broken for all time to come.

Typing in a Action: Two Case Studies

No text regarding the art and science of typing would be complete without a clinical example of typing in action on real people. The following two patient studies represent my actual experience with two of the most common clinical problems I've encountered as a professional nutritionist. Naturally, these patients wish to be kept anonymous, and I will not bridge the confidentiality gap. For the purpose of simplicity and brevity—and to spare readers tedious details—I have condensed my findings into an easy-to-understand discussion format. Let me therefore refer to these patients as Person A and Person B.

Person A

Person A first came into my office looking for a fast way to lose body fat. She had gained almost 50 pounds during a period of depression, brought on by a prolonged divorce process. She desperately wished to lose this excess poundage . . . yesterday! We began a medical history on her, where nothing serious in the way of identifiable organic disease was present according to previous doctors. In fact, there was a total absence of nutritional intervention by any previous health professionals because, as Person A stated, "I really didn't need nutritional help before I gained all this weight. Just six months ago I looked and felt great." Consequently, she had not sought nutritional help. Now this middle aged woman wanted to lose weight naturally and without any drugs. Her existing supplements consisted of a one-a-day type of vitamin and mineral tablet, an extra capsule of vitamin C (500 mg), and a standard 400 mg calcium supplement with 200 mg of magnesium. My patient had also recently begun exercising three hours per week on the treadmill at moderate intensity.

Person A complained of fatigue, restlessness during sleep, more indigestion than "normal," occasional constipation, sore feet, aching knees and back, mental haziness, shoulder rashes, no energy, headaches, and suicidal tendencies. She ate whatever was at hand and had a food history that looked like she lived in several countries at the same time. One day it was McDonald's, the next day it was sushi, and the next day it was a gallon of ice cream—you name it, it was there—with no distinct rhyme or reason. Just looking at Person A's routine diet even made my iron stomach queasy!

A physical exam revealed slightly elevated blood pressure, a low back spasm, good reflexes, and mostly normal conventional findings, although her body fat percentage was a lot higher than the statistical average. We took a conventional blood and urine sample, which after analysis revealed very little other than a high-normal concentration of cholesterol and triglycerides in the blood, and a tiny bit of blood in the urine (later determined to be non-pathological). We finished our first consultation and conventional exam sessions with high spirits and future hopes. The third appointment was set and Person A canceled it having left a message that she was going on vacation for about three weeks and would resume her typing visits after that time.

As it turned out, **three months** passed before I saw Person A again. Into my office she walked, about 25 pounds lighter! At first I was pleasantly surprised . . . until I studied my patient further. Her face and skin were very pale and saggy, her eye whites had a pinkish tone, her allergy spots and kidney reflex points were darkened under the eyes, her tongue was whitened, and her manner was very sullen with less expression than on our first visits.

Person A proceeded to tell me how she had gone on a pure vegetarian diet (no meats, fish, dairy, poultry, etc.)—only vegetables, grains, and fruits. She had joined a network marketing group and took certain herbs and vitamins that they recommended and provided. This group also helped her stay on a strict vegetarian diet, which they consensually felt was healthier than diets containing meat, fish, and dairy products.

At first, when Person A "converted" to vegetarianism and started on the "special" herbs and vitamins, she felt great. A lot of her former symptoms—in particular the constipation—seemed to disappear. She began losing weight rapidly and felt excited about her new lease on life. Then about five weeks into her new program, the weight loss slowed, energy levels dropped, and the old symptoms came back while some new symptoms arose.

To add to the old list of symptoms, some brand new symptoms appeared during her vegetarian experience, including a chronic mild diarrhea problem, terrible fatigue (she seemed to sleep forever), some "touch and go" abdominal pain; to this were added some hair loss and thinning, dizzy spells, bad gas, and frustration with her new lifestyle. Person A's only recognizable and consistent symptomatic improvements during this time were less restlessness at night, no more constipation in favor of mild diarrhea (which she was told was normal by network marketing friends due to her body "detoxing"), less observable body fat, although she felt untoned and saggy, and a shoulder rash which seemed to have disappeared. One concern that she expressed regarding her new host of symptoms was a newfound and extreme craving for chocolate and an ongoing unquenchable thirst for fluids. Person A also seemed to have a mild cold she couldn't shake.

Given these symptomatic changes, I reexamined her and added new, though still conventional, blood and urine tests to rule out thyroid dysfunction and diabetes (fatigue, thirst, sugar cravings, gas, mental confusion are all textbook symptoms for diabetes and thyroid imbalance for forty-year-olds and older). Sure enough, her thyroid function had slowed from her last blood test, but readings were still within the lower limits of normal.

According to the blood tests, she was on the verge of microcytic anemia and had more white blood cells in her blood than normal. The glucose tolerance test given did not reveal full blown diabetes of any kind so I suspected other problems in this regard that were nutrition related (perhaps deficiencies of chromium, boron, selenium, and vanadium). I then proceeded to "type" her in order to reveal other underlying metabolic factors relative to nutrition. I quantified and qualified (Step 1) a theoretical nutrition plan for her after considering all reported lifestyle factors and body fat test results. After shelving this rough plan (temporarily), I proceeded to body type her (Step 2— Pure Metabolic Typing). Her round features, feminine hourglass shape (wide hips, soft skin, etc.), and other categorizable physical and psychological factors, blood type (O), and physiological measurements (blood pressure, heart rate, body fat percentage, etc.), scored her as a

Pancreatic Dominant Type with a secondary Gonadal Dominance. According to typing science, her recessive glands were the liver and pineal gland. Her nerve type was a Type B (Endotonic) with a Parasympathetic Autonomic Dominance and Low Medium Oxidation amount and rate (refer to Tables 5, 5A, 6, 7, and Appendix A and B). Her psychological profile was that of being food-oriented and generally happy with a very social and sensual orientation. Given these factors and others, I categorized her as a "carnivore—vegetarian," carni-vegan for short. (Refer to Appendix B: Blood Type Diet Categories for Blood Type O to get an indication of what the best food selections would be appropriate in her case; as you will find in Appendix B, red meat is necessary for this "type," as is the majority of alkaline vegetables and fruits found in nature.)

We then proceeded to Step 3 (Laboratory Assessment aka Profiling) and I designed a battery of laboratory evaluations based on where I felt the most metabolic upsets would be found given the information from Step 2 (Pure Metabolic Typing). So we took blood, urine, saliva, feces, and hair samples for the non-conventional metabolic tests that I decided on. The results are summarized below:

- Full blown deficiencies of iron, B12, B6, folic acid, tyrosine (an amino acid), calcium, magnesium, manganese, and many trace minerals.

- Marginal deficiencies of chromium, selenium, vanadium, boron, copper, zinc, molybdenum, and lipoic acid (a fatty acid).

- Higher than normal tissue lead levels and free radical stress.

- Delayed response allergies to milk, potato, tomato, garlic, citrus fruits, and sesame.

- Bowel parasites, leaky gut syndrome, low stomach acid, and poor fat digestion.

- Depressed DHEA levels (dehydroepiandosterone)

- Higher than normal creatinine (urinary) level.

The metabolic evaluation of Person A revealed a complete mismatching of diet and body type. This person was not designed to eat only vegetables and fruits. Not eating red meat had created deficiencies of iron, copper, zinc, B12, folic acid, and tyrosine which led to thyroid dysfunction, anemia, and fatigue. Having deficiencies of chromium, manganese, selenium, and vanadium could well cause chocolate cravings due to their effect on insulin function and the fact that Person A's body type is more prone to diabetic disorders than other types. The increased white blood cell count was a direct indication of her cold's systemic presence. The deficiency of lipoic acid undermines essential fatty acid metabolism in regard to the immune system increasing recovery rate time from colds and all disease and symptoms. No wonder this current cold was hanging on for so long! Depressed DHEA levels are indicative of accelerated aging, adrenal stress, and endocrine imbalances (along with hypothyroidism). Bowel parasites and free radical stress were due to a depressed intake of immune related factors and an increased intake of raw and improperly cleaned foods. Parasites also rob the body of essential nutrients and resultantly add to deficiency states as well. Heretofore undetected allergies to foods Person A craved and ate regularly (including garlic) only served to further complicate her health status.

Delayed food allergies overload the body with even more stress which leads to further imbalances and disease as well. Person A required more calcium in the diet in combination with higher amounts of magnesium proportionately, and boron to improve upon these deficiencies. Betaine hydrochloric acid is also helpful in this regard. With all this metabolic "chaos" going on, its no wonder Person A was suffering from chronic diarrhea which further hampered her body's ability to absorb proper nutrients (especially electrolytes) and therefore worsened her condition. Good and bad metabolic balance is created by a cause and effect chain reaction of metabolic and nutrient factors. Person A's condition reflects the chain reaction of poor health and further validates Dr. Vander's quote preceding Chapter I (If you look at Appendix B for Blood Type O as reference, you will see that Person A demonstrated sensitivities to foods that according to typing science should theoretically be bad for her. This is where laboratory assessment comes in very handy so that we can fully understand where a metabolism truly stands up to the moment.)

In Step 4 (Diet and Supplement Customization) I compounded all of the above information and designed diet and supplements accordingly.

From a disease standpoint, Person A was on the verge of full blown osteoporosis, heart and circulatory disease, osteo-arthritis, adult onset diabetes, and a handful of other diet-related diseases. From a symptomatic standpoint, this person lived in a chronic state of dis-ease, suffering a very uncomfortable day-to-day existence. As she walked out of my office with her brand new custom diet program and laboratory manufactured custom supplements, my prayers went with her.

Upon Re-Evaluation (Step 5) after four months, when I retested Person A, much to my pleasant surprise the majority of the laboratory tests were clear. She had lost another sixteen pounds and she looked and felt, as she put it, "better than ever before" and had that special sparkle in her eyes that I equate with good health. Even though Person A went on a short term detoxification and cleansing food rotation regimen to clean out and overcome food sensitivities, she still showed some lead deposition in her hair (to be expected for a while) and some mild allergic responses to tomato and eggplant (night shades), sesame, and milk.

All of her levels were down from the initially moderate and high sensitivity readings. Person A was gradually becoming less sensitive to these foods. She still had a slight calcium/magnesium deficiency but all other tests were perfectly normal including the parasite profile. Even the back spasms were gone after adjusting her spine and pelvis only three times in conjunction with our house massage therapist working on her soft tissues a total of eight times during the previous four-month period. In less than another six months, Person A tested negative to all her other deficiencies and imbalances including the occurrence of lead in her system. She also lost another eleven pounds and 6% more body fat to look, as she put it, "like a teenager again." She had fully recovered in less than ten months and reached all desired objectives.

Person A's story was one of total success. I chose to describe this case because of its commonality with many others I've treated. Here we have a typical person desperate to lose some weight and feel better. Instead of following through with me from our first visit, she falls into the trap of completely changing her diet on the basis of one-size-fits-all as reinforced by the political manipulation of pseudo-nutritionists whose motivation at bottom was to sell her their products and get to her sign up more people to their network—all without a true understanding of or honest regard for her health. These networkers further mislead Person A by reinforcing her vegetarianism, telling her what she wanted to hear about its benefits. They also lead her to believe that the chronic diarrhea problem was just a normal detoxification response to their herbs, when in fact it was a warning sign that something more serious was wrong. Along with her new network marketing "friends," Person A piecemealed assorted supplements from their marketing inventory (multivitamin-minerals, calcium, vitamin C, and others), which did little to nothing to properly nourish her metabolism.

As for the supplements they had given her, when I examined them I found them to be of low quality, generally unbalanced, and very overpriced. When Person A first began her new vegetarian diet and network marketing supplements, she felt better because of the immediate reduction in saturated fat calories in her new vegetarian diet (her body type does not do well with too much dietary fat), the natural cleansing, detoxification and laxative effects of a mostly raw, completely vegetarian food intake, her extreme compulsive excitement about losing weight and artificial feelings of wellness due to the highly stimulating effect the network marketing herbs had on her body and mind (they contained MaHuang, guarana, caffeine, and other stimulants).

Within four to five weeks, though, her new vegetarian-based nutritional program had bottomed out, having failed to fully meet her metabolic needs. Her body chemistry was unable to make up the difference from its reserve nutrient storage. This was the time when Person A really began to feel poorly and reluctantly deduced that something was wrong—perhaps even more so than before she actually started her vegetarian diet. But it took almost three more months before she contacted me because of her network marketing "support" group, who continuously convinced her that everything was okay in spite of her feeling bad and that her overall response was actually quite normal. After all, she had lost some weight, right? It must be working! This was their basic argument for their program's viability.

Luckily, Person A finally got fed up with feeling progressively worse and overcame the false belief-fostering and brain-washing network support group mentality about her diet and supplement plan and finally contacted me once again. Unfortunately for Person A, like many typical Americans she was willing to wait until a crisis situation developed before taking action. In this case, Person A constantly ignored the way her body felt because she really wanted things to work out socially with her new "friends." She consequently suffered through more than what most people would put up with, finally contacting me only when it became truly unbearable. She conveyed to me that because her vegetarian-herb program was a form of "natural" healing, she wanted to give it every benefit of the doubt and therefore hung in there as long as possible. It's all-natural—so it must be good, right? At that very moment in our conversation, she had just realized the important fact that her body is so unique that even "natural" things not right for her body type can cause problems. Just because a product or program is sold or touted as being all "natural" doesn't mean that it's right, or even safe for you (or her).

Typing worked exceedingly well for Person A and her true health potential was restored with many positive lessons learned. Probably most important, she realized that one-size-fits-all nutritional programs were no good, and that you shouldn't believe everything you're told— especially when the people talking are in a big hurry to sell you something.

Person B

Person B is an interesting case when it comes to demonstrating the inadequate nature of mainstream medicine (and sometimes even alternative medicine), and how novice and even professional non-typing nutritionists can inhibit a **person's** attainment of good health instead of promoting it.

Person B first came to my office after having been to at least fifteen other health practitioners within about three years (this was and still is a record in my mind.) She had contacted various mainstream doctors, none of whom could find any organic disease present upon examination. Person B brought in piles of medical records, which contained little evidence of any disorders—at least by conventional testing and exam parameters—other than some slightly elevated liver enzymes (showing liver stress), depressed iron levels, disproportionate ratios between two blood proteins, and a slight viral infective process that seemed to have cleared up long ago and which may have caused all of these findings in the first place (except for the low iron levels).

The last three conventional MD's whom she had visited weren't able to help her significantly, so they told her that her 30 or so presenting symptoms were essentially "all in her head." This erroneous diagnosis was probably made because (after all) these doctors could not find anything "concrete" using their standard examination and laboratory evaluation procedures. Actually, one physician wrote in his notes "Munchausen Syndrome," which is fancy terminology for hypochondrism.

Out of frustration and desperation, Person B fell in with a mail order scheme that guaranteed a cure for all her ills with that one magical product (you know the one—aloe). There's that old "silver bullet" or "magic bullet" mentality again—one healthy thing that does it **all**, which, of course, is impossible. This silver bullet, aloe, naturally didn't help her in the least, so she sought help from a novice nutritionist who proceeded to give her a canned diet and supplementation program with (of course) no exam or lab analysis other than some basic screening questions.

This one-size-fits-all approach didn't work either, except that my new patient liked a highly stimulating supplement she had bought from this particular nutritionist—a special herbal blend of MaHuang, caffeine, guarana, and yerba mate. She liked it because this supplement was the only thing that seemed to fully wake her up (other than coffee). Person B actually became addicted to the mixture and took it seven to ten times per day (the label recommended two doses per day). Without the supplement, she said that she'd have had to sleep 24 hours a day; and, despite the herbal boost, she was still in bed fourteen hours a day on average, due to her general fatigue.

Out of continued desperation, Person B decided to go to a university medical center, where she spotted a wall advertising a new community nutrition clinic. She visited a doctor there who put her through more conventional tests that showed nothing remarkable, and then one "unconventional" metabolic test, which yielded three new clinical insights. (The treating physician must have just learned about this particular test and didn't fully understand its implications, because his written and verbal recommendations taken from records continue to puzzle me to this day.) Person B was found to be fructose-sensitive, although no therapeutic diet was given to help her with this. Also, there was "some" disorder in protein metabolism noted, for which she was given a single, very expensive amino acid as treatment (I still don't understand why!). Then she was referred back to her regular family physician because her blood lipids (fats) were found to be elevated above normal. Person B revisited him with her new reports and the tests from the nutrition clinic, and he in response told her to eat less fat and that everything should be okay. The family doctor also recommended that she try the Pritikin diet, but didn't have a copy of the manual on hand to give her.

By now, Person B was mad as a hatter and completely abandoned the thought that mainstream medicine could help her. She just seemed to get bounced around from doctor to doctor with nothing much accomplished! Consequently, she went to an Iridologist, who provided a huge written report and told her that she possessed a Lymphatic body type. Unfortunately, only about three of the total 50 pages in her Iridology report provided any real information that she could use. Most of it was just background information. Person B, however, was given a list of foods that—according to iridological findings—should be good for her, as well as a list of foods to avoid. That was it.

Person B was not really feeling any better at this point, and felt instinctively that there was still a lot missing from what she really needed to be well. The Iridologist's food list seemed to help her energy a little now and then, but Person B was still confused about whether this was going to be the end of the therapeutic line for her, or whether she should look further for help. Acting on the advice of a friend, she consulted a nutritional allergist (M.D.) who gave her some non-conventional food allergy tests (some that I use in my practice), and came up with a much more definite list of foods to avoid. Thanks to these new tests, Person B felt that she was actually getting somewhere. Unfortunately, just following the "eat this" and "don't eat that" list from this doctor was not helping her much either, although she did experience some definite, if mild, improvements in her symptoms.

Following an advertisement in a natural healing magazine, my patient then contacted an N.D. (naturopathic doctor), who proceeded to perform a hair analysis. More significant information came out of this procedure. Person B showed a tissue iron deficiency, a large imbalance in electrolytes (sodium, potassium, etc.), candidiasis (yeast infection), an abnormal amount of aluminum tissue deposition, zinc and chromium imbalances, and a very high tissue calcium concentration. She was then put into one of three body type classifications based on oxidation rates alone. She was found to be a slow oxidizer (Kelley and Watson System).

Person B thought to herself, "Now we're finally getting somewhere!" Everybody before had missed these new findings. But, unfortunately, due to this most recent doctor's heavy reliance only on hair analysis and its nutritional implications, the total typing process was still not complete. Person B's subsequent lack of full symptomatic relief demonstrated this during therapy. Even with the naturopathic doctor's prescribed supplements and her new diet recommendations, the majority of symptoms remained. Now Person B was thoroughly perplexed, so out of pure desperation she went once again for another opinion of her case . . . this time to a famous "nutritionist to the stars."

Her new novice nutritionist (this person has no discernible degrees) had the self-proclaimed distinction of being a celebrity—a pioneer in nutrition—because she worked with some celebrities. Person B was given an extended (rather egotistical) verbal synopsis of the novice nutritionists' self-proclaimed greatness, which she simply found to be disgraceful. Person B also didn't like the fact that this nutritionist, much as all of her previous practitioners, didn't look the part. All of her previous practitioners, including this one, didn't look particularly healthy or fit—disturbing indeed! The celebrity nutritionist was overweight and undertoned, and looked older for her age than Person B had expected. The phenomenon of the "armchair expert syndrome" was beginning to take hold in Person B's consciousness.

Looks aside, the celebrity nutritionist briefly reviewed Person B's medical/nutrition records and told my patient that she just needed to "touch up" some areas of nutrition for her and then Person B would be fine. She charged Person B $150 for about 15 minutes of her time and told her to schedule another appointment. On the second visit, Person B was given a slightly more detailed diet plan than the previous naturopathic doctor, but it was written using only information from her hair analysis report. The celebrity nutritionist recommended that Person B take "hand selected" supplements in addition to those Person B was already taking, and then come back in one month. Person B was charged another $150 for her fifteen-minute visit, and then another $150 for the supplements.

During the ensuing month, Person B faithfully followed this program—gained 4 pounds and experienced severe headaches. She returned and reported this information to the celebrity nutritionist. The nutritionist reassured her that everything was fine and that the weight gain was normal during her body's metabolic rebalancing process. The celebrity nutritionist then gave Person B white willow bark extracts for her headaches, promising that they would go away. The nutritionist also replenished the supplement supply for another 60 days, at an overall total cost of $475 including the visit.

Her symptoms only worsened over the next two months, to the point where Person B was truly fed up. Just before the 60 days were up she saw a TV program that I happened to be on and decided to seek my help. So, in she came, totally disgusted, with piles of reports, generic diets, and bags of supplements—all of which landed on my desk with a resounding crash. (Almost as if it was my fault that she had gone through so much time and money and that I was the last straw.)

Sparing most of the tedious typing details, let me tell you what I discovered about Person B, as amazing as it is. First of all, nobody had ever quantified and qualified (Step 1) her diet for her, nor fully body typed her. Not even a fraction of the evaluative metabolic instruments that I have at hand were used. These were her presenting symptoms and my initial diagnostic impressions:

Anger	Headaches
Anxiety	Allergies
Poor Muscle Tone	Depression
Defensive Posture	Fatigue
Gastritis	Candida
Liver Spots (brown age spots)	Edema
Indigestion	Coated Tongue
Ears ringing	Irritability
Behavior Problems	PMS
Loss of Concentration	Low Self-esteem
Suicidal Tendencies	Mood Swings
Weak Nails and Hair	Muscle Weakness
Premature Graying	Itchy Skin
Progressive Stress Syndrome	Halitosis
Negative Emotionality	Poor Memory
Generalized Myalgia	Nutrient Deficiencies
Intermittent Diarrhea	Toxic Accumulation
and Constipation	Nutrient Imbalances

This was quite a list of problems Person B was still experiencing, especially if you consider all the professionals who had treated her up to this point.

Her only stated objectives were to feel well again, to get her energy back, and tone up her body. My body typing process revealed her to be a slightly Gonadal Dominant Type, followed closely by Secondary Pituitary Dominance, with a strong showing as a tertiary Thyroid Dominant classification. Her liver, pineal gland, and lymphatic system were all recessive. Her blood Type O classification designated Person B as a carni-vegan "type" of eater with a special need for dark green leafy vegetables. (As a matter of interest—Person B shied away from leafy greens due to digestive discomforts she experienced and because of her inability to taste them—zinc deficiency? Could be!)

This patient craved beans and garlic (she reeked of garlic when I saw her), both of which were contained in high doses in the celebrity nutritionist's diet. In a previous allergy test by doctor number thirteen, she was found to be allergic to milk, yeast, pork, concentrated fructose, and dextrose. This allergy profile fits right in with what you'd expect for this body type. In Step 3 (Laboratory Assessment) of her typing, I tested her further and found that she was also allergic to garlic and all kinds of beans.

The garlic sensitivity we would theoretically expect for this body type, but it hadn't shown in the previous test by doctor number thirteen, so I had to assume that she had developed a garlic sensitivity since that time (or a possibility that the first test was inaccurate). Person B's sensitivity to beans was somewhat unexpected, except perhaps due to strong thyroid gland influences; again (like the garlic sensitivity), something that either had developed or was missed by previous allergy tests for technical reasons. Going by pure typing science tenets, you'd expect sensitivity to nightshades (potatoes, eggplant, etc.). but this didn't show up in my tests. perhaps due to good thyroid strength within her metabolic system. (Thyroid Dominant Types do well with nightshade vegetables in general.)

Interesting to note here were Person B's garlic and bean cravings. Here she showed a delayed allergic response to both foods, and yet she constantly craved them. Dr. Braly's "allergy-addiction syndrome" was plain to see in this case. These particular foods created an allergy-initiated stimulatory effect in Person B's body, which actually helped to keep her awake and energetic. This type of stimulation is much like a person's "wake up" response to a cup of coffee. This wake up effect was part of her body's resultant defensive sympathetic response to the allergenic invaders in synergistic combination with the highly stimulating herbal supplements she had become addicted to. In fact, her nervous system was being simultaneously jolted by the IGg4 allergen response and the strong herbal stimulants.

Person B also suffered (according to my tests) from a full-blown thiamin (vitamin B1), magnesium, and iron deficiency, and from mild to moderate functional deficiencies of all B complex vitamins, magnesium, manganese, lipoic acid, L'Carnitine, CoQ10, chromium, vitamin C complex, L-tryptophan, N-acetylcysteine, and more.

I wondered how these deficiencies could continue, given all the supplements and the special celebrity diet? Could it all be due to her metabolically "hyped up" state, buzzing on allergens and stimulants in spite of the "special" nutrition program? Even Person B's blood amino acid profile showed a huge protein imbalance with some notable deficiencies. Tests demonstrated huge malfunctions in digestion and absorption, and her liver detoxification pathways were completely overloaded. This unfortunate woman also had a marked aluminum deposition in her tissue samples. How could this be, in consideration of all the professionals who have treated her?

Truly, she was not suffering from Munchausen Syndrome—this patient had many obvious physical problems. Even the specialized metabolic assessment laboratories were strongly indicating the presence of many more potential health problems and were suggesting that I use other tests to rule them out. One lab even suggested that she might have incipient cancer that was developing into a serious condition.

Person B's urinary organic acid profile demonstrated a huge outpouring of just about every metabolite and metabolic intermediate from the primary enzymatic pathway that produces energy in the body. There were so many enzymatic upsets present that I could barely count them. No wonder she needed stimulants to keep her awake— there was hardly enough energy production by her body to keep her awake naturally. Saliva and urine pH's were so low, considering her rather alkaline diet . . . it all just didn't seem to make much sense.

It took me a few long restless nights to realize that Person B was suffering from a huge "megadosing and allergenic syndrome." She was taking so many of the wrong supplements, in such staggering amounts, that her body was registering them as toxins and shutting down defensively in an effort to throw them off. I now call this "nutrient-megadose-toxin overload." She must have had the most expensive urine, feces, mucous, and sweat known to humankind! Person B was so completely overloaded with supplements that normally valuable nutrients at these super-high dosage levels prescribed were now actually considered to be poisons by the body.

Just think, too much of a concentrated intake of the same vitamins, minerals, and other nutrients that normally preserve our wellness can actually very seriously damage our bodies. This is why I always say, "Megadosers and shotgunners beware!"

We dumped all of Person B's former diets and supplements, directly into the trash can. We rebuilt her from scratch, orthomolecularly, according to my more complete typing and profiling program.

At first my patient went through a special fast and detox program before she got into the main part of the customized eating and supplement program. This initial accelerated cleansing program reduced stress on her system and allowed the liver and other elimination organs to clean out and regain their functions; at this stage, the body was given just enough nutrients to sustain itself under these special detoxification conditions. Even the initial fast helped Person B feel better as her body started to come out of its huge vitamin and mineral overload syndrome. Just throwing off the excesses of what we normally value as essential nutrients within our bodies made her feel better. In this case, less vitamins and minerals taken in made her feel better.

Needless to say, as Person B proceeded through the typed program she happily experienced gradual improvements, although she did have some occasional symptomatic flare-ups—to be expected in any natural healing process. To Person B's surprise, those green leafy vegetables that she had previously avoided quickly became a strong part of her diet, and she actually looked forward to eating them once her zinc level was in balance.

At the Step 5 (Re-Evaluation), Person B showed substantial improvement in all lab tests, especially those to do with the liver and other eliminative systems. The lack of measurable toxic stress alone, as seen in the retests, demonstrated that taking away the shotgunned and megadosed nutrients had allowed the liver and body at large to recover very rapidly.

This clinical story is proof positive that too many vitamins can damage your liver and body just like alcohol or any recognizable toxin. I guess my mother was always right when she said "moderation is the key," and Person B knows this much better now than ever before. Person B was completely back into metabolic balance within one year of eating and supplementing specific to her biochemical uniqueness and metabolic type. She is a case in point when it comes to discussing the dangers of megadosing and shotgunning. It should be noted that many more additional conventional tests were recommended to further investigate the patient's problems by the nutrient testing labs. There was so much "metabolic chaos" present in her body that the testing labs felt that this patient should be investigated further for more serious disease patterns. Consequently, generalized mainstream clinical logic in this case was directed towards finding more evidence of serious organic diseases such as cancer, autoimmune disorders, chronic fatigue syndrome, digestive inflammation, connective tissue disorders, and others. In effect, Person B's vitamin-mineral overload syndrome was causing changes within the body construed as serious disease possibilities by conventional and unconventional medicine. These disease possibilities all disappeared once metabolic rebalance was nutritionally reestablished.

This serves to exemplify the awesome power of individualized nutrition over one-size-fits-all, piecemealing, shotgunning, and symptom relief drugs. If any of Person B's metabolic symptoms were leading her down the path to any one of the serious diseases suspected by the labs and myself, all clinical concern has now been put to rest— thanks to typing for "nipping it in the bud." Typing is the ultimate system of disease prevention!

Metabolic Maps—A New Diagnosis Frontier

You will be hearing a lot more about Metabolic Mapping as the art and science of typing expands throughout society. Metabolic Mapping is a specialized form of typing used specifically to detect diseases long before **conventional** disease detection and laboratory techniques reveal their presence. Early disease detection has always been heralded as the premier lifesaving "factor among factors" in man's wellness struggles. In scientific fact, the earlier a disease process is known about, the greater the chances to reverse its progression **before** it impairs the quality and quantity of one's life.

The conventional approach for detecting disease states throughout the various laboratory specimens available is to look for body chemistries which are clearly "out of range" when compared to what is considered "normal." Normal is defined as chemistry measurements which fall within established reference ranges which, in turn, are based on many thousands of people studied over the years.

An example of this reference range phenomenon can be seen when you consider your own personal numerical blood cholesterol levels. If your blood cholesterol sample shows a reading of 115 mg/dl (dl = deciliter), it may actually be considered to be too low and can be correlated with some potential disease states. (Although, I would personally favor a lower versus a higher cholesterol any clinical day of the week.) If you were tested at 140 mg/dl, you would fall into the optimally healthy range, which categorically falls numerically towards the center of the cholesterol reference range based on human standards. If your cholesterol sample tested at 260 mg/dl, your cholesterol level would be considered dangerous (or pathological) because research samples have demonstrated a very strong correlation between high cholesterol readings such as this one with the presence and/or development of heart disease and other health deteriorating disease as well. (An interesting side note is that **indiscriminately** lowering cholesterol levels too much statistically increases the incidence of death from suicide and cancer.) Cholesterol samples that are clearly out of range, either too high or too low within the standard reference range, construe a diagnostic "red flag," which generally indicates the need for treatment because the measurement is considered to be abnormal.

There are many body chemistries based on this reference range system of diagnosis and evaluation that, when out of range, strongly or weakly demonstrate disease presence. Different chemistries reveal different metabolic information, but when any chemistry is out of range it constitutes a problem which may or may not be life-threatening, depending on which chemistry we are considering at the time.

TABLE 11
REFERENCE RANGE FOR CHOLESTEROL

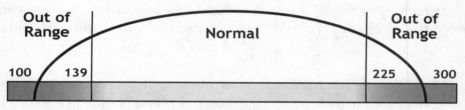

Cholesterol Reference Ranges (mg/dl):

AGE	Low (10th percentile)	High (90th percentile)
00–19 YR	120	191
20–29 YR	130	209
30–39 YR	139	225
40–49 YR	154	247
50 + YR	162	261

Cholesterol ranges based upon data from Lipid Research Clinics Population Study (Schaeffer & Levy, *NEJM*, 312:1300, 1985)

The inherent problem with this "in or out of range" evaluative system is that there is no allowance for metabolic chemistries which only slightly shift position within the established reference range but are still within the normal range, or those that may be only slightly out of range. Just being within range for a given chemistry is simply an atrocious diagnostic understatement when it comes to assessing an individual's optimal health range. This approach may work to pick up full-blown sicknesses, but that's about it. The real story behind one's true health status can be found by defining these ranges more closely and in their relationship to one another on a much more specific level. Unfortunately the "standard" metabolic chemistry panels in conventional diagnosis do not define nor reflect the critical significance of these subtle relationships and their varying numerical shifts on the reference scale.

When shifts occur in multiple metabolic chemistries from any or all body mediums (and especially blood), it is nearly impossible to accurately measure. This is because the numerical values of these metabolic chemistries and their true biological meaning as related to their shifts on the reference scale cannot be directly compared or correlated in conventional medicine. This seems ludicrous in light of the fact that each variable (cholesterol, triglycerides, HDL's, uric acid, creatinine, etc.) exists "interdependently" and is functionally inseparable from a metabolic standpoint. As stated above, this results in a pathology that will only become noticeable after its progress is full-blown, because conventional medicine has resigned itself to perceiving only the out-of-range chemistries as significant.

A new technology known as **balascopy** completely changes the way we can examine the values of an individual's chemistry profiles. Using balascopy, we can detect and precisely measure metabolic relationships between chemistries on a profoundly sensitive scale never before thought possible. Consequently, the way an individual's metabolism is functioning can be better viewed as an integrated whole and not just as a list of fragmented and isolated variables. In fact, these metabolic variables are now being integrated into an understandable network of interrelationships termed **metabolic network**.

Metabolic networks can be extrapolated from individuals and thanks to years of research now observably demonstrate balance or imbalance, which reflects specific metabolic patterns. Many of these have simply been derived by nutritionally analyzing (i.e., lab profiling) millions of people already suffering from medically diagnosed diseases and notating their mathematical proportions in quantums. When we "backtrack" this information into non-diagnosed seemingly healthy individuals we find these same biochemical patterns presenting before the disease process becomes diagnosable through conventional assessment. It can take many years for these patterns to worsen, which eventually brings on the full-blown disease state.

The bottom line on this process is that we can finally diagnose a disease (by name) many years before conventional medicine can detect it. Once diagnosed in this manner, we can reverse the disease-diet connection **before** diagnosable sickness takes hold. Plus, we can generate dramatically more information and a better contrasted perspective on the body's true health status. Furthermore, Metabolic Mapping can monitor the progress of a disease as well as its response to treatment.

Metabolic Mapping is a very powerful tool within the art and science of typing, which will someday become conventional, as will all aspects of typing.

Summation One

From this point forward, as a person who's been "typed" properly (that is, as my hypothetical patient), your life's quality and quantity will improve dramatically. Many aggravating aches, pains and symptoms will disappear forever. Energy levels will increase and persevere as fatigue dissipates into nothingness. You will find that fewer drugs (or none at all) will be necessary for your comfort and living functions. No one will ever say to you again that "it's all in your head" (or chalk whatever symptoms you may have up to Munchausen Syndrome in your medical records). Sickness will rarely affect you and a more positive attitude will follow. Your lifespan will move closer to its full potential, and fat will melt off your body and stay off.

Perhaps one of the greatest benefits from typing will be the one you take most for granted—a lack of serious disease—because you may never come down with any. Just think, in your lifetime you will not have come down with cancer, diabetes, heart disease, or some other life-threatening condition! You will come to truly understand that your lack of disease, the absence of daily discomforts, and a low-fat body is the direct reward for staying on your typing program.

You are now well into final frontier of nutrition, for your body only. You'll never again have to guess about what is and is not right for you (and perhaps damage yourself in the process)! Here's to your health and longevity!

CHAPTER FIVE

The Final Frontier of Nutrition

Nature Cannot Be Fought.
—**Ladislav Pataki, Ph.D.**

Studies show that every one dollar spent on preventive care saves ten dollars in medical costs later on.
—**Barbara Austin**

Healing is a matter of time, but it is sometimes also a matter of opportunity..
—**Hippocrates**

There are no riches above a sound body.
—**Biblical Apocrypha**

A new scientific truth does not triumph by convincing its opponents and making them see the light, but rather because its opponents eventually die. and a new generation grows up that is familiar with it.
—**Max Planck**

By now, you should have a conceptual grasp of what's involved in the art and science of Typing and Profiling. You have already seen how complex this process can be, but also how concisely typing and profiling investigates biochemical uniqueness. No other nutritional approach makes this proper acknowledgment, nor is there another system capable of specifying human uniqueness to this degree.

The purpose of this book is to help you clearly see that one-size-fits-all thinking is functionally obsolete and is quickly becoming extinct. In its place we find the final frontier of nutrition: Typing and Profiling. Known as "TPing" for short, this process is available at long last, ready to help you in all of your health needs. TPing provides our only effective weapon against diet-related dis-ease and diseases. It helps us realign with the natural chemistry of the universe, tapping into the nourishing elements from within our environment and in accordance with how God and nature have designed us individually. The chemistry of life is contained within the chemistry of the land, air, water, and all that thrives upon it. Our ancestors lived in harmony with the land and its nourishing elements, and in time our bodies became an even closer reflection of those nourishing elements found in our particular areas of origin phenotypically compounded over many thousands of years.

Only in recent times has man blatantly defied the rules of nature (and God). He has dramatically rearranged the environment and those nourishing elements derived from it—doing things "his way" in obstinate defiance of the natural order. Man-made environmental alterations are most apparent within the more civilized nations and in places where people pay the least attention to their traditional ways of living. We cannot rapidly change the natural order of human life, which has been established over the last 40,000+ years, in a century or two, without severe consequences. Our genetic constitution simply cannot accommodate radical changes in short order.

When it comes to diet-related health, it is blazingly clear that we are living with a modern epidemic of diet-related degenerative disease, which plagues our society like nothing ever before. Even the ancients didn't have it this bad! Consider modern-day "primitives" who live double our effective, "civilized" lifespans, and those less civilized and more ritualistic countries who far outperform the U.S. in diet-related good health—yet spend a mere pittance on healthcare by comparison. It should be so dramatically obvious to each of us that the answers to our diet-related disease epidemic cannot be found in some magical drug, pill, potion, or lotion, the one-size-fits-all approach or a sophisticated surgery that allegedly "does it all."

Instead, it is only through the clearer understanding of what specific nutrients (from minerals and vitamins to amino and fatty acids), each of our bodies needs to consume in order to optimize the way it was designed to function healthfully. Our bodies are designed to last **healthfully** for at least 100 years, disease-free. We are not designed to be sick or dependent on non-nutrient/non-life-essential drugs for comfort. Our bodies are dependent on the natural order of essential-for-life and life-quality nutrients given to us by God and nature. All we need do to be virtually disease-free is to take what God has given us (that is, our bodies and minds) and match them back to the environment from which they were derived. The three factors of diet, exercise, and lifestyle are the controlling forces of good health that need to be "matched back" to the environment, because this is where we have most radically strayed away from our roots. TPing shows the way back to what's right for your biochemical individuality.

Modern Man's Seven Biggest Wellness Mistakes

1. Not being TP'd for diet, exercise, and lifestyle—one-size-fits-all is dangerous to our health.

2. Continuance of the ongoing decimation of our topsoils through mass production, high yield quotas, and the push-it-to-the-limit for profits nature of modern farming philosophies, which includes genetic engineering.

3. Belief in the "magic bullet" of good health. You know, that special pill, potion, lotion or devotion to the program or treatment that in and of itself "does it all," and is therefore the final answer to all of our wellness problems and body design needs.

4. Self-destructive behavior and lack of personal responsibility. Doing what's obviously bad for us and/or just not taking responsibility for ourselves and taking things for granted (especially diet).

5. Carelessly polluting our environment and adding more, unnatural chemicals to our foods. We really don't need any more toxins than those already overloading our bodies and world we live in.

6. Having a "sickness system" of medicine rather than a "wellness system." Betting on getting sick and then heavily rewarding physicians for "curing" our illnesses is costing us too many lives and too much money.

7. Blindly trusting our government, drug companies, insurance companies, and mainstream doctors when they all have far too many ulterior motives to be fully trusted.

Let's Get You Started

In order to become a full-blooded "TPer," you first need to modify your attitude about some things. The preceding chapters have given you some special insights about the attainment of good health, how society is duplicating instead of eradicating nutrition-related disease, and what can be done about our current "health crisis," using precisely applied nutrition as our primary methodology. The scope of what you've read so far may have been further reaching with greater implications than you ever imagined—but it needed to be said.

I hope that this book is really "striking home" for you. With any luck, the ideas presented here have really gotten you thinking . . . free of one-size-fits-all's brainwashing. The information presented has been scientifically generated, is continually being proven time and time again on thousands of people, is purely logical, and simply makes sense. Hopefully you are happy and relieved about finding something that takes the guesswork out of attaining wellness through nutritional programming on the most personal level. To officially begin this process for yourself certain baby steps need to be taken.

Taking the Guesswork
Out of Attaining Wellness, Step One

Truly understand and faithfully believe that your body is designed to be disease- and pain-free, full of energy and life, and synergistically receptive to all that you want to experience and accomplish in your lifetime.

You are not meant to be sick, crippled, lethargic, depressed or to settle for second best in life. Stop betting on getting sick (like our health insurance industry does) and start betting on being well. To be well, you must not take stock in anybody or any medium that tells you that you can't be your healthy best (as many doctors do, unfortunately). Don't depend on your doctors and others for health needs that you can take control of yourself. In ancient China, the doctor was paid only when the patient was well and did not receive payment during sickness.

The general wellness status found in China today far exceeds that of the U.S., even though the Chinese spend only a tiny fraction of our healthcare budget. In our society, we actually reward doctors for our sicknesses by paying them huge amounts of money only when we are sick! Why would a doctor work hard to get us well when he's paid only when we're sick? Why should he or she even attempt to convince you that you can be well, when he or she makes more money when you are sick (or when you think you're sick)? Why not use "quick symptom fixers" to temporarily cover up the real problems?

Is it any wonder then that our 1.4+trillion dollar per year healthcare budget (the largest in the world) is making so very few inroads into resolving the majority of disease processes and especially diet-related diseases which account for 80% of all U.S. diseases?

If everyone was able to stay well on their own, many doctors and the industries that support doctors' drug and surgical therapies would not be necessary. Do you honestly believe that these groups of people would tell us how to be truly healthy even if they really knew? They'd be out of a job! We're not only paying for their high-profit support with money that can be spent on better things, but we're paying them and continually repaying them with our persistent sicknesses which ultimately decimates the quality of lives (not to mention breaking all of our financial "backs").

Step number one, then, can be summed up thus: **don't be fooled** again! Don't fall for one-size-fits-all rhetoric ever again! Take control of your God-given ability to prevent and reverse disease with TPing, and from your heart believe that you can and will be well!

Taking the Guesswork Out of Attaining Wellness, Step Two

Don't believe that your genetics "doom" you in either life's quality or quantity. First of all, you have no real way to measure what your genetics are all about without TPing. So you really can't be all that sure that you're "doomed" to be fat, or die young, or learn slowly, or whatever, just because some family member with a completely different lifestyle and biochemical identity has suffered.

Secondly, researchers commonly believe that genetics account for about two-thirds of what becomes of you physically (and mentally) over the first forty years of life, with one-third physical effect coming from your environment. (There is a genetically determined nutrient reserve that provides a certain measure of "metabolic insurance.") But in the next ten years or so after your fortieth birthday, this genetic-to-environmental ratio reverses to the point that overwhelming effects of environment can catch up with you and either wear you down or kill you off quickly—if you haven't taken care of yourself over time. If you have taken adequate care of yourself, these positive environmental effects will guarantee you the longest lifespan possible.

The bottom line "baby step" here is to utilize TPing to help you work in harmony with what you possess genetically, so that you may stand up to the moment metabolically in order to optimize and maximize your life. In this way, you will overcome many of the genetic blocks you may only **think** you have. You will also extend and maintain nutrient reserves at more optimal levels.

The secret is simply to make what God has blessed you with work for you—and that's what TPing is all about. And, by the way, one of the doctors heading the "Genes 2000 project" in a recent TV interview said that environment can counteract "bad" genes to a large degree. So, food can remove much of your weak genetic tendencies when it is precisely measured.

Taking the Guesswork
Out of Attaining Wellness, Step Three

Begin to remove the most obvious health barriers from your lifestyle. Some of these barriers may seem generic to a TPer but, for example, there would be no doubt to anyone in the world that if you put your unprotected hand in the fire you'll get badly burned—so why do it? Unless you absolutely have no respect for yourself or are just totally naive, why should you defy all reason by placing your hand in the fire and suffering? I don't believe that anyone really wants to suffer, whether you're from Tibet, China, the U.S., or wherever.

These seven barriers in particular need to be eliminated:

1. **Drinking inadequate amounts of water.** We all need to drink pure, "chemical-free," high energy water for the best health results. Distilled, pure spring or adequately filtered water is the healthiest. Do not rely on impure water beverages to account for your water intake. Soda pop, juices, tea and coffee don't count here. A good rule of thumb is to drink one ounce for water to each pound of bodyweight divided by three. If your weight is 100 pounds, you should drink at least 33 ounces of water per day. A good clinical tip many of my patients are pleased with is to drink as much of your daily water as you can the moment you wake up in the morning. At this time, your body is the most dehydrated that it will be in a 24-hour period. And drinking the water upon rising hastens and increases bowel movements. This beneficial "megadose" of water also helps to dissolve membranous solids hastening waste elimination through the genitourinary and bowel systems. Always use pure or distilled water to help filter wastes out of your body—do not use your body to filter wastes out of impure water!

2. Smoking. At least 36 of the 2,000 compounds found in tobacco smoke and nicotine are known carcinogens. The nicotine found in smoke is truly addictive and also physiologically stressful. Tobacco smoke paralyzes the cilia in your respiratory system allowing particulate matter to slide back into the lungs instead of "brushing" it out of the trachea. Heart, lung diseases, cancer and other conditions have been medically linked to smoking. Each body type has a different capacity to resist the negative consequences of tobacco smoke. Some will tolerate it better than others with some lucky individuals beating the statistical odds of smoke-related premature death.

But why play Russian Roulette with something that is a basic strain on all body types in the first place? Why put your hand in the fire again and again and again with each new cigarette? Your particular body type may be the one that smoke hits the hardest! From a nutritional standpoint, tobacco and other types of smoke act as potent anti-vitamin substances which strip your body of many essential nutrients and especially anti-oxidants. It also depletes the body of much needed oxygen. When one wishes to stop smoking but doesn't know how to, there are numerous options and TPing will clearly help in this regard. As an example, some scientists have postulated that nicotine dependence is related to nutrient deficiencies. Although this connection is not fully understood yet nor the exact nutrient factors which are involved, "TPing" will faithfully restore across-the-board person-specific nutrients that are essential to good health. Because TPing automatically restores needed essential nutrients to a specific individual and concomitantly balances the metabolism, theoretically, any nicotine dependence created from an unbalanced metabolism should dissipate as a result. I have experienced this phenomenon clinically. Some "TP'd" patients actually quit smoking because their nicotine cravings dissipated over time as their "TP'd" program was put into practice. To this day I'm not exactly sure which aspect or aspects of the TPing program were responsible for this turnaround. In the case of pica and sugar craving syndromes, deficiencies of chromium, selenium, and manganese have been implicated and I have observed notable improvement in patients with these disorders after TPing them. I anticipate that someday, thanks to continued TPing research, we will reveal the nutrient-nicotine connection for each body type and/or all body types. Perhaps when this happens, smoking as a common habit among humans may disappear altogether--or maybe not, because of man's incessant desire for stimulants. Even among high longevity societies and ancient "naturally pure" societies, there is always something around that people smoke as part of their religious and social rituals or simply as common practice. At this moment in time, it's very difficult to tell if the smoking habit is here to stay and what overall impact "typing" will eventually have on it. If you are a smoker, for best health results, make sure that your body type's nutritional program is in order to help protect your health and if you consequently lose your nicotine craving—so be it!

3. **Long-term drug dependence of any kind to maintain non-pain comfort levels.** In the first place, long-term drug use for pain inhibition of any kind has serious health-deteriorating side effects. In the second place, if you keep experiencing pain and discomfort repeatedly, your body is telling you that something is wrong and that the pain-blocking drug you're taking really has **no curative effect** because the physical problem returns once the medication wears off or when you again duplicate the irritation that instigates the pain in the first place.

   Example: People chronically take antacids to eliminate stomach pain that could be avoided in the first place with better food combining, appropriate digestive enzymes, slower more relaxed eating, and the use of natural curatives like aloe vera or bismuth, d-glycerrhizerated licorice or *nux vomica* (a homeopathic formula). Once you're fully "TP'd," most if not all pain relief medications become a thing of the past and are no longer necessary because the body will heal itself as a result of the TPing program. Remember that your body is designed to heal itself (termed homeostasis) and that pain-relief drugs do not heal anything when they merely block the conscious symptoms of pain messages your body is sending the brain. If anything, this pain-blocking effect disconnects consciousness from the reality of your body's health condition which in turn may seriously undermine your attempts to keep from damaging yourself further at work or play.

Natural curatives like herbs, vitamins, minerals, homeopathics, etc., work in chemical harmony with the body to actually stimulate the healing process. Sometimes natural curatives do not remove the pain as quickly and may take a while to turn the condition around—so patience may be required. However, when the pain is gone under natural healing conditions it's because the body has actually healed itself and not because the sensation of pain is artificially blocked off as in the case of pain-relief drugs. When you're TP'd and metabolically balanced in the first place, the need for any curative will lessen. If a TP'd person does require a natural curative for a short period of time, we will typically find that it works much faster and completely than on a "non-Typed/Profiled" person.

4. **Physical inactivity.** Regular physical activity is a healthy common denominator for all body types whether you're from Old World or New World Georgia. The full TPing process matches specific physical activity to specific body types. Some types simply do better with some forms of exercise than others. TPing takes this into account.

As an example, Adrenal Types require very vigorous, heavy, and high intensity exercise to feel, look, and be their best. On the other hand, Thyroid Types do better with slow, methodical stretching and yoga, Tai chi, dance and aerobic dance, and light aerobics.

By the way, Adrenal Types usually scoff at this "sissy stuff." They categorically believe that you have to lift heavy weights or beat yourself into a pulp to get anywhere in life. On the other hand, Thyroid Types tend not to be the best weight lifters and tend to shy away from heavy weight training.

Until you personally reach an advanced stage of exercise "typing," just start to move in whatever way that even remotely appeals to you. Walking regularly is a good way to get started on your personal war against inactivity and it just so happens that walking, as an exercise, is beneficial to all types so you can't go wrong. Remember that greater amounts of physical activity require an even more nutrient dense and balanced nutrition program for best results. The higher the intensity of physical activity, the faster your body metabolizes food, vitamins, and minerals. If you already have nutrient deficiencies and/or imbalances to begin with, exercise will only serve to worsen these metabolic inconsistencies. For all of the goodness regular exercise affords the body, there is this "downside" to consider.

It has reached a point where articles are being written to warn people about this problem; for instance, Dr. Joel Wallach, B.S., D.V.M., N.D., in his article "Exercise Without Supplementation Is Suicide" (mentioned previously). TPing yourself properly will completely eliminate any concern that you may have about exercise undermining your wellness status, because it precisely accommodates the body's metabolic requirements under all conditions. A properly TP'd person will obtain only maximum benefits from their exercise program. In my mind, "exercise without typing is suicide."

5. **Inadequate sleep, improper relaxation.** A lack of proper rest and relaxation over time puts a severe and cumulative stress on the body that will only serve to lessen the quantity and quality of life. Consistent exercise activity will always help in the promotion of better sleep patterns. According to TPing science, sleep patterns are very individualized. We don't each need the same amount or quality of sleep. Dream and sleep states vary among types and are loosely categorizable to some types.

Overall, however, due to the many complexities in our lifestyles it's very difficult to generalize from person to person. In our own individual cases, it is always better to sleep a little more than to sleep a little bit less than what we each perceive our actual sleep needs to be.

TPing, in my clinical experience, has served to lessen insomnia for some patients. and has eliminated it altogether for others. TPing's metabolic rebalancing process can only help improve sleep's healing functions. Both consistent sleep patterns and regular relaxation periods are found amongst long-living contemporary "primitive societies." These peoples are without many of the sleep limitations imposed on us by modern society. Besides eating and drinking properly, sleeping properly is probably the next most important health-promoting factor in life followed closely by regular exercise.

The three essential components of eating sleeping, and exercise represent our foundation of life and should never be taken lightly, overlooked or carelessly disrupted. A true typer will never undermine nor undervalue these three factors.

6. **Don't take responsibility for yourself.** Blame everyone except yourself for your problems in life. Believe that you are always right and everyone else is wrong and when something goes wrong in your life, it's due to a conspiracy against you. This way of looking at life only serves to depreciate your wellness and happiness. Life is about learning. Take control, overcome obstacles, and learn from your mistakes. Do not be closed-minded or stubborn about this. TPing involves taking steps to learn how to be in living synchrony and harmony with the universe. We are using art and science to accomplish this natural state of being and are hoping to enhance spirituality in the process.

TPing helps to better align your physical and (resultant) mental energy to the energy within the environment that's best for you. It helps you use the proper foods and lifestyle to align yourself. This alignment process will in turn impact on the way you think about spirituality. In fact, the science of psychoimmunoneurology is endeavoring to outline our "food-body-mind-body connection." This new science has revealed that the foods we eat have a direct connection to the way we think which in turn has another connection to our body functions. It all starts with the foods that we consume which is where TPing is the most focused. It's no secret that many of our living primitive societies and other native societies all have a spiritual conviction to the natural order of the land. This is part of their healthy secret to a long productive life. It needs to be ours as well. TPing helps to take us one step closer to this natural way of life on the smallest molecular order—food. We are what we eat, what we think, and everything we do. We are part of the spirit of life.

7. **Obsessiveness and extremism.** My mother always told me, as did my favorite biology teacher, that moderation is the key to life and that too much of one thing or another can "do you in." Obsessive and extremist behavior is yet another obstacle to good health one needs to confront and conquer.

Whether you suffer from fits of anger and rage, all work and no play or the reverse, eating a lot of one thing and very little else (megadosers, take note), constant over-exercising, vicarious thrill seeking (living through other's actions), a state of all talk and no action and no listening, excessive complaining, too much rest, too much sun tanning, constant impatience, overt narcissism, unbridled ego or any other excessive tendencies—they all need to be reckoned with for proper balance. We need to stay in our center. From a nutritional and lifestyle standpoint, TPing is the primary catalyst for life's balance.

The seven health obstacles that we've just reviewed really must be overcome for best TPing results. Your next step is to start applying the TPing process to yourself in the Workbook Chapter, "How To Quantify and Qualify Your Diet."

As you have already seen, TPing is a very complex process and needs to be dealt with in its simplified entirety in the *For Your Body Only* Workbook Chapter for maximum self-accuracy; an expanded version of this workbook is available from Dragon Door Publications. For those who want to go deeper, the help of a highly skilled metabolic typing nutrition specialist can be used to complete this process. Because not everyone has the benefit of someone like myself to work with, many people may not be properly typed and profiled. The

TEFFT System For My Body Only self-help workbook, available from the A.S.A.P. (see Chapter 8) will help to simplify this process drastically. For now, I have found a way to bring typing immediately into your life without having to read more books or concern yourself with any accuracy or motivational issues you may have about your ability to TP yourself. I have found a way to have all of the TPing work done for you automatically while you sit back and enjoy the rewards.

If there's one thing that Americans enjoy, it's keeping things simple. The TPing program you are about to be introduced to is a miracle of modern technology and research. It is what I respectfully refer to as the "New World" within the final frontier of nutrition. This is my most exciting discovery yet! It can ensure everyone in America and throughout the world a vital opportunity to maximize his or her individual wellness through metabolic Typing and Profiling.

This New World is known as *Personalized Nutrition*. Personalized Nutrition is the last word in Metabolic Typing and Profiling systems, and will allow everyone the superior health advantages TPing has to offer.

What, Exactly, is Personalized Nutrition?

Personalized Nutrition is a special program of TPing, which combines the five steps of typing—Quantification/Qualification, Pure Metabolic Typing, Laboratory Assessment, Diet and Supplement Customization, and Re-evaluation—into one simple procedure. It requires no real learning effort or self-determinations about bodytypes by the user, so there is little room for human error. There are no expensive doctor or nutritionist fees, no middlemen, no multiple office visits, and no unnecessary procedures or requirements. It can be put into effect in the privacy of your own home. It is predicated upon typing and profiling and ongoing laboratory research and up until recently was only available through clinical nutritionists. Personalized Nutrition has been "precisely" designed to take the guesswork out of TPing for each and every one of us.

The Research Behind Personalized Nutrition

The development of this program was motivated by Metabolic Typing and Profiling research (much of which is mentioned in this book), research regarding the phenomenon of "Zeta Potential" (a law of biological ionization), new laboratory technologies and other adjunctive research, and agricultural and soil research. Personalized Nutrition's research and development began over sixty-six years ago and involved the combined efforts of MD's, ND's, DSc.'s, DO's, Ph.D's, and other professional nutritional, chemical, agricultural and metabolic specialists. It has been tested on millions of people in clinical studies and has healthfully served many millions more who have generated data for Personalized Nutrition by being in the program. The refinement of this program continues up to the moment, to say nothing of the influence this research has had on all those programs derivative of it—the overall wellness benefits people enjoyed by using the program are countless.

Personalized Nutrition and Our Topsoil

There has been a wealth of information generated by the government (U.S. Department of Agriculture) and private enterprise about the changing status of our topsoil. As far back as 1938, in Senate Document #264, scientific evidence regarding our nutrient depleted topsoils was presented to Congress for consideration. Again, in 1971, when the U.S. Department of Agriculture published *An Evaluation Of Research In The U.S. On Human Nutrition*, the research revealed inconsistent and severely depleted mineral concentrations in the soil throughout the U.S. These findings have generated extreme governmental concern and the subsequent use of millions of dollars more to study this phenomenon further. These 1971 and 1938 studies, along with others, including Senate documents 264 and 268, have revealed that our topsoils are thinning out and losing their nutrient density over time and that this trend is intensifying at an alarming rate.

During the time of the 1971 U.S. Department of Agriculture study mentioned above, there were a number of "soil deficiencies" noted throughout the U.S. At that particular time, the primary soil deficiencies were cobalt, copper, phosphorus, and iodine. Although there were selenium deficiencies noted during the 1960s, there also were many toxic levels of soil selenium and molybdenum demonstrated. Selenium and other minerals are in more of a deficiency state nowadays than ever before while soil toxicities of these minerals are much less common unless artificially induced.

The agricultural industry's immediate response to soil depletion studies and the increasing nutrient deficiency states demonstrated therein was to employ the use of more petrochemicals and other synthetic soil additives to "enrich the soil." These supplemental petrochemicals were primarily supposed to improve mass-production yields but not necessarily the quality of the foods grown in the soil. Certain minerals do increase produce yields and these are the only ones found within these "soil supplements." The other minerals necessary for complete soil balance and consistently nutrient dense foods are purposely left out due to their added cost and minor effect upon yield **quantity**. Unfortunately, food's **nutrient quality** takes a "back seat" to profits every time in mass-production agriculture. Our continued use of synthetics in soil has its own unique set of problems all in addition to the farmers' ongoing struggle to keep the soil functional for better yields under the constant deterioration of soil conditions and other inconsistent variables such as weather and parasites.

Nutrient inconsistencies, deficiencies, and imbalances found in the soil are passed down through the food chain to you and I. All that grows in the soil is affected, as well as that which consumes what is grown.

Much of what has spurred the explosive growth of the nutritional supplement industries are the publicized accounts of the appearance of wide variations among nutrient densities in our foods. Does that orange your holding actually contain any vitamin C? Maybe or maybe not. Only a food assay can tell for sure. For vitamin C insurance, we'll typically take some supplemental C as compensation for nutrient-sparse oranges. Packaging, storage, processing, genetic alteration, additives, preservatives, pesticides, pollution, varying weather patterns, and over-cooking only serve to deplete food nutrients even more. These processes and conditions add many chemicals to food that are unnecessary for good health, are very difficult to metabolize and, in many cases, may be harmful.

Over 60 years ago, an agricultural specialist who worked as a consultant for the federal government and for the U.S. agricultural industry at large studied this soil and food depletion phenomenon. This man was an agricultural engineer, chemist, biophysicist and mathematician who had 34 agricultural engineers working with him on his projects. Interestingly, he was actually a student of Albert Einstein, with whom he openly discussed his biological ionization theories with on many an occasion. This particular scientist was contracted to assist farmers in rebuilding their soils for better product yields. He felt that much of the information revealed in his work should benefit humans. Our researcher saw imbalances in the pattern of nutrients within the soil that was transferred to the fruits, vegetables and grains which grew upon it, and in turn transferred to the animals that were fed these staples, along with the humans who fed upon both sources.

This scientist was able to see that if there was no copper present in the soil then there would be none in the plants or the animals that fed upon these plants. His quick reference check into diseases affecting people eating these foods on a regional basis statistically retained by the U.S. government demonstrated a greater incidence of heart and circulatory diseases, which is linked to copper deficiency, in the same specific regions of soil copper deficiencies.

These soil deficiency patterns and food-to-human regional connections were more statistically evident years ago, but are increasingly more difficult to decipher nowadays due to year-round growing seasons and the way foods are shipped into every state and country without the marketing limitations or boundaries present 30+ years ago. In previous days, a much greater proportion of the foods available in your neighborhood market was from local farms indigenous to your area. In our time, it's very difficult to tell just where people are getting their food from so statistics are difficult to compile in this regard. The bottom-line result is that the number of deficiencies across-the-board found in people is exploding. A recent statistic on minerals alone shows that the vast majority of people in industrialized countries (especially the U.S.) do not even come close to reaching 75 percent of the RDA level for numerous trace minerals taken into their bodies from food. Our trend-setting scientist, known as "C. R." (short for Dr. Carey Reams), would consider the previous statistic as only "tip of the iceberg" information compared to his overall findings.

An agriculturist, C. R. had once wished to remain mostly anonymous, desiring to help people compensate for nutrient inconsistencies that he found in food and to benefit from his knowledge of agriculture and livestock. C. R.'s scientific interests and medical background helped initiate the research and development of the program now known as Personalized Nutrition. His work helped infuse the system with all its fabulous nutritional discoveries, such as diamtomaceous earth, special mineral colloids, calcium's potent role within human metabolism's balance, and individualized metabolic patterning and customizing technologies. He used this special program to assist diseased patients sent to him from three hospitals within the state of Florida, which kept his independent laboratory operation very busy for many years. These hospitals relied exclusively upon C. R. for nutritional healing therapies. His success rates were nothing short of remarkable!

A follower of this metabolic scientist, "Farmer John" Aguila, also an agricultural engineer, has taken this scientific information to an advanced level of organic farming technology that insures nutrient densities in food at the levels typically present fifty to one hundred years ago. The nutrient-dense foods mentioned in Chapter IV, also known as "supernutritious foods," are adjunctive to the Personalized Nutrition program.

Personalized Nutrition, Heart Disease, and Zeta Potential

In 1968 a physical chemist, Thomas M. Riddick, authored *Control of Colloidal Stability Through Zeta Potential*. In 1970 he published another work, entitled *Heart Disease, A New Approach to Prevention and Control*. He examined the initial discoveries of the chemist Reuss Over 160 years before Riddick began his study, Reuss had found that, when a ball of clay was placed underwater in a glass jar with two glass tubes extended from above the water surface into the clay ball, and then DC (direct current) voltage was passed through electrodes placed in the tubes, the water's surface would be elevated in one tube and depressed in the other.

Riddick could not find an explanation for this phenomenon, until he came across the work of the German physicist Hemholtz (the father of Zeta Potential); the answer had been published by this scientist in 1878, where a scientific explanation for the phenomenon was at last put forward. Hemholtz's work laid the foundation of a natural law called *Zeta Potential*, which was furthered by his disciple, Smoluchowski. Today, the fundamental formula for cell electrophoresis still bears both of their names.

At the time, the work of these two German physicists was limited by incomplete experimental data, due to inadequate instrumentation. Riddick developed a technologically advanced instrumentation to more precisely examine this chemical phenomenon and continue the Germans' work (as well as that of others) on into its human metabolic implications and applications. He found that the Zeta Potential phenomenon works within the body as much as within the universe outside of the body, and this helps to explain the ionic nature and energetic properties of all metabolisms.

He was inspired by personal health needs: Riddick desperately suffered from seriously advanced heart disease. and in the process of his work learned how to apply his research on Zeta Potential to himself in the hopes of staying alive long enough to finish his research projects (and his life). He lived day by day, using nitroglycerin to stay alive, afraid that he could die at any moment—a constant prediction made by his medical doctors. Riddick was literally fighting for his life as he learned to apply the concepts of Zeta Potential to the stability of the human metabolism. His scientific revelations and survival results were and still are truly amazing, far exceeding the expectations of all concerned. His insights into heart disease and all diet-related diseases are revolutionary. He has inspired countless biologists, chemists, mathematicians, physicists, and physicians who fully subscribe to his ionic principles of wellness.

Besides dramatically extending his life and fortifying its quality by stabilizing and reversing his own advanced heart disease, Thomas Riddick revealed many certainties that physicians today accept as such. He fully demonstrated that:

1. Our major hospitals and their medical doctors do not have the proper equipment to demonstrate intravascular coagulation—a phenomenon of Zeta Potential that produces morbidity and death. (Dr. D'Adamo also examined this in his research.)

2. There is an insufficient medical recognition of the role of dissolved mineral salts when it comes to overloading the human blood system which consequently produces intravascular coagulation because of the age—progressive inability of the kidneys to clear these mineral salts from blood, most noticeably at the very low "pure" water intake typical of Americans.

3. Our conventional understanding of the ECG (electrocardiogram) which we see as a function of polarization, depolarization, and repolarization is inaccurate because its true function is based upon inverse electroendosmosis.

4. The radial pulse should be simultaneously monitored with a contact microphone when taking a patient's ECG to better interpret the elasticity of the aorta.

Riddick believed that if physicians took the four previous points into consideration, "it would be virtually impossible for a person to be judged well today, then die of a heart attack tomorrow." Unfortunately, current reality demonstrates that many have died from heart attacks within a few hours of having been examined medically (including an ECG) and consequently pronounced as being in good condition.

Using the properties of Zeta Potential as measured within the human body, Riddick was able to see the whole picture of all those individual facets involved in the cause of cardiovascular disease. Over 35 years ago, he concluded scientifically that the causes of cardiovascular disease are:

1. Basic misconceptions and lack of knowledge on the part of the Food and Drug Administration (FDA) concerning the physical chemistry of food processing.

2. Excessive input of mineral salts into the human system (especially table salt).

3. The inversion of normal sodium to potassium ratios in foodstuffs through processing.

4. The gradual overload and eventual overwhelming of the kidneys due to ingestion of excessive mineral salts.

5. Trivalent cations (minerals with three negative charges per atom—aluminum compounds fall into this category, as well as other heavy metals) ingested by humans. These are also known as 321 electrolytes. Also, a deficiency of copper causes degeneration.

6. Cigarette smoking, most particularly due to its gummy and coating nature as a two micron carbon colloid and, of course, due to nicotine and other toxins found in smoke.

7. Alcohol consumption beyond one two-ounce drink of 90 to 100 proof per day.

8. Lack of daily exercise.

9. High fat input and weight. (Interestingly, from a Zeta Potential standpoint, Riddick postulated that the cause of death from fats was from a phenomenon present in physical chemistry known as "critical micelle concentration," whereby critical fat concentration in blood or CMC—a chemistry term—effects significant precipitation which clogs arteries and capillaries.)

Much of Riddick's Zeta Potential research revelations came long before medical doctors and the general population acknowledged the need to lower salt intake, drink more high energy "pure" water, avoid silver fillings (mercury), aluminum containing cookware, drugs and toxic food containers, emphasize fewer canned and processed foods in their diet, understand the FDA's shortcomings and its politics, minimize alcohol consumption and smoking, exercise regularly, cut fat consumption, and reduce stored body fat levels—all in the name of preventing and reversing heart disease (and other diet-related diseases).

Utilizing tens of thousands of urine samples collected from test subjects and himself, Riddick was able to fully measure and understand urine's direct relationship to the Zeta Potential of blood and to the entire ionic water medium of the body. He was effectively able to measure chemical states within the body and control them nutritionally in the prevention and reversal of heart disease and other related disorders. Riddick was ultimately able to closely monitor Zeta Potential and its nutritional variables using standard laboratory technology which he helped to calibrate accurately.

In time, the natural law of Zeta Potential may well prove to be the most fundamental of all insights into metabolic balance (aka good health) and is in complete congruence with C. R.'s biologic theory of ionization. For now, Personalized Nutrition's CLIA laboratories and software experts have adopted and refined further the Zeta Potential concept and C. R.'s biological ionization principles within its chemical profiles and metabolic algorithms and equations.

These are primary factors in TPing that can only be found within Personalized Nutrition's individualized process of nutritional intervention. You might say that Personalized Nutrition's program is "all heart," when you consider that a significant part of its origin was derived from the scientific quest to eliminate heart disease—our number one killer—from the human race.

Personalized Nutrition's Goals

The original goals of the Personalized Nutrition program are listed below:

1. To incorporate our scientist's (C. R. and others) agricultural and livestock nutrition information and his biological ionization principles into a human user-friendly program of diet and supplementation.

2. Utilize all generic nutritional research done on farm animals and humans where applicable. (For those concerned about research on animals, please note that the majority of this research was devoted to making the animals healthier and not hurting them in the process.)

3. To incorporate the understanding of all the known metabolic TPing programs available in the research including all the ancient and modern systems mentioned previously, into the Personalized Nutrition project.

4. Maximize the role of individualization in the deliverance of Personalized Nutrition to its consumers.

5. Adjunctively combine the new and rapidly developing laboratory technologies focused upon metabolic uniqueness with Personalized Nutrition wherever applicable.

6. Employ the full implications of the Zeta Potential phenomenon to the TPing process.

7. Link diet and supplements to each person on the most specific levels possible and in accordance with testing procedures and information which everyone can relate to and apply.

8. Develop a computer software package that will streamline the entire process of Personalized Nutrition.

9. Clinically validate the program on thousands of people.

10. Minimize costs to the consumer wherever possible so that Personalized Nutrition can reach as many people as possible.

11. Take the guesswork out of and put science back into the pursuit of nutritional perfection to allow each of us to become our healthy best.

12. Effect a major impact on the prevention and remediation of diet-related disorders in society.

How I Discovered Personalized Nutrition

I first came upon the Personalized Nutrition program in the early 1990s, when I was practicing in Malibu, California, at the Malibu Health and Rehabilitation Center. At this time, the majority of my healing focus was centered on all drugless healing techniques and most specifically clinical nutrition. I had access to a specimen collection laboratory on the premises and the camaraderie of other "natural-oriented" health practitioners representing various disciplines (MD's, other D.C.'s D.Homm's, ND's Ph.D.'s and RPT's) who shared the center with me. Having this variety of different yet synergistic health practitioners on site made for a very progressive and all encompassing healing climate for patients. This was an atmosphere I truly enjoyed.

On the staff of Malibu H & R, I was considered to be the in-house "metabolic nutritionist," primarily specializing in clinical nutrition. I had the responsibility of completely customizing individualized nutrition programs specific to patients' needs. I employed the five step typing process consistently (overviewed in Chapter IV). Whether in the treatment of diet-related disease, weight loss, subclinical ailment syndromes, soft tissue injuries, media appearance preparation for celebrities, body detoxification, total lifestyle makeovers or peaking for world-class athletic competition, some or all of my five step process was utilized. This process is now known as the Tefft System of Personalized Nutrition or to some as the Tefft Alternative Nutrition System.

In Malibu, my responsibilities to my patients as the "house nutritionist" included being aware of every clinical nutrition breakthrough in existence. I wanted to remain on the "cutting edge" of nutritional sciences at large; therefore, I was always looking for new information and procedures.

I came upon Personalized Nutrition after talking with an investment banker from Beverly Hills who told me about its existence. He felt that I should research Personalized Nutrition to see if it would be of benefit to my patients. I assured him that I would and immediately followed up with a thorough investigation.

As my investigation process was being completed, I became pleasantly surprised. This program was the granddaddy of all individualized nutrition programs to follow. Personalized Nutrition's program provided a succinct way of categorizing 14 to 25 metabolic patterns (or types), including seven male and seven female basic "types," from a uniquely different standpoint than any other assessment tool in my possession. (Actually—and amazingly—this program in pure form is capable of recognizing up to 2,600 metabolically distinct types.) This essentially took the five steps I have been using to TP my patients and wrapped them up into one simple, streamlined procedure, which covered about 50% of what my $10,000-per-patient makeover program covered (at a dramatic cost savings for the patient), and meant much less tedious work for me.

What's Different About Personalized Nutrition

Aside from being much more cost effective for clients than other typing programs that I had been used to utilizing, Personalized Nutrition provides an approach to nutrition that many typing purists would almost consider "putting the cart before the horse."

Instead of beginning the typing process with Step 1 (Quantification and Qualification) and then proceeding through Steps 2 (Pure Metabolic Typing), Step 3 (Laboratory Assessment), Step 4 (Diet and Supplement Customization), and Step 5 (Reevaluation), Personalized Nutrition begins in Step 3 and then corrects for Steps 1 and 2 culminating in a completely custom nutrition plan (Step 4). It then moves on to Step 5 to re-check results within a three- to six-month period. From a clinical standpoint, Personalized Nutrition "cuts to the chase" right from the start by starting with profiling. It typically moved patients through to nutrition program completion in seven to fourteen days—with two visits instead of my usual six- to eight-week term—with seven total visits.

Starting in Step 3, Personalized Nutrition is designed to generate laboratory data which immediately groups patients into one of fourteen primary metabolic types. or what I now call "patterns" in reference to Personalized Nutrition. There are more than 28 metabolic patterns that this program routinely classified for men and women. Personalized Nutrition is actually capable of classifying thousands more, as I've mentioned. It also immediately provides long and short-term data on the immediate metabolic status of the individual.

In other words, with Personalized Nutrition, I can immediately decipher an individual's strengths and weaknesses as a metabolic type and also have a direct measurement (profile) of how much in or out of balance an individual is at the moment in relation to their type and in relation to overall body functions (digestion, assimilation, absorption, and elimination). The Personalized Nutrition (P.N.) system provides me with an instantaneous overall picture of nutrition-related metabolic function in one full sweep. This was not possible for me prior to my discovery of Personalized Nutrition.

Clinically, PN's process is extremely efficient. Personally, I liked Personalized Nutrition's simplicity from the start. I've employed many different lab procedures based on various specimens like blood, urine, saliva, feces, hair, and tissue, all of which provide different informational fragments. Each lab procedure measures certain metabolic factors and has its own inherent limitations. I used to be required to combine and correlate this information through my TPing procedures in order to finish the custom program for the patient. Personalized Nutrition, on the other hand, isolated key metabolic factors from urine and saliva and measured and correlated each factor individually and in relation to one another as it deductively formatted an entire therapeutic nutritional intervention. It literally connected-the-dots of information automatically. This all-in-one efficiency saved me a lot of time, and any of the other tests I used or procedures I performed at the time layered easily into this fundamental program.

Using the original *Personalized Nutrition's Doctor's Handbook* which I further improved upon in Malibu, I was able to closely follow and interpret what the test results meant with their furthest-reaching health implications. Also, this professional manual enabled me to concisely explain all aspects of the program to my patients. The Original Personalized Nutrition group even supplied me with a special manual to train me (as a doctor) thoroughly in the use of this program with optional training seminars if I desired even more information. Personalized Nutrition clearly wanted there to be no gaps in my understanding of this program so that I could fully serve my patients with it. From a clinical nutritionist standpoint, it's nice to know you have a support team like this behind you.

Unfortunately, none of the other laboratory programs or procedures I was utilizing then could compare to Personalized Nutrition in terms of overall frontline thoroughness. All in all, Personalized Nutrition was just what the doctor ordered. The biggest difference between Personalized Nutrition and other laboratory typing and profiling procedures is in where it fits on the priority list of what needs to be done first through last. In the overall process of TPing, the researchers at Personalized Nutrition positioned it as first priority. In relation to other laboratory procedures it occupies a special position of first priority as well. The Tefft Alternative Nutrition System expands further upon this approach using hair and other adjunctive evaluations.

Personalized Nutrition's Priority Position

Part of the TPing process requires selecting the most pertinent laboratory tests that need to be performed on an individual. Step 2 (Pure Metabolic Typing) provides insights into the trouble areas of metabolism, which need to be further investigated by body type. Knowing these trouble areas helps to narrow down the field of laboratory testing to only those tests that are most important to perform.

Given the typing insights afforded by Pure Typing, it just doesn't make sense to order all of the possible tests in a shotgun approach. "Shotgunning" lab tests can be very expensive, is not scientific, and will yield a preponderance of negative test results. A test result is positive when there is something found that indicates a problem. A negative test result demonstrates no disorders found. A larger amount of test negatives demonstrates a wasted effort and this simply is not necessary when you understand how to type properly. If I were to put myself in the patient's chair, having just given "gallons" of blood, urine, feces, and saliva and then had a bunch of my hair plucked out, I'd want to see some significant results without any unnecessary or costly tests. Furthermore, when positives do appear on lab tests, I'd want them to disappear by the time of my next laboratory evaluation because the custom diet and supplements had actually worked. (Retesting, of course, is the only scientific way that you can truly monitor progress.)

This is where Personalized Nutrition comes into play. First of all, its value/expense ratio is the highest amongst all TPing procedures. Its value to the patient as compared to its expense is the highest for all typing and profiling. It costs the least and yields the most information. This system also helps to keep the "horse in front of the cart." From a nutritional science standpoint, Personalized Nutrition's lab assessment provides the first line of laboratory generated metabolic data which we would want and need to know up front.

Not only does Personalized Nutrition's data cover most of the Pure Typing (Step 2) for an individual but it also provides up-to-the-moment metabolic information that really is necessary to have before selecting any other laboratory procedures. In effect, it is a first priority in lab testing, as well as in overall TPing because it provides immediate, future, and on-the-spot insights into what other TPing procedures may be necessary in the short and long term. If we were to skip the Personalized Nutrition procedure altogether and move into another lab assessment procedure we'd mistakenly eliminate valuable information that other tests don't provide. Consequently, because we didn't choose our lab procedures wisely, we would end up with many more negative test results, wasted time, increased costs and impertinent procedures, which to me, as a professional, is intolerable.

Personalized Nutrition's second greatest distinction as a TPing procedure in relation to other lab procedures is that it measures nutritionally correctable metabolic inconsistencies which when corrected may absolutely negate the need for many of the other lab tests. In other words, if we initially use Personalized Nutrition's assessment and customization, it will automatically fulfill a person's nutrient needs which if left uncorrected would show up as inconsistencies in other tests.

A good example of this can be seen when you consider the pH testing portion of Personalized Nutrition. If one takes the Personalized Nutrition test which in part measures the pH differential between saliva and urine, we can tell if the body is operating on an acidic or alkaline level. This information is invaluable when it comes to understanding what the tested person is going to need nutritionally to correct problems. As with the soil, a person's body in being too acidic or alkaline has a direct impact on which vitamins, and especially which certain minerals, the body will metabolize properly and which macronutrients it has too little or too much of. The Personalized Nutrition program customizes diet and supplements to correct pH problems and the nutrient inconsistencies that go with them. If we were to skip this frontline procedure and go straight to a blood deficiency analysis for example, we would find deficiencies that would be considered common for acidic or alkaline metabolic imbalances. When certain demonstrable deficiencies are known about, but not corresponding pH levels, we could go ahead and give an individual more of those same vitamins and minerals they were found to be deficient in, in the first place, and then retest in a while and surprisingly find that the initial deficiencies have not changed significantly or may have even worsened.

Why? Because we didn't first correct the pH balance which would have removed the deficiencies that the second test picked up. When pH is out of balance, no matter how many vitamins or minerals you feed the body, some will just not assimilate well in an acidic or alkaline medium. But if you correctly balance the pH first with Personalized Nutrition, those same micronutrients lost when the body is too acidic or those lost when too alkaline will then assimilate and metabolize correctly, effectively eliminating deficiencies. Therefore, you can inadvertently put the cart before the horse if you don't measure and correct pH balance first, before looking for nutrient deficiencies, and then attempt to treat deficiencies having skipped this pH evaluation and correction.

The originators of Personalized Nutrition have isolated certain key chemistries in urine and saliva, which serve to measure "front-line metabolism," and when found to be unbalanced, these are directly correctable with individualized nutritional intervention. The program was designed to be put into effect long before delving into other potentially inappropriate and sometimes expensive laboratory procedures. The customized nutrition program designed from these chemical test results effects metabolic rebalancing with a minimum of any further testing or typing. Consequently, this program can stand alone both as the means to a therapeutic end in and of itself and as an entry-level program front line to all TPing procedures. From "cause to correction," it is highly efficient.

Personalized Nutrition Stands Alone

As we have seen in the prior discussion, Personalized Nutrition stands alone in many ways:

1. Ease of usage for both patient and clinical nutritionist.
2. Shortness of time required assessing and correcting metabolic inconsistencies.
3. Minimum number of visits, procedures, and complexities for all concerned.
4. Direct relationship to all TPing procedures. It fits right in, helps clarify the TPing regimen, and can be layered upon by other TPing procedures.
5. All-in-one assessment—to—correction procedure with no gaps, gray areas or guesswork, and with professional backup for both nutritionist and client.
6. Highest value/benefit ratio due to its fundamental importance to all TPing in combination with exceedingly low costs.
7. Ability to help narrow down the need for and selection of other laboratory procedures, and in helping to sequence their order within the testing regimen more appropriately.
8. Capacity to act alone in the detection of metabolic inconsistencies and institute the appropriate nutritional intervention without having to add extra procedures or other corrective nutritional factors.
9. As first frontline priority in the undertaking of any and all TPing procedures whether from Steps 1, 2, 3, 4, or 5.

TABLE 12
PERSONALIZED NUTRITION OVERVIEW

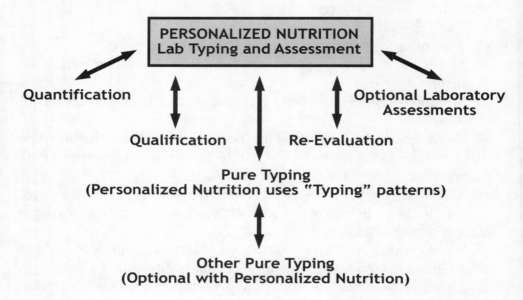

PERSONALIZED NUTRITION
Lab Typing and Assessment

Quantification

Optional Laboratory
Assessments

Qualification   **Re-Evaluation**

Pure Typing
(Personalized Nutrition uses "Typing" patterns)

Other Pure Typing
(Optional with Personalized Nutrition)

Big Added Benefit: Personalized Nutrition Puts the Cabosh on Docterly Invasions of Your Private Body—Just "Say No" to the Scrapings, Cuttings, Puncturings and Pluckings

One feature of Personalized Nutrition that most TPers favor is the complete lack of invasiveness to the body. The fewer invasions to the body for any reason, the better. There are no needles, biopsies, complicated stool samples, skin scrapings, hair (through pluckings), blood drawings, special fasts, anything to swallow or any pain in the collection of the necessary specimens (urine, saliva and hair). No laboratory visits, cold hands, nurses with plastic gloves, long road trips, or extended visits are part of Personalized Nutrition's program.

As of late, Personalized Nutrition has further simplified its specimen collection procedures so that it is exceedingly simple with "home kits" for use in the privacy of one's home. The person providing the specimen sample just follows a couple of steps for collection and then puts the specimen box into the mail and Personalized Nutrition does the rest. All of my Personalized Nutrition patients have enjoyed the privacy, ease, comfort, and simplicity of this program.

In the earlier days of Personalized Nutrition, both blood and urine were used as the primary evaluative specimens. As time progressed, research and development continued and new technologies came up allowing Personalized Nutrition to drop the blood component of its assessment and derive the information it required from urine, hair, and saliva alone. (Hair is used for differential mineral comparisons.) This has served to make Personalized Nutrition the least invasive and easiest-to-use of any lab procedures I've ever employed.

Why Urine and Saliva?

Why completely center a nutritional program on urine, hair, and saliva assessments?

Aside from being non-invasive, there are other, more technical reasons why Personalized Nutrition processes urine samples (known as metabolic urinalysis), hair analysis (known as Tissue Mineral Analysis), and saliva (pH tests) in its TPing system.

Two-and-a-half thousand years ago, Hippocrates instructed his pupils in the use of urine as a basis for predicting the course of each illness. Less than a century ago, physicians would taste urine to determine the presence of sugar and to aid them in their diagnosis of diabetes. From a conventional medical standpoint, urinalysis is the most important test for the evaluation of kidney and urinary tract diseases.

Moreover, urine accumulates throughout the body, coming in contact by one means or another with virtually every cell in the body and carries away the byproducts of each cell, tissue, and organ. It starts as urea in the blood and becomes urine after reaching the kidneys which add even more body waste components to it. The toxic residues of the body and its overall metabolic byproducts are filtered out by the renal system and concentrated as urine.

The concentration of metabolic waste products in urine reveals the amount of toxins and byproducts that are being dumped by the body. The measurement of this waste material in urine can be equated to the amount of stress being applied to the various body systems. The central concept of Metabolic urinalysis is akin to examining the mouth of a river in order to identify chemicals and other toxic products derived from upstream sources. Emptying the bladder is a natural and necessary process that removes excess water, salts, and the numerous waste products derived from metabolism. If something is wrong with metabolism the composition of urine will reveal it. Personalized Nutrition's particular program is designed to detect and elaborate upon urine's inconsistencies in terms of their metabolic implications and then effect the proper nutritional adjustments necessary to correct these inconsistencies.

In the medical and nutritional world, saliva is fast becoming "hot" for assessing a multitude of metabolic functions and nutrient/toxin status ranging from the functional states of intestinal mucosa (internal lining of intestines), to parasitic infiltration, to certain hormonal chemistries of stress within the body. Some of the assessment criteria revealed by saliva are strictly for medical use, like cultures while other criteria is non-medical and has metabolic implications which can signal the need to modify diet accordingly. In the case of Personalized Nutrition's program design, only the pH of saliva is necessary to correlate with urine in determining acid and alkaline states of metabolism. When compared to urine pH, the actual pH of saliva reveals a wealth of information, which Personalized Nutrition utilizes to help formulate corrective diet maps and supplements.

The Tefft Alternative Nutrition System is expanding further upon the use of saliva and breath analysis for other nutritional and toxic measurements heretofore only thought attainable with any accuracy from blood, urine, and hair specimens. Saliva may one day provide the majority of metabolic information needed to perfect nutrient balance, further simplifying TPing still more, while reducing the cost further.

Compared with urine's constituents, blood has its own set of metabolic implications and limitations that most people are not aware of. To take a quote from Mark Stern, M.D., of Utilization and Review Associates, Inc.:

"It is not uncommon to have normal blood studies as evident in many of the cases reviewed, and yet have imbalances associated with metabolic urine studies. This reflects the fact that the blood is well protected in the homeostatic mechanism of the body with the directive to maintain the integrity of normal blood components many times at the cost of tissue, lymphatic or urinary homeostasis. The marvelous aspects of the body to concentrate or dilute through many of the processes of biochemical dynamics, represents some of the fascinating realities of how man has been created."

In essence, Dr. Stern is here extrapolating upon the fact that blood is a highly controlled body medium. It acts as a messenger service for hormones, is a nutrient delivery system, provides immune and protective functions, and is a waste remover and transporter.

In relation to each of these functions, there are certain built-in tolerances or limitations and blood tissue – specific needs. An example of this can be seen when it comes to glucose (sugar) levels in the blood. When sugar rises too quickly and goes beyond a certain level in blood (specific to each individual), the body adjusts hormone secretions to quickly turn the blood sugar into muscle and liver glycogen, converts it into fat, and eliminates it through the kidneys. All of these physiological adjustments have to be made before the blood sugar level rises too far and causes physical damage. This automatic homeostatic control factor in blood is especially dramatic when it comes to keeping metabolic waste product blood levels low because of their concentrated toxicity. An increase in toxic factors will cause physical damage long before a similar rise in blood sugar would. A pH shift of just a couple of tenths of a point could bring on immediate death, as one example. As a blood tissue-specific need, iron is more concentrated here than in any other body fluid or tissue and it doesn't give it up easily.

The body, therefore, has to utilize the urinary system to quickly and effectively dump waste products before blood levels change significantly damaging the organism at large. In effect, the urine is a perfect contrasting indicator for the actual proportion of metabolic waste products that the body is creating. Urine takes up the "homeostatic slack" for blood by serving as blood's own personal waste dump, which the blood can use at any moment to help maintain its own "critically tight" tolerance ranges (homeostasis) for each metabolic byproduct. The result of this process is that the urine gives an up-to-the-moment reflection of the balance of many metabolic processes we need to know about in order to adjust nutrition properly.

A good example of this can be seen in one of my own clinical experiences. I had a patient with a normal calcium concentration in the blood, yet suffered from a raging case of osteoporosis. A comparison between urine and blood tests revealed there was an extremely high concentration of calcium in the urine. Blood calcium levels were normal because homeostatically and reflexively it dumped excess calcium directly into urine to help moderate its own tolerable levels. Therefore, in this case urine was the primary indicator of osteoporosis, while blood indicated normalcy. Using this valuable urinalysis information in my TPing procedures with this particular patient allowed me to nutritionally correct the condition right away.

Hair analysis is extremely reliable to demonstrate average mineral levels present in the body. Because nutrient minerals are atomic in size (the smallest complete particles found in nature), they are most important to assess within the body. Our personal atomic structure and everything found in the universe is predicated upon the differing weights and attractive and repulsive properties. The way these tiny particles stack up within us not only determines our most fundamental constitution, but also reveals weaknesses and strengths within our bodies relative to sickness, wellness, and energy production. Vitamins (short for "vital-minerals") are molecular minerals derived from atoms, connected in many ways to the presence of minerals within our bodies. But it all starts with minerals—they are the building blocks of all life and must be equated in our metabolism for best TPing results.

Neither non-hair tissue nor fecal analysis fully measures up to urinalysis as a front-line metabolic evaluation methodology. Each has certain strengths and weaknesses in what they reveal about metabolism. These particular evaluation methodologies are better capitalized once metabolic urinalysis, hair, and saliva analysis are performed, after which a clearer determination of their actual need in the TPing program can be made.

A redeeming characteristic of Personalized Nutrition is that any adjunctive information about metabolism added in from other TPing procedures comfortably layers onto Personalized Nutrition's program. Other adjunctive TPing information can be added into Personalized Nutrition's software features for further nutritional refinements when and where needed.

A Special Feature

Personalized Nutrition's program provides a special measurement of metabolic efficiency that I've never seen formally represented before in any laboratory typing procedure. This measurement is based on what biochemists call the "Theory of Ionization and Metabolic Balance," and is of great value to both patient and clinician.

The Theory of Ionization and Metabolic Balance, as it relates to our health status and metabolic balance is expressed in the following simplified mathematical formula.

TABLE 13
PERSONALIZED NUTRITION
EQUATION OF GOOD HEALTH

$$H = E \div R$$

(Health Index equals Energy divided by Resistance)

H = Health Index   E = Energy   R = Resistance

The following information will help you to understand the meaning of this formula.

1. **State of Health** (also known as "Health Status")—the constant variable adaptation of the overall metabolic chemistry between the internal environment and the external environment of a human organism relative to its coefficient of activity.

2. **Coefficient of Activity**—the measurable level of the sum total of all biochemical processes in relation to the process of ionization which forms the nature of one's metabolism.

3. **Ionization**—the process by which nutrients are moved from one place to another by ions.

4. **Ions**—positive or negative charges or charged particles.

5. **Nutrient**—any naturally occurring substance that provides or catalyzes energy production for the growth and maintenance of the human organism.

6. **Metabolism**—the total profile of all biochemical activity required to maintain life.

7. **Resistance (overall)**—the electrical and chemical inhibition of "free" energy production within the body due to the presence of inadequate nutrition, pathological disease states, physical degeneration (including premature aging), and/or injury to either the physical, mental, or spiritual condition of the individual.

8. **Resistance (electrochemical)**—the effect produced when atomic particles of varying energy potentials encounter one another and produce energy.

9. **Metabolic Balance**—the relative path of least physiological resistance to energy production in the body. In the case of Personalized Nutrition's biochemistry profiles, a perfect state of balance occurs when all measured body chemistries are within approximately 5%, plus or minus their optimal range for each metabolic pattern.

10. **Health Index**—the degree of metabolic balance within the body expressed by the mathematical ratio of Energy to Resistance and represented as a probability factor. This number is expressed as a percentage of metabolic efficiency.

11. **Nutrition**—the process by which nutrients maintain the life of the body and mind.

12. **Free Energy**—the lifeforce available to the body above and beyond that which is being consumed to counteract Resistance (overall) within the body and mind.

Mathematically speaking, the Health Index represents the fact that there is a direct health correlation between an individual's biochemistry and the condition of their body (the physical), the soul (mentality, will, and emotions), and the spirit (wisdom and understanding).

This relationship is demonstrated below:

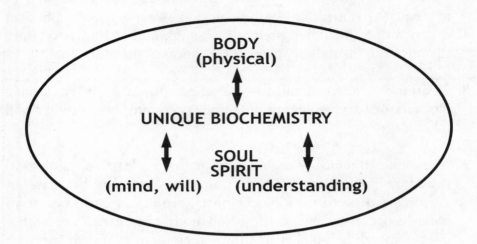

The law of cause and effect is a law of nature which controls the dynamically interacting relationships between health, energy, and resistance in the body, the soul, and spirit. The next table will help to clarify the various cause and effect relationships.

TABLE 14
CAUSE AND EFFECT RELATIONSHIPS

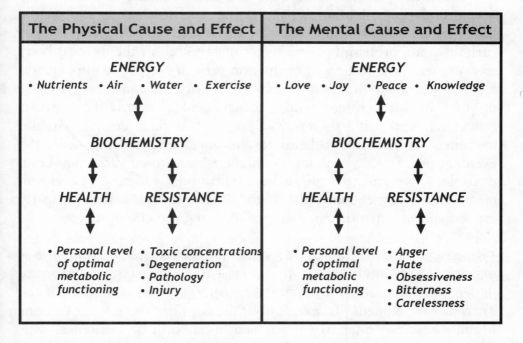

The Physical Cause and Effect	The Mental Cause and Effect
ENERGY • *Nutrients* • *Air* • *Water* • *Exercise* ↕ **BIOCHEMISTRY** ↕ ↕ *HEALTH* *RESISTANCE* ↕ ↕ • *Personal level of optimal metabolic functioning* • *Toxic concentrations* • *Degeneration* • *Pathology* • *Injury*	**ENERGY** • *Love* • *Joy* • *Peace* • *Knowledge* ↕ **BIOCHEMISTRY** ↕ ↕ *HEALTH* *RESISTANCE* ↕ ↕ • *Personal level of optimal metabolic functioning* • *Anger* • *Hate* • *Obsessiveness* • *Bitterness* • *Carelessness*

The mathematical expressions of the "Physical Cause and Effect" and the "Mental Cause and Effect" are therefore embodied within the H = E divided by R formula.

Each biochemistry measured within Personalized Nutrition's "metabolic test" (hair, urine, and saliva evaluation) has its own degrees of balance or imbalance, whether high or low, which can be expressed as a percentage of optimum, but in addition, all the biochemistries used in a person's metabolic test are factored in together for an overall combined percentage of nutrient efficiency. The Nutrient Efficiency Level reported to an individual can be expressed as a percentage. This percentage represents one's particular body's rate of converting food into energy, also known as metabolic efficiency, and is a direct reflection of his or her own particular health index from a nutritional standpoint. In other words, the proportions of nutrients, given one's personal metabolic state, which directly influence one's measured biochemistries will demonstrate an in or out of balance food intake pattern.

In effect, the Personalized Nutrition's metabolic test is a laboratory analysis of specific hair, urine, and saliva chemistries examined for the purposes of evaluating the acid/alkaline, electrolyte, mineral, vitamin carbohydrate, protein, fat, and water metabolism of the internal body environment. The test result evaluation provides scientific information as to which metabolic chemistries are out of balance in comparison to optimal or ideal ranges and mathematical patterns. The precise nutritional corrective therapeutic protocol is then determined and instituted to restore biochemical and metabolic balance with the eventual outcome of attaining the highest Nutritional Efficiency Level possible. Once reached, the highest Nutritional Efficiency Level will create as a consequence the highest Health Index that properly individualized nutrition can deliver under all given circumstances.

Referring back to Table 13: Cause and Effect Relationships, it is important to understand that various body organs generate "adaptable chemistry" to compensate for the given condition of the internal environment. To exemplify this, consider the effect of toxins brought into the internal environment as a form of resistance. This resistance factor causes the body to generate an abnormal body chemistry. The resulting biochemical changes are reflected primarily in urine and saliva, although some chronic conditions will also appear in blood, tissue, and hair. Personalized Nutrition picks up and correlates this metabolic information and then interprets it nutritionally, that is, it alerts the person being tested that there is a problem and then automatically changes the diet and supplements to effectively remove or reduce the resistance.

The body must always be fed the right nutrients, the right amount of water, and be given the right type and amount of detoxification before metabolic balance can be fully restored. Metabolic balance (shown as $H = E/R$) is reflective of the internal environment's status. Once it is re-established into proper balance from a state of imbalance, the body chemistries measured by Personalized Nutrition will automatically adjust on their own, revealing this newly achieved metabolic balance.

Using the Personalized Nutrition Equation of Good Health, the primary objective of Personalized Nutrition is to help an individual attain the ideal Nutritional Efficiency Level of 100%, which in turn will, when it occurs, reflect the attainment of perfect metabolic balance (i.e., perfect wellness), which again represents the ideal Health Index or 100% energy production with no resistance. This relationship is demonstrated in the following table:

TABLE 15
PERFECT WELLNESS

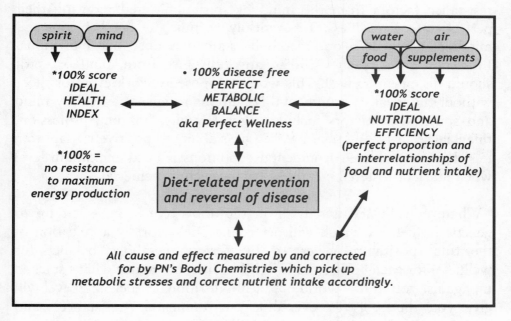

It should be apparent by now that one's Nutritional Efficiency Level is a mirror of their nutrient induced potential to achieve 100% metabolic balance, which in turn is either reinforced or reduced by mind and by spirit generated resistances not directly affected by nutrition.

If an individual takes Personalized Nutrition's metabolic test and his or her reported Nutritional Efficiency Level is 65%, this means that they are removed from their full nutritional potential by 35%; this gap must be bridged in order to achieve 100% of their metabolic efficiency and full balance. In essence, when the patient then follows his or her prescribed Personalized Nutrition's Custom Diet Map and consistently consumes their Personalized Nutrition's Customized Supplements, their personal Nutritional Efficiency Level increases towards the 100% level. When achieved, this level is considered to be perfect for their type of body.

Let's say hypothetically that one reaches 100% of nutritional efficiency, then this person theoretically would achieve 100% wellness (or Perfect Metabolic Balance) provided no non-nutrition-related resistance factors from the mind or spirit interfered reducing their perfect state of wellness. Theoretically, so much of our behavior and mindset is linked to our metabolic state that once our Nutritional Efficiency Level reaches 100%, any resistance from mind or spirit should disappear as well. This would supposedly work even for those without the ideal environmental conditions to ensure a healthy mind and spirit; such factors include a good family, fulfilling profession, financial security, and secure love. One's ability to positively adapt to a less than favorable environmental conditions is at its maximum level when nutrient-fostered metabolic balance is fully achieved.

Whatever isn't accounted for in the above equation is left up to genetic influences, which will determine one's worldly application of the total positivism generated by perfect metabolic balance (or wellness) for each body type. In other words, no matter what's stacked up against you in this world, an ideal Nutritional Efficiency Level will give you the tools to overcome environmental "resistance" and succeed in life in your own nutritionally maximized positive manner.

When my patients take the Personalized Nutrition metabolic test, the percentage scores of nutritional efficiency give them a starting number to work from, in order to challenge themselves to improve their health status; this is a great feature. In effect, Personalized Nutrition takes a complicated assessment process, sums it up, and gives each individual tested a simple number (as a percentage) of the "ideal." If an individual scores 65% upon initial testing, they'll hope to see perhaps a 70 or 75% retest score, which would be scientific proof that they are indeed improving in simple and easy-to-understand terms, not in fragmented and complicated jargon.

This scenario is similar to taking body fat tests in order to monitor body fat loss and receiving a simple number, which reflects your body fat status (expressed as a percentage) and the amount of improvement that you achieve as you progress through a weight loss program. TPing has never before had such a precise and poignant mathematical tool that would help each person understand where they metabolically stand at the moment and where they must go nutritionally to be fully well, in accordance with their biochemical individuality. When that 65% score goes to 70%, the results are truly felt by the individual as free energy production explodes, body fat melts off, and uncomfortable symptoms disappear forever. When you think about just how much our well-being rests upon that tiny Personalized Nutrition test number, it staggers the imagination and excites the spirit. To think that just increasing that number can mean so much to the quality of life . . . .

From the very start, it became obvious to me that Personalized Nutrition was not just another "typing" test; rather, it was a special process born out of an all-encompassing, therapeutic philosophy designed to simplify, clarify, and potentiate the universal key to wellness—balance. Personalized Nutrition's Nutritional Efficiency Level is the balance "zone," mathematically derived, that we all need to be our healthy best. Without it, we can't be sure where we stand, metabolically and nutritionally.

In Clinical Retrospect

In my work as a professional nutritionist, it became evident to me from the start that the Personalized Nutrition program was a "home run" when it came to fulfilling my needs and my patients' needs. I did a lot of background research on this program so that I would have no doubts about its therapeutic validity and wouldn't miss any of its special features or useful implications within the process of TPing.

Many times I've seen practitioners with invaluable healing tools in hand which they did not fully comprehend in both theory and application. Their demonstrable lack of understanding only serves to limit the potential use of a given methodology in providing the most benefits possible to the patient. Taking nothing for granted, I guess you can say that I have become an outright expert on this particular program and all of the other programs used for my patients and myself.

As much as I've wanted to help my patients throughout my years in practice, I've always started with my own self-experimentation. In this way, I can say confidently that **I practice what I teach!** I have received much praise from my patients to this effect, and I've always felt rewarded in setting a good example for them. I've always been (thankfully) rewarded with extremely good health and fitness levels for myself, except for my bout with asthma, and mercury and arsenic poisoning. I have found that taking boundless health and fitness to some of the extreme levels that I have achieved, especially in athletics, has served to help me challenge myself; more importantly, my own example can help to inspire patients to challenge themselves.

As a clinician, I have never considered myself—nor been considered by my patients—to be merely an "armchair expert." Getting down into the trenches with everyone else has its true-to-life advantages when it comes to fully embodying the principles and application of nutrition and exercise. It also increases my ability to personally relate to the information that I am presenting to others. It helps me relate to what other people are doing and telling me about their particular health practices. Practicing what you preach (or teach) perfects your ability to empathize and synchronize with patients. Without exception, all doctors should do this.

From the moment I found the original Personalized Nutrition program, my wife and I tried it and were pleasantly rewarded. I then incorporated it into my TPing procedures (i.e., The Tefft System) with never a complaint, only praises and positive testimonials from my patients. You can say that because of this positive response, I've always been on good terms with Personalized Nutrition, and consistently utilize the program in practice—both with my family, my patients, and myself.

What about the rest of you who aren't my patients or who don't know a clinician who uses Personalized Nutrition? Those of you who are not working with someone who employs the Tefft System? This question brings us to my final discovery about Personalized Nutrition—what I refer to as my biggest surprise! This special surprise is what I term as the "New World" within the final frontier of nutrition.

The New World...At Last

Personalized Nutrition scientists came up with certain questions over time throughout the advancement of the program. How do we bring the nutritional advantage of Personalized Nutrition to everyone? Why shouldn't everyone have the TPing advantage Personalized Nutrition has to offer, regardless of income, their own nutritionists' knowledge parameters, convenience of clinical settings and living location—or any other factor that could potentially limit their ability to access Personalized Nutrition in order to customize a nutrition program scientifically? How can we contribute to the large-scale extinction of the clearly obsolete one-size-fits-all mentality and its related products in society once and for all (before it does any more damage)? In answer to these questions, Personalized Nutrition faced its task force of health professionals and specialists with this ultimate challenge.

The results of their work are a custom-tailored program specifically for those outside of the clinic setting—what I refer to as the New World. The impact of this work has been overwhelmingly successful from every standpoint. This program is now designed so that anyone can access it, and it has been even further streamlined to more precisely meet the overall needs of each and every person who uses it.

The current Personalized Nutrition program excites me more than ever because I've always felt that good health as related to nutrition should never be exclusively the domain of only those who can pay an exorbitant price for it (like many of my Malibu patients). The rich and famous should not be the only ones who can comfortably afford the specialized process of being TP'd. Every man, woman, and child in our great country deserves to be as healthy as possible. The U.S. needs to turn around its poor health standing in the world, ending needless nutrition-related suffering and once and for all! We can lead the world in good health. You and I can only accomplish this if nutrition is utilized for your body only . . . with the help of Personalized Nutrition.

CHAPTER SIX

A New Beginning:
The Recreation of the
"Good Old Days" in Modern Times

Nature cannot be fought.
—Ladislav Pataki, Ph.D.

It may have occurred to you by now that Metabolic Typing and Profiling is an art and science completely dedicated to resurrecting from "olden times" the concept that each one of us requires an ideal lifestyle, with unique requirements for optimum wellness. Some of these ideal wellness lifestyles still persist among a handful of modern-day "primitive societies," such as the Hunzas, Tibetans, Aborigines, Titikakas, and so on. Very little has changed within these societies over thousands of years, and the net health result is the (almost) complete absence of diet-related disease among these peoples.

Each of our bodies would have experienced many of the same wellness benefits that these primitive groups enjoy, had we been born earlier in man's history. In our day, however, these "primitives" and other staunchly traditional yet somewhat modern societies lead the world in overall good health, complete with an undeniably apparent lack of diet-related disease. These particular cultures thrive healthfully, while highly sophisticated, extensively modernized, weakly traditional or non-traditional "melting pot" societies suffer the consequences of a never-ending plague of diet-related disease.

In lieu of this phenomenon, much can be said in favor of "the good old days and the good old ways" when it comes to fostering perfect wellness. It's really no wonder then that so many modern day health practitioners are traveling full circle—straight back into the therapeutic application of ancient health wisdom in synergistic combination with modern healing science. This old and new blending of health-promoting philosophies is helping people to more effectively and comprehensively balance wellness naturally. But only TPing can fully restore past history's most healthful virtues and conditions to modern society precisely—and in "modern terms" that we all can easily relate to. It accomplishes this by utilizing the most sophisticated science and technology, skills never before present in our history, to fully restore our primal wellness to its full potential.

Even though we may no longer have the pristine and unpolluted environment of old—nor the nutrient-dense foods, low stress, family-oriented values, high activity levels, and genetically matched living conditions that our ancestors once enjoyed—TPing can accurately calculate, completely restore, and even improve upon our current lifestyles and wellness states with more precision than our ancestors ever experienced.

Thanks to the development of TPing's expansive knowledge base, cutting-edge technological breakthroughs, and most of all, the desperate state of mankind's need to overcome diet-related and degenerative disease, Metabolic Typing and Profiling has now attained its most supreme form. TPing is ready to be used **right now**—the most potent weapon against disease that we possess! In the final analysis, Metabolic Typing and Profiling allows us to effectively synergize old and new wisdom on the most highly individualized level, to bring back life's perfect balance as God and nature intended it to be.

Body type by body type, uniqueness by uniqueness, TPing offers each of us our very own, custom-designed wellness lifestyle, which guarantees us eternal health on the orthomolecular level (i.e., molecule-by-molecule), in perfect alignment to the universe **within and without**. Employing the Typing and Profiling process to eliminate health resistances and to restore wellness catalysts avails to each of us all the benefits life has to offer.

As TPing becomes increasingly more conventional and accepted by mainstream society, life for each and every one of us, no matter what our differences, will become worth living more than ever before. . . we are entering mankind's most exciting historical period! In this coming period of national and global well being:

- Our energies will flow freely, fatigue and fatness will dissipate, total fitness will become the norm, and once and for all, wellness will eternally prevail over sickness.
- Our healthiest genetic codes will be fortified throughout future generations, and life as we know it will become **even better** for our children.
- Our close attention to the TPing details of wellness will pervade the world's collective mindset as we purify our environment, intensify our productivity (instead of destructive tendencies), optimize our nourishment, maximize our personal and collective ecology, and bring back once and for all the natural balance of our entire planet so that we can finally thrive in peace, harmony, happiness, and wellness.

We really have **no other alternative**. Typing and Profiling is that important!

CHAPTER SEVEN

Direct Genetic Testing: The Next Generation of Profiling Has Arrived

A whole new dimension to the Typing/Profiling process has just been added. This exciting profiling procedure is so new that it is not actually available to the public at the time of writing but is becoming available within the next few weeks. This test layers right into the Typing process most significantly by contributing essential information at the level of the gene, with undeniable accuracy. Although direct genetic testing has been described "generically" throughout the text, further explanation is necessary to give you a clear picture of this cutting-edge science.

Most profiling techniques measure your internal biochemical environment (metabolism) to find harmful nutritional and toxic inconsistencies so that we understand how to rebalance the chemical system into a disease-free, optimal functioning state, which matches your genetic ideal. In other words, whatever you've inadvertently done to your body, right or wrong, for your true genetic "desires" is revealed through typing/profiling and precisely corrected, leading to an eventual biochemical steady state which is exactly the place your genes wanted you to be in the first place for maximum wellness. This steady state also represents your exact genetic individuality as expressed through metabolism and constitution. (Refer to Table 3, Categories of Human Uniqueness).

Does your body automatically maintain more tryptophan in the blood, a lower average pH, a higher vitamin C retention, or perhaps more digestive proteases—according to your genetically calibrated uniqueness? All will be completely revealed, in time, as you approach your optimal balance level. This is that special place that your genes want you to be in for your absolute best health.

However, this latest profiling procedure is a **direct genetic test** based upon actual DNA evaluation. This DNA test actually identifies onsite genetic defects that contribute to disease. It reveals what are known as single nucleotide polymorphisms. These SNP's, as scientists call them, are single point mutations in the genetic code which impair certain protein and enzyme production in cells and are associated with many chronic diseases.

So, what's the practical implication of this direct genetic profiling test for the other Typing/Profiling procedures? Simply put, the test picks up existing genetic defects while the other Typing/Profiling picks up environmentally induced biochemical inconsistencies, which, in many cases may have caused the genetic defect in the first place. At the same time these other non-gene direct Typing/Profiling procedures pick up what these genetic defects are doing to your biochemical consistency, with and/or without consideration for environmental influences.

In effect, we're burning the metabolic candle from three ends to the middle. First, we're showing what's already in that special body of yours—all things considered. Second, we're discovering what your genes really want in your unique body. Third, we're determining what's genetically and metabolically repairable and what may not be. The sad news is that some genetic defects and their consequences are not repairable by Typing/Profiling. But, the good news is that most **are** repairable.

For the first time in history, we will be modifying and repairing the phenotypic expression of many SNP's with Typing/Profiling-based personalized nutrition, customized lifestyle, and last but not least, individualized pharmacological intervention. Many people are still going to absolutely require some drug intervention in their lives in spite of where Typing/Profiling comes in—now, the doctor won't have to guess about what will work best.

"The final frontier within the final frontier" is now attainable through this special profiling procedure so that each of us can finally know: the diet we were born to eat, the life we are meant to lead, the relationship to all others that we can have, and how best to relate to our innermost selves and the outermost universe in its entirety.

CHAPTER EIGHT

Dr. Tefft's *American Society for the Advancement of Personalization*

"The environment is considered a candidate for healing alone with the individual person."
— David J. Hufford

"Who would believe that so small a space could contain the image of all the universe."
— Leonardo Da Vinci.

"Unless we put medical freedom into the constitution, the time will come when medicine will organize into an undercover dictatorship."
— Benjamin Rush, M.D.
   (Surgeon General of George Washington's armies)

The **American Society for the Advancement of Personalization** (**ASAP**) has been formed by people who understand that the science and art of metabolic typing and profiling is the only sure means to insure maximum health, fitness, and longevity for each and every one of us. This association will help to accelerate the advancement of personalization throughout society with the expressed purpose of one day making typing/profiling a conventional health promoting instrument for use at home, in the doctor's office, by educational institutions, and wherever else the health and well-being of humans is a concern. **ASAP** is devoted to expediting the extinction of one size fits all health and nutrition practices in favor of the early detection and natural correction of health disturbances on only the most highly individualized basis.

ASAP acts as an information dissemination vehicle, a consumer awareness and protection agency, and serves as a direct link to all products, services, and legislation associated with the typing/profiling process. This association will continue to keep its members on the cutting edge of research and innovations, nutrition and lifestyle politics, Personalized Nutrition (as reviewed in Section V), and all other relevant typing and profiling procedures.

The Metabolic Typer, which is **ASAP** 's official newsletter, keeps members closely attuned to the progress science makes as we master the final frontier of wellness. This newsletter keeps members aware of upcoming events the **ASAP** sponsors organize, including informational seminars, radio and television events, community programs, and other special events that have been planned. Most of all, *The Metabolic Typer*, issue by issue, will bring each reader step by step through the world of metabolic typing until each member is fully "typed and profiled".

I urge you to become a "typer" (and profiler) now by becoming a member of **ASAP** and receiving it's many benefits. Your support of our cause will reward you with the best of health and a complete perspective on life's greatest opportunity for fulfillment.

To become a member simply turn to the Typer's Checklist (Chapter Nine), or you can simply call **1-800-899-5111** to get started.

"As soon as possible we must reverse the nutrient deprivation and toxic accumulation mankind has wrought upon the individual, the environment, and the collective consciousness of the world at large... before it is too late to help ourselves..."

—Dr. Greg Tefft—Founder ASAP

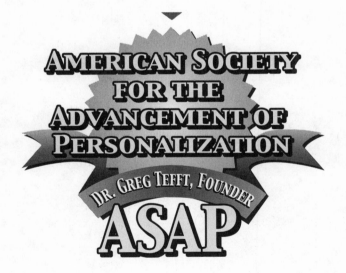

CHAPTER NINE

The "Typer's" Checklist and Action Plan

"No two people are alike - not even twins."
—**Peter Smerick, FBI Investigator**
  (Commenting on the Jon Benet Ramsey case)

"The greatest homage we can pay truth is to use it."
—**Ralph Waldo Emerson**

To help you "type and profile" yourself, we have compiled a checklist for you to follow:

1) Read *For Your Body Only* thoroughly.

2) Calculate your Total Caloric Need Per Day from Step 1 in the Workbook, and use the sample worksheets and food exchanges to create a "rough" dietary plan. (Remember—this is only a theoretical plan which must be adjusted to further TPing specifications.)

3) Quick Check yourself in Step 2 of the Workbook to find your genetic/Metabolic Type and match yourself to the appropriate food patterns and nutrient zones.

4) Work through Step 3 and call **1-800-899-5111** to arrange mail order tests and/or doctor referrals.

5) Become a part of the **ASAP** and use its resources to precisely build your own Typed/Profiled nutritional program.

Typing Checkllist of Completed Objectives

(The expanded Quick Check Program is available through the *ASAP* newsletter/workbook or by calling **1-800-899-5111**.) The short version is in the Workbook.

• **Quantification** of theoretical nutritional plan

• **Qualification** of theoretical nutritional plan

• **Pure Typing** (follow our Quick Check System)

Lab Typing/Profiling

Personalized Nutrition—Workbook following for details

1. Urine, Saliva, Hair Foundational Metabolic Balancing Program.
2. Blood Type, "Blood Spots" and Hidden Allergy Tests
3. Human Metabolic Map derivations

Optional Procedures
(Based on Personalized Nutrition Analysis and Recommendations)

1. Other Digestive, Absorptive, Assimilative, and Elimination Profiles (blood, urine, saliva, hair, feces)
2. Detoxification Panels—(blood, urine)
3. Hormonal Profiles (DHEA, testosterone, estrogen, etc.) Can be performed in first step of Personalized Nutrition if desired.

Steps 1-4 performed over time will ensure your precise metabolic/genetic uniqueness and help to further customize your diet, supplementation, exercise, and personal ecology accordingly.

Education

Use ASAP's educational materials and services (books, newsletters, videos, audios, and seminars) to help you become an expert Typer/Profiler *For Your Body Only*.

Ecological Purification

Use **ASAP's,** *For Your Body Only* guidelines for air, water, hygienic, living and working environment detoxification.

To simplify the process of Typing and Profiling for yourself, please call **1-800-899-5111**.

ASAP and Dragon Door Publications will directly assist you in obtaining Dr. Tefft's, *The Tefft System For My Body Only expanded workbook*, including Quick Check, a **Personalized Nutrition Program** as described in Chapter Five, other nutrition/metabolic tests you can order for home use, special product directories, doctor referrals in your area if you need extra assistance, and a library of materials to help you perfect your personalized nutrition program.

WORKBOOK

Step 1: Compute Calories How to Quantify and Qualify Your Diet

I. You must estimate your BMR first.

Note: The following mathematical computations represent results derived from multiple studies on direct and indirect calorimetry

Males burn 1.0 Calories per kilogram of body weight per hour, which equals

24 Calories per kilogram of body weight per day.

Females burn 0.9 Calories per kilogram of body weight per day, which equals

22 Calories per kilogram of body weight per day.

So take your **weight in pounds** and **divide by 2.2** (pounds per kilogram).

A) Your weight_____ divided by 2.2 = _____Kgs.
   *Example: Robin's weight **122** divided by 2.2 = **55** Kgs.*

B) Your weight_____multiplied by 22 or 24 = _____calories / day.
Example: Robin's weight 55 multiplied by 22 = 1,210 calories /
day = BMR (Multiply your weight in kilograms by 24 for males
and 22 for females.)

Note: Subtract 10% of this figure (BMR) if you are over 40 years of
age. Add 10% of this figure (BMR) if you are under 21 years
of age. Remember: Kcal = Calories

II. Next, you must calculate your Daily Physical Activity Need (DPAN) by choosing one of the following categories:

_____Bedrest   = 0 Kcals or Calories

_____Very Light Activity or Sedentary   = 1/4 BMR (25% of BMR)
(Light work, no formal exercise)   0.25 multiplied by BMR

_____Light Activity =   1/3 BMR (30% of BMR)
(**Light Duty Job** combined with
30 minutes of exercise 3—4
days/week)   0.33 multiplied by BMR

_____Moderate Activity   = 1/2 BMR (50% of BMR)
(**Light Duty Job** combined with
5 to 9 hours of exercise/week
or **Moderate Duty Job** combined
with 2—5 hours of formal
exercise per week)   0.50 multiplied by BMR

_____Light Heavy Activity   = 3/4 BMR (75% of BMR)
(**Light Duty Job** combined with
10 to 15 hours of exercise/week
or **Moderate Duty Job** combined with
5 to 10 hours of exercise/week)   0.75 multiplied by BMR

_____Heavy Activity   = 1 BMR (1 full BMR)
(**Heavy Duty Job** combined with
5 or less hours of exercise/week
-armed forces recruits; or national
and professional athletes 15 or
more hours of exercise/week)   1 multiplied by BMR

Light Duty Job—very light activity, such as a sitting or standing with minimal walking; examples include a desk job or light housework.

Moderate Duty Job—moderate activity, where one is moving or lifting most of the time; examples include a waitress or warehouse type job.

Heavy Duty Job—heavy activity on one's feet most of the time, regularly required to carry heavy objects; examples are found in trades such as construction or masonry.

Note: Except for professional athletes, most of my patients fall into the first four categories of DPAN. Aerobics instructors should fit into DPAN categories on the basis of how many hours they teach per week (usually Moderate to Heavy Activity or 50–100+ of BMR).

Example: Your hypothetical category is Moderate Activity
            which = **1/2 BMR**
1/2 of Robin's BMR = 605 = DPAN
Your BMR (plus) DPAN = _____
*Robin's BMR + DPAN (1,210 + 605) = **1,815 calories***

III. Last, you must add in your Specific Dynamic Activity (SDA).

This measurement represents energy spent on food digestion, absorption, and assimilation including energy spent by **brown adipose tissue or BAT**. To calculate SDA:

Take 6% of your combined BMR and Daily Physical Activity Need (DPAN) measurements:

Your SDA equals:

		Robin's SDA equals:
BMR + DPAN = _____Kcal		$1,210 + 605 =$ **1,815 Kcal**
.06 X _____Kcal = _____Kcal		$.06 \times 1,815 =$ **109 Kcal**
SDA = _____ Kcal		SDA = **109 Kcal**

Then <u>add</u> all numbers together:
  BMR + DPAN + SDA = TCND (Total Caloric Need Per Day)
  For Robin: **1,210 + 605 + 109 = 1,924 Kcal = TCND**

IV. The last figure represents your energy need per day.

The next step is to make a decision about whether you want to lose, gain, or maintain weight. To maintain weight, do not change the Total Caloric Need Per Day figure (TCND). To gain weight healthfully, add 500 Kcal to this figure. To lose weight efficiently, subtract 500 Kcal from this figure to determine your <u>Target Calorie Level (TCL)</u>:

Your TCND + or—500 = _____Kcal = Target Calorie Level
Robin's TCND = <u>1,924 Kcal</u>—500 = 1,424 Kcal = Target Cal. Level

Note: This 500 calorie addition or subtraction per day translates into a 3,500 calories' gain or loss per week, or 500 Kcal multiplied by 7 days = 3,500 Kcal. Since 3,500 Kcal is equivalent to 1 pound of fat, *you will lose approximately 1 pound of fat / week on a weight loss program* (Negative Calorie Balance). On weight gain programming (Positive Calorie Balance), you will gain approximately 1 pound of mostly muscle if you exercise hard enough, although some of this gain may be from fat as well.

To avoid risking any fat gain whatsoever, it is best to stay on a *Neutral Calorie Balance* which is your Total Calorie Need Per Day and let the exercise program "harden up" your body by building muscle as your body naturally reduces its body fat composition concurrently. Those under 18 years old should add 300 calories (if one weighs under 150 pounds) or 500 calories (if one weighs over 150 pounds) into their Total Calorie Need Per Day to allow for normal growth patterns; this assumes that one is exercising regularly.

V. Now that you know your Target Calorie Level (TCL) , we must compute your macronutrient balance based on each macronutrient calorie percentage scientifically recommended for good health.

This remains a *rough* figure until the "typing" process is completed. The National Academy of Science (NAS) recommends the following calorie percentages:

Protein	20%
Carbohydrate	60%
Fat	20%

Now that you know the ideal (NAS) generic calorie percentages, calories can be converted into food weight so that you can precisely measure food intake. The Atwater Coefficients are used to accomplish this:

1 gram protein	= 4 Kcal (or calories)
1 gram carbohydrates	= 4 Kcal
1 gram fat	= 9 Kcal (highest energy yield)
1 gram ethanol	= 7 Kcal

So, in Robin's case: 1,424 multiplied by .20 (20% protein) =
285 Kcals protein

In Your Case (substitute your own figures): (TCL)   _____

1,424 multiplied by .60 (60% carbs) = **854 Kcals carbs**_____

1,424 multiplied by .20 (20% fat)   = **285 Kcals fat**   _____

The above equals the *Target Calorie Level* (TCL) for each macronutrient.

VI. Now convert percentages of food weight (in grams):

285 (Kcals protein) divided by 4 Kcals (per gram
= 72 grams of protein / day   _____

854 (Kcals carbs) divided by 4 Kcal (per gram)
= 214 grams of carbs / day   _____

285 (Kcals fat) divided by 9 Kcals (per gram
= 32 grams of fat needed / day   _____

Robin needs:
   71 grams of protein   _____

   214 grams of carbohydrates   _____

   32 grams of fat   _____

The above macronutrients must be spread out over 3 meals / day.

VII. Now we must obtain the right amount of protein, carbohydrate, and fat from "real foods."

Here is a basic food-grouping chart to help you to understand where to obtain these foods.

Protein Sources

Eggs (especially egg whites)   Turkey (especially white meat)
Milk (and milk products)   Pork (lean)
Cheese (Low fat is best)   Beef (lean)
Non-Fat Yogurt   Soy (Tofu, etc.)
Chicken (especially breast meat)   Legumes
Fish (especially white fish)   Grains
Seeds

Carbohydrate Sources

Calorie-Dense (high calorie starchy vegetables and grains)
Brown Rice   White Rice
Pasta   Cereals
Breads   Peas
Whole Grains   Corn
Yams   Beans
Potatoes   Legumes

Calorie-Dilute (very low calorie vegetables)
Green Leafy Vegetables (greens, lettuces) = Sprouts

Squashes	Peppers
Cucumbers	Mushrooms
Tomatoes	Broccoli
Cabbages	Asparagus
Cauliflower	Beets
Celery	Carrots

Simple Carbohydrates (natural sugar)

Citrus (oranges, lemons, grapefruits)	Peaches
Pineapples	Pears
Melons	Dried Fruits
Bananas	Grapes
Apples	Apricots
Berries	Kiwi Fruit
Raisins	Plums

Fat Sources

Meats	Vinegar
Dairy Products	Avocado
Nuts	Butter
Egg Yolks	Margarine*
Oils (Flaxseed, Olive, Sunflower, etc.)	Mayonnaise

*Keep intake to a minimum due to trans fats.

VIII. Next, we go to the food lists to obtain the precise amount (weight) of each food we wish to include on our diet so that they can be "programmed in" most efficiently.

We will build your "rough" diet as a working model from the following:

Food Exchanges

Milk Exchange:	1 Milk Exchange = 12 grams carbohydrates, 8 grams protein, trace of fat, and 80 calories. 1 cup skim milk 1 cup plain yogurt 1/2 cup canned evaporated skim milk

Vegetable
Exchange:

1 Vegetable Exchange = 6 grams carbohydrates, 1 gram protein, and 25 calories.

1/2 cup of the following:

Asparagus	Eggplant
Beets	Mushrooms
Broccoli	Onions
Cabbage	Pepper
Carrots	String Beans
Cauliflower	Tomato (1 small)

1 cup of the following:	2 cups of the following:
Celery	Lettuce (any kind)

Meat
Exchange:

Meat, Fish, Poultry Exchanges. Based on lean meat.
One lean Meat Exchange = 7 grams protein,
3 to 5 grams fat, and 55 calories:
1 ounce most fish
1 ounce skinned chicken
1 ounce turkey

1 ounce lean beef (most lean cuts)
1 ounce cheese with less than 3% butterfat
1/4 cup 2% butterfat cottage cheese
1/4 cup crab or shrimp

Fat Exchange:

One Fat Exchanges = 5 grams fat and 45 calories.
1 teaspoon butter or margarine
2 tablespoons sour cream
1 teaspoon olive oil (sunflower, safflower, etc.)
10 whole almonds
6 small walnuts
1 teaspoon bacon fat
1 tablespoon cream cheese
1 tablespoon French dressing
1 teaspoon mayonnaise or 2 teaspoons light mayonnaise

Fruit Exchange:

One Fruit Exchange = 10 grams carbohydrates and 40
1 small apple
1/2 cup apple juices
1/2 cup blueberries
1 fresh fig
1 small grapefruit
1/8 medium honeydew
1 pear
2 tablespoons raisins
1 medium orange
3 ounce (1/3 cup) orange, grapefruit or pineapple juice

Bread Exchange:

One Bread Exchange = 15 grams carbohydrates, 1 gram fat, and 70 calories.
1 slice wheat or whole grain bread
1/2 English muffin
1/2 small bagel
6" tortilla
6 saltines

1/2 cup cooked or dry cereal
1/2 cup rice or barley (cooked)
1/2 cup (pasta)
1/2 cup beans
1/2 cup corn
1/2 cup lima beans
1/2 cup mashed potato
1 small baked potato (2 small = 1 large)

Medium Fat Meat Exchange:

One Medium Fat Meat Exchange = 1 lean Meat Exchange plus 1/2 Fat Exchange = 7 grams of protein, 6 grams of fat   =78 calories
1 ounce (15% fat) ground round or rib eye
1 ounce pork, loin, boiled ham, Canadian bacon
1 ounce liver
1 ounce most cheeses
2 tablespoons peanut butter (plus 2 extra Fat Exchanges)
1 large whole egg (no more than 2 per day) until typed

Egg Exchange:

Eggs are an independent exchange.
We recommend no more than 2 whole eggs per day at this time until further "typed" or very athletic. Egg whites are used to "bump up" protein levels slightly usually by adding to the morning meal or snacks (hard-boiled egg whites are best).
1 large whole egg = .5 grams of carbohydrates, 6.6 grams protein, and 82 calories.

1 large egg white = 0 grams of carbohydrates, 3.8 grams protein, 0 fat, and 17 calories

IX. At this point, we must incorporate 71 grams of protein, 214 grams of carbohydrate and 32 grams of fat into 3 meals/day using the food lists. Each meal should consist of foods from each exchange (excluding eggs) which only needs to be in one meal/day.

It is best to evenly spread the macronutrients out over the course of the daily meal plan. So divide by 3:

71 divided by 3 =	24 grams of protein per meal
32 divided by 3 =	11 grams of fat per meal
214 divided by 3 =	71 grams of carbohydrates per meal

Now we must choose the proper foods:

Robin's Diet for Tuesday

Note: The following computations are based on the food exchanges mentioned earlier.

	Grams of Protein	Grams of Carbs	Grams of Fat	Calories or Kcals
Meal #1				
1 large soft boiled egg	7	5	4	82
2 large boiled egg whites	8	0	0	17
8 ounces skim milk	7	12	0	80
1 cup bran flakes	1	30	0	70
1 slice whole grain toast	1	15	1	70
1/3 cup grapefruit	0	10	0	40
2 teaspoons butter	0	0	5	45
TOTALS	25	68	10	404

Meal #2

3 1/2 oz. Tuna in water	24.5	0	2	105
1 squirt lemon juice	-	-	-	-
2 teaspoons "light" mayo	0	0	5	45
2 slices pumpernickel bread	2	30	2	140
1 cup raw celery	0	6	0	25
1 cup raw carrots	0	12	0	50
1 small apple	0	10	0	40
1/2oz. Ice tea	-	-	-	-
TOTALS	**26.5**	**58**	**9**	**405**

Meal #3

3 1/2 ounce skinless chicken breast	24.5	0	2	105
1 large baked potato w/skin	2	30	2	140
2 tablespoons sour cream	0	0	5	45
1 medium salad:				
2 cups lettuce	1	6	0	25
1 large tomato	2	12	0	50
1/2 cup cucumber	1	6	0	25
1/2 cup broccoli	1	6	0	25
1 tsp. safflower oil	0	0	5	45
6 tsp. red wine vinegar*	0	5	trace	20
2/3 cup pineapple juice with 1/2 cup water	0	20	0	80
TOTALS	**31.5**	**85**	**14**	**560**
DAILY TOTALS	**83**	**211**	**33**	**1,369**
ORIGINAL TARGET	**71**	**214**	**32**	**1,424**

Special Note: There is roughly a 10% protein loss (1 gram out of each 10 grams ingested) due to a protein quality factor in foods. As a result, the daily protein total seems a little larger than it actually is. Subtract 8 grams (10% of 83) from this figure for a more realistic factor and add 8 grams to the daily carbohydrate total, which reflects this protein's use as sugar by the body. A few extra grams of protein for extra "exercise insurance" is desirable. Calories don't change.

*Vinegar can be used as shown in the nutrient amounts. It is an excellent "fat mobilization factor" for the body and should be used on salads to aid in body fat reduction unless further typing and profiling procedures negate its usage.

	Grams of Protein	Grams of Carbs	Grams of Fat	Calories or Kcals
Daily Totals	83	211	33	1379
New Totals	75	219	33	1379

SAMPLE DIET WORKSHEET

Meal #1

Exchanges	Grams of Protein	Grams of Carbs	Grams of Fat	Calories
Egg Exchange				
Milk Exchange				
2 Bread Exchanges				
Fruit Exchange				
Fat Exchange				
TOTALS				

Meal #2

Exchanges	Grams of Protein	Grams of Carbs	Grams of Fat	Calories
Meat Exchange				
Fat Exchange				
2 Bread Exchanges				
2 Vegetable Exchanges				
Fruit Exchanges				
TOTALS				

Meal #3

Exchanges	Grams of Protein	Grams of Carbs	Grams of Fat	Calories
Meat Exchange				
Bread Exchange				
2 Fat Exchanges				
5 Vegetable Exchanges				
TOTAL				

Daily Totals				
Original Target				
New Totals (after protein				
Protein loss correction)				

X. So now you have your own "Rough" Diet Map. You have to go through the "typing" procedures of Step 2 ,3, and 4 to further refine this map using correction factors that further "Typing/Profiling" reveals.

If Steps 2, 3, and 4 are not taken, for now, simply alternate foods from the food lists for daily variety using the same format as Robin's Diet. Use this simple rule of thumb for strategizing food exchanges on a generalized level:

1—2 Milk Exchange / day (unless you are known to be allergic or can't digest)

3—6 Bread Exchanges / day

1—3 Fruit Exchanges

4—8 Vegetable Exchanges

1—3 Meat Exchanges (1 egg exchange)

The above expresses minimum amounts of each exchange.

REMEMBER: *Robin's Diet* and your "rough" diet as obtained from this system is a *high carbohydrate, high fiber, moderate protein, low fat, low sodium, diet plan.* According to the most contemporary research (NAS), this generic type of eating is considered best for maximum health, fitness, and longevity for the average person . . . but not necessarily for you. Typing and Profiling will adjust this rough format according to your specific needs. In effect, your final Custom Diet Map may look very much different than this initial "Rough" Diet Map. The sections below are just generic suggestions for all body types just to get you started.

XI. Food Preparation: It is best to prepare foods in such a way as to not add extra fat-calories or salt and to minimize nutrient losses from heat. It is best to eat foods prepared in the following ways:

• Raw	• Stewed
• Steamed	• Microwaved
• Baked	• Sautéed
• Broiled	• Simmered
• Poached	• Pressure-cooked
• Boiled	• Stir-fry

AVOID: **Fried, salted, and highly processed foods** (The more natural the food state, the better!)

SEEK: **Fresh foods!** (and super-nutritious foods)
Do not overcook—heat destroys vitamins, minerals, and enzymes in food. Use freeze-dried, frozen, and canned foods to a very limited extent. These foods have lost nutrients and can have many chemical additives.

I. Liquids
A.   Drink 1/3 of your body weight (in pounds) as ounces of "good" water. (Example: if you weigh 100 pounds, drink 33 oz of water per day.)

B.   Use teas and carbonated water to accompany meals if so desired or add water to your fruit juices to dilute slightly. Use a minimum of water with meals.

AVOID (in general):
- More than 2 cups of coffee per day
- Carbonated soft drinks

- Gravies and sauces due to hidden calories
  and questionable ingredients
- Alcoholic beverages (up to one glass
  of wine per day with meals is okay, *in general*)
- Tap water (use filtered, distilled or pure spring water)

XIII. Recommended Dietary Allowances

Specific vitamin, mineral, and protein amounts proven to keep the body free of deficiency diseases or conditions in general as determined by the Food and Nutrition Board of the U.S. Government. These amounts may have no relationship to your specific needs and are just giving a "rough" foundation for your perusal:

Protein	65 g
Vitamin A	5,000 iu
Vitamin C	60 mg
Vitamin B1	1.5 mg
Vitamin B2	1.7 mg
Vitamin B3	20.0 mg
Vitamin B5 (Pantothenic Acid)	10.0 mg
Vitamin B6	2.0 mg
Folic Acid	0.4 mg
Biotin	0.3 mg
Vitamin B-12	6.0 mcg.(micrograms)
Calcium	1.0 g
Iron	18.0 mg
Vitamin D	400 iu
Vitamin E	30 iu
Phosphorous	1.0 g
Iodine	150 mcg
Magnesium	400 mcg
Zinc	15 mg
Copper	2.0 mg

You have now gone through Step 1: Quantification and Qualification, to create a rough and working theoretical diet pattern. Next, you need to be metabolically "typed," which is the focus of Step 2: Pure Metabolic Typing. After Step 3: Laboratory Assessment (Profiling) is completed, Step 4: Diet and Supplement Customization consists of coming back to Step 1 and modifying it according with the individualized information revealed in Steps 2 and 3. In essence, Step 4 consists of adjusting macro- and micronutrient "inter" and "intra" proportions (or zones) according to the biochemical uniqueness revealed Steps 2 and 3.

An example of this would be in the deletion of beans from your diet because you were found to be allergic in Step 3, decreasing starch amounts in your diet because you are a carni-vegan (Step 2 and 3) and adjusting your supplements because you were shown to have severe subclinical deficiency patterns. The inter proportions or "zones" of macronutrients (protein, carbs, fats) recommended by the National Academy of Sciences (60/20/20) are just a standard foundation from which to construct you own "typed zones." Typed zones can range from 70/20/10 to 40/40/20 with many more combinations according to typing and profiling specifications.

WORKBOOK

Step 2: Quick Check
(Pure Metabolic Typing)

The next step in the typing process is Quick Check, the non-laboratory-mediated step that helps you match your physical, intellectual, personality, ethnic, and religious characteristics as closely as possible to your primary metabolic type. Quick Check helps you to recognize your genotrophic category (or metabolic type) to better clarify how your body and mind works. It reflects how your ancestral environment has shaped you and indicates your ideal environment and lifestyle.

It would be so much simpler if we could just identify you as a Hunza tribesperson, for example, with a pure genotrophic category that has not been historically impacted upon by other people's cultural and genetic influences or man-made environmental changes. Then we could send you to your homeland or at least simulate its living conditions in order to optimize your wellness level. Unfortunately, this is rarely possible in this day and age, so instead we must compile your personal data into a metabolic profile from which we can "match" your nutritional, environmental, and lifestyle needs. The end result is what the Hunza already know—100 plus years of quality (disease-free) life.

There are eight genetic patterns that I encounter regularly. Using the Quick Check typing system you will quickly and easily identify that primary dominant patterns and any secondary patterns that relate to you as well. Your blood type is matched to a basic food profile, while your endocrine gland balance as determined in Quick Check refines this information further and also outlines special supplemental needs and ranges in subsequent chapters.

On a side note, it is true that there are many more types than the eight basic ones presented here, such as exocrine types, sensory types, nerve types, oxidation types, somatotypes, constitutional types, etc. But these are of secondary (or lesser), incremental importance to the controlling, "primary essence" metabolic types presented here. These eight types are in effect based solely upon the most powerful biochemical-physiological-psychological regulators of the body, and not the secondary or tertiary ones. In other words, the metabolic types presented here represent the essence of one's genetic/metabolic design, which sets the pattern from which the other types as mentioned above (really minor subtypes) manifest over time. The "functional distinctions" of these other significant minor subtypes is covered *only* for the most discriminating typer.

For now, do not concern yourself with the smaller details. Rather, fit yourself into your metabolic types as described in the following pages. There is a chart and a table that are included which will minimize any chance for mistakes. The goal of the Quick Check System is to take what would otherwise be a rather complicated procedure and simplify it so that anyone can find his or her type quickly.

In order to properly type yourself, you must first scrutinize your body and mind closely. For some this may seem the hardest part because your awareness of self is put to the test. It's time to face up to what you look like and who you really are.

First you need to find out what your blood type is from your doctor, blood test (obtainable from Dragondoor Publications) or relatives. Your blood type is a must because it helps identify your basic food pattern as a meat eater, vegetarian derivative, or omnivore. Are you blood type O, A, B, or AB? Are you Rh negative or positive?

Next, you must obtain your height in feet and inches in bare feet. For typing purposes tall men are considered to be six feet and over, tall women are considered to be five feet seven inches and over. Average height for men is considered to be five feet seven inches to five feet eleven inches; for women, five feet three inches to five feet seven inches is the norm. Short men are under five feet seven inches, while short women are considered to be under five feet three inches in height.

Your body shape, fatness, hairiness, and muscularity must also be characterized. Are you round, fatty with very soft muscles? Are you long, thin with average looking musculature? Are you naturally muscular with an athletic appearance such as toned muscles and a very sturdy look to you?

Ladies, do you have an hourglass figure with large breast and/or hips, soft muscles and cellulite tendencies when you gain a few pounds? Gentlemen, do you have a barrel type chest with abundant hair and/or extra large shoulders, small hips, and average to better than average muscle tone? Do you have a large prominent forehead or a large round occiput (rear of skull)? Or are you one of those rather rare individuals that is just symmetrical—the human average—not particularly fat, tall, short, overly muscular, round, square, triangular, voluptuous, hairy, and with no features that are seemingly out of proportion?

Two easily identifiable psychological traits also need to be characterized. Are you only happy when you are the leader or when in front of an audience? Are you extremely charismatic? Are you highly sensitive and intuitive to the point of being a psychic or clairvoyant? Think about it.

One word of warning: do not make the typing process more complicated than it really is by over rationalizing your descriptors. Simplicity is the key. Pick your blood type first then obtain your height, then visualize your shape and next consider your personality in terms of being a leader or highly sensitive/intuitive. The rest will fall into place as typing proceeds forward.

Super Quick Check

About 40% of the civilized world is blood type O. This is the oldest of the blood types. If you are a blood type O there is only one of four primary metabolic types that you can be. The metabolic types are named after the strongest functioning gland in the body (except for the balanced type where all is equal).

For "O" blood these types are:

1. Gonadal Type or T4 (type 4)—Gonads are the sexual glands.
2. Pancreatic Type or T5 (type 5)—Pancreas controls blood sugar/digestion.
3. Thymic Type or T 6 (type 6)—Thymus effects growth/immune system development.
4. Pituitary Type or T 7 (type 7)—Pituitary is the master gland over all others.

Dead Giveaways—To quickly discover which metabolic type you are based on blood type O match yourself up with the four physical and/or psychological descriptions listed for each of the types T4, T5, T6, and T7 below:

Gonadal   *Women:*   Curvaceous
(sexy)   Hourglass type figure (large breasts/hips)
                            Cellulite tendencies
                            Up to 5'7" tall (rarely over 5'7")
                            Slight weight gain tendency

         Men: Male pattern baldness
                            Barrel chest/pot-bellied over time
                            Hairy body especially chest
                            Up to 5'11" (rarely over 5'11")

Pancreatic *Women:*   Always overweight or obese since childhood
(overweight)   Chubby features/very round body and face
                          Can be big eaters
                          Any height

        Men: Always overweight or obese since childhood
                          Chubby features/round body and face
                          Can be big eaters
                          Any height

Thymic *Women:*   Taller than average usually 5'7" or more
(tall)   Long limbs
                          Long face shape
                          Knobby joints and/or large rib cage

        Men: Taller than average usually 6' or more
                          Long limbs
                          Long face shape
                          Knobby joints and/or large rib cage

Pituitary *Women:*   Large prominent forehead in width, depth, height
(leader)   Slightly receding frontal hairline
                          Has to be the leader
                          Extremely charismatic

        Men: Large prominent forehead in width, depth, height
                          Slightly receding frontal hairline
                          Has to be the leader
                          Extremely charismatic

The second oldest of the blood types is blood type A. If you are a blood type A there are only one of four metabolic types you can be. These types are:

For "A" blood these types are:

1. Thyroid Type or T1—Thyroid controls metabolic and oxidation rate.
2. Pineal Type or Subtype T1A—Pineal sets wake/sleep hormone cycles.
3. Thymic Type or T6—Thymus effects growth/immune system development.
4. Balanced Type or T3 (this only applies to men)—No dominant gland.

Dead Giveaways—To quickly discover which metabolic type you are based on blood type A match yourself up with the four physical and/or psychological descriptions listed for each of the types T1, TA, T1A, T6, and T3.

Thyroid   *Women:*   Always on the thin side
(thin & quick)   Up to 5'7" in height
                            Small bones/delicate features
                            Move quickly and/or restless

               Men: Always on the thin side
                            Up to 5'11" in height
                            Small bones/delicate features
                            Move quickly and/or restless

Pineal   *Women:*   Large occiput (rear skull area)
(intuitive)   Usually thin/sometimes frail
                            Extremely aware/sensitive/intuitive
                            Any height

               Men: Large occiput (rear skull area)
                            Usually thin/sometimes frail
                            Extremely aware/sensitive/intuitive

Thymic (tall)	*Women:*	Taller than average usually 5'7" or more Long limbs Long face shape Knobby joints and/or large rib cage
	Men:	Taller than average usually 6' or more Long Limbs Long face shape Knobby joints and/or large rib cage
Balanced (average)	*Men:*	No overpowering physical characteristics Medium body shape and features 5'6" to 5'11" The statistical human average (1% to 3% of world population)

Blood type B is the next oldest blood pattern that occurred from a genetic mutation allowing for better milk digestion. These types are:

For "B" blood these types are:

1. Adrenal Type or T2—Adrenals control amount of oxidation and metabolism.
2. Thymic or T6—Thymus effects growth/immune system development.
3. Balanced or T3—(primarily women) No dominant gland.

Dead Giveaways—To quickly discover what metabolic type you are based on blood type B match yourself up with the four physical features listed under each of the types T2, T6, and T3.

Adrenals (muscular)	*Women:*	Prominent muscles/stable weight Good muscle tone Strong, dense bones Any height but usually 5' to 5'8"

	Men:	Prominent muscles/stable weight
		Very good muscle tone
		Strong, dense bones
		Any height but usually 5'2" to 6'
Thymic (tall)	*Women*:	Taller than average usually 5'7" or more
		Long limbs with above average muscle tone
		Long face shape
		Knobby joints and/or large rib cage
	Men:	Taller than average usually 6' or more
		Long limbs with above average muscle tone
		Long face shape
		Knobby joints and/or large rib cage
Balanced (average)	*Women*:	No overpowering physical characteristics
		Medium body shape and features
		5'3 to 5'7"
		The statistical human average
		(1% to 3% of world population)

Blood type AB is the newest and rarest of the blood types, which mutated approximately 1,000 years ago from blood type B and blood type A interbreeding (this according to geneticists). If you are a blood type AB there you can be only one of two primary metabolic types.

For "AB" blood these types are:

1. Balanced Type or T3—(men and women)—No dominant gland.
2. Thymic Type or T6—Thymus effects growth/immune system development.

Dead Giveaways—To quickly discover what metabolic type you are based on blood type AB match up with the four physical descriptions listed for T3 and T6.

Balanced *Women*: No overpowering physical characteristics
(average)   Medium body shape and features
                         5'3 to 5'7"
                         The statistical human average
                         (1% to 3% of world population)

          Men: No overpowering physical characteristics
                         Medium body shape and features
                         5'6" to 5'11"
                         The statistical human average
                         (1% to 3% of world population)

Thymic *Women*: Taller than average usually 5'7" or more
(tall)   Long limbs with above average muscle tone
                        Long face shape
                        Knobby joints and/or large rib cage

          Men: Taller than average usually 6' or more
                        Long limbs with above average muscle tone
                        Long face shape
                        Knobby joints and/or large rib cage

NO DOUBT ABOUT IT FLOW CHART

Blood Type O

T4	T5	T6	T7
Gonadal Type	Pancreatic Type	hymic Type	Pituitary Type
F: Curvy, to 5'7"	M&F: Round and	F: Long, over 5'7"	M&F: Huge forehead
M: Balding, to 5'11"	Overweight	M: Long, over 5'11"	Leader mentality

Blood Type A

T1	T1A	T6	T3
Thyroid Type	Pineal Type	Thymic Type	Balanced Type
F: Small features,	M&F: Lrg occiput,	F: Long, over 5'7"	M: 5'7" -5'11"
Under 5'7"	Frail, intuitive	M: Long, over 5'11"	Human average
M: Small features.			Medium features
Under 5'11"			

Blood Type B

T3	T6	T2	
Adrenal Type	Thymic Type	Balanced Type	
M&F: Muscle tone,	M&F: Muscle tone	M&F: Med. features	
Athletic appearance	Long limbs	Human average	
F: 5'0"–5'8"	F: 5'7" plus	F: 5'3"–5'7"	
M: 5'2"–6'	M: 5'11" plus		

Blood Type AB

T3	T6		
Thymic Type	Balanced Type		
M&F: Long limbs	M&F: Med. features		
F: Over 5'7"	Human average		
M: Over 5'11"	F: 5'3"–5'7"		
	M: 5'7"–5'11"		

If you find yourself confused at this point, don't fret: you will make your personal metabolic connection by the end of this chapter.

Typing At a Glance

Typing At a Glance will help the reader to better visualize the redeeming physical feature for each metabolic type. Rough illustrations are used because detailed photographs of the different types tend to be confusing.

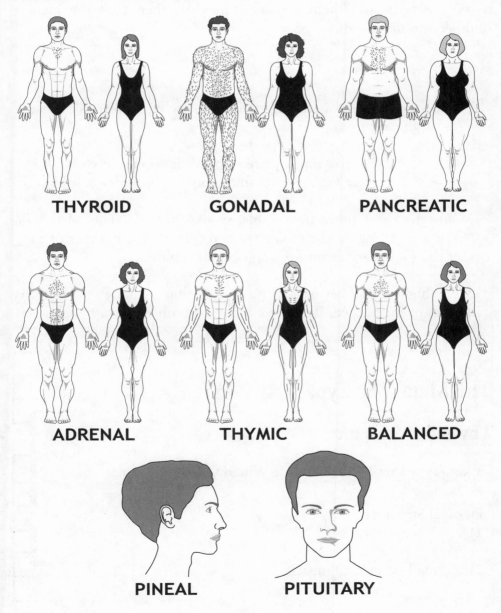

THYROID   **GONADAL**   **PANCREATIC**

ADRENAL   **THYMIC**   **BALANCED**

PINEAL   **PITUITARY**

Super Duper Quick Check

The Super Duper Quick Check is for only the most discriminating typers or that small percentage of readers who need a little more reassurance about which type they are. It's based on counting the asterisks attached to the following descriptions that most closely apply to you. Simply add them up for each type, then pick the highest number and that is your type.

Rules

1. When you find a matching description with an asterisk place a "+" sign next to it.

Example: Under Thymic Type descriptors:
    +   * Creative Intelligence (+means it applies to you)
               • Over 6' tall (it doesn't apply to you so leave it blank)

1. Turn to the Completion Table at the end of "The Metabolic Types" starting on the next page and transfer the number of each of the +'s you made into the appropriate column.

2. The highest number of +'s in a given column relative to others is *your* primary type. The next highest number is *your* secondary type.

The Metabolic Types

Thyroid Dominant

a.k.a. Type I or T1 "The Quick-Witted Gazelle"

Physical Structure
1)   Thin appearance*

2)   Small bones and muscles*

3) Delicate features*

4) Engages in quick movement*

5) Can have good muscle tone but small muscles, hard white teeth and nails, and finely molded features and hands

6) Generally has low body fat but it can slowly increase with age

7) Small to medium height with lower body weight

8) Generally profuse amounts of hair

Intelligence
1) Good technical abilities*

2) Works quickly and handles detail well

3) Workaholic tendencies

4) Can be obsessive when searching for information

5) Very intelligent and can be extremely creative

Personality
1) High-strung*

2) Generally nervous, sometimes irritable

3) Highly meticulous at work and at home

4) Generally well organized

5) Can suffer from insomnia

6) Usually dreams in vivid detail and easily remembers dreams, starting in childhood but usually fading as one matures

7) Can become frustrated and dissatisfied easily

Energy

1) Fast oxidation rate (keeps the body thin)

2) Lack of sustained endurance unless created by regular aerobic exercise at high intensity levels

Blood Type
1) Usually A, sometimes O, but very rarely B or AB*

Exercise
1) Does well with dancing, swimming, yoga, jogging, and relaxing exercise such as Tai Chi or Feldenkrais or hiking/walking and aquatic therapy

2) Does poorly with activities based on strength, large size, and power, although can do well at gymnastics

Ethnicity
1) European and Asian (especially) dominance, although very common among black, red, and brown races from higher altitudes and coastal areas. Many Christians, Buddhists, and followers of Native religions, such as Aborigines, American Indians, Eskimos, etc.

Miscellaneous
1) May be prone to acne and rashes (especially in youth)

2) Tends to have low stomach acid and commonly low chromium, zinc, copper, iron, vanadium, and B-vitamin deficiencies along with hypoglycemic tendencies

3) Generally high pulse rate (73–86 bpm at rest). Can awaken in morning with approximately 80 bpm regularly. Low blood pressure (approximately 85/50–105/65)

4) Tends to have a sensitive digestive system

5)   Can have a V-shaped jaw (not as apparent in Asian races)

6)   Females: pregnancies are usually shorter term than for other types.

7)   Women tend to be slightly more thyroid than men.

8)   Female: usually possesses fine, silky, straight hair and very thin delicate skin.

Animal Kingdom Examples
1)   Thoroughbred racehorse

2)   Greyhound dog

3)   Gazelle

4)   Cheetah

Celebrity Examples:	Female	Male
	Twiggy	Bruce Lee
	Meg Ryan	Don Knotts
	Gilda Radner	George Takei (Star Trek)

Pineal Dominant

a.k.a. Subtype 1A or T1A "The Ultra-Sensitive Knower"

Note: The Pineal type is categorized as a subtype of the Thyroid type because of many similarities to Thyroid types. There are, however, classic distinctions that need to be made for maximum accuracy. There are rarely exceptions to the rule, where blood type AB or O is present.

Pineal types can be thought of as a more psychic or intuitive form of Thyroid types, with less interest in exercise unless it is very peaceful or in a natural setting.

Physical Structure
1) Small to medium size*
2) Large occipital region (rear of skull), characterized by dome-shaped head (like a bird's head minus the beak) *
3) Generally thin, sometimes frail looking*

4) Other physical features similar to Thyroid types

5) Delayed puberty

Intelligence
1) Highly intuitive (may be "psychic" or clairvoyant) *

Personality
1) Very sensitive and aware*
2) Generally high-strung and nervous*

3) Usually very intuitive dreamer, dreaming of future events that often come true or receiving the thoughts of others in the dreams

Energy
1) A medium to very fast range of oxidation, although generally a lower amount of overall oxidation (Keeps body relatively thin and the bones and muscles small)

2) Does not do well with strenuous exertion

3) Very prone to nervous exhaustion

Blood Type
1) Usually A

Exercise
1) Does well with yoga and Tai Chi or light intensity activities

Ethnicity
1) Equal showing in all races and religions although many Asians and Indian/Buddhist people fit into this category, as do a fair number of holy men and women and healers

Miscellaneous
1) Low pulse rate (usually about 65-85 bpm) with blood pressure at low to medium levels (85/60-115/75)

2) Generally weak digestive systems

3) Can have very large piercing or sad eyes

4) Not a primary type—more a subtype of Thyroid or a secondary pattern for other metabolic types

5) Extra sensitive delicate skin

Animal Kingdom Examples
1) Bird

2) Tree lizard with a third eye (like a chameleon)

Celebrity Examples:

Female	Male
Usually method actresses that play psychics, witches, and fortune tellers	The Dalai Lama
	Asian method actors or actors playing old "wise men"
Mia Farrow	Joel Grey
Kristin Scott Thomas	

Adrenal Dominant

a.k.a. Type II or T2
"The Invincible Jock"

Physical Structure
1) Prominent muscularity*
2) Thick or dense, hard bones*
3) Good muscle tone *
4) Jaw and teeth are large and round or squarish*
5) Larger features*
6) Dry, thick, warm skin*
7) Shorter and thicker neck and fingers*
8) Hair tends to be coarse and curly*

Intelligence
1) Very practical*

2) Usually not very abstract, prefers concrete knowledge

3) Prefers careers in professional sports, the military, the police, business, or skilled trades

4) High degree of coordination (high motor IQ)

Personality
1) Physically oriented and athletic*

2) Fairly easy-going although slightly insensitive

3) Female: Tend to be more reserved, less verbal and more physical
   Male: The strong, silent, physical type

4) Competitive, aggressive, slow to anger, although can become violent when aroused

5) Experiences little fear and anxiety; feels invincible

6) Generally loves to exercise vigorously

Energy
 1) Medium oxidation rate with a larger amount of oxidation overall (allowing the muscles to be larger)

2) Great strength and lasting endurance

Blood Type
1) Usually B for the more "pure" Adrenal Dominant types, though sometimes O*

Exercise
1) Enjoys vigorous exercise; well-suited to weight-training and high intensity sports like wrestling, martial arts, and lacrosse

Ethnicity
1) African and European dominance, although still somewhat common among brown and red races, least common among Asians

2) Usually lower altitude people

3) Many Christians, Muslims, and Jews

Miscellaneous
1) Head and face shape usually square with a round jaw and an overall body shape that appears compact (not linear or round)

2) Medium pulse rate (62–74) with an average to high blood pressure (120/75–140/85)

3) Rarely ill

4) Tends to develop heart and circulatory problems from running themselves down due to feeling of invincibility

5)   Good protein digestion but sensitive to concentrated sugar

6)   Needs large amount of free radical fighters in the system, such as the antioxidants C, A, and E

Animal Kingdom Examples
1)   Tiger
2)   Bulldog
3)   Draft horse

Celebrity Examples:

Female	Male
Martina Navratilova	William Shatner
Jessica Lange	Wesley Snipes
Angela Bassett	Rob Lowe
Cory Everson (Ms.	Peter Strauss (actor)
Olympia, top female	Michael Paré
pro bodybuilder)	Lawrence Fishburne
Jackie Joyner Kersee	Mike Tyson

Male-Female Comparative

1)   Men tend to be more adrenal than women
       I. There are more men than women in this type

Balanced

a.k.a. Type III or T3

"The Average One"

This type represents the human average of all metabolic typing characteristics—not too fat, not too muscular, not too small, not too hairy, not too round, square, etc. This type represents approximately 1–3 percent of the human race, but is more common as a secondary pattern with a slight adrenal predominant tendency for men and a slight thyroid predominant tendency for women.

Physical Structure
1) Medium features*
2) Medium body shape*
3) No overpowering characteristics (balanced blend of all metabolic types) based on endocrine glands*
4) Very symmetrical (medium bones, muscle, face—no overpowering characteristics)
5) Stable weight, medium frame, average to moderately tall

Intelligence
1) Flexible intelligence and can adapt to a variety of situations*

2) Knowledgeable on a large variety of topics

3) Tends not to specialize—more of a "know-it-all" mentality (example: a Balanced type is more likely to be a general medical practitioner than a neurosurgeon)

Personality
1) Affable and adaptable*

2) Moderate disposition

3) Able to easily shift between entire range of emotion without losing balance or poise

4) May be without direction or clear purpose

Energy
1) Low-medium to high-medium body oxidation rate and amount (keeps body "average" looking)

2) Medium endurance and strength capacities

Blood Type
1) Female: Usually AB, but may be B
   Male: Usually AB, but may be A

Exercise
1) Does well with all types of exercise but doesn't generally excel in any one area

Ethnicity
1) Rare as a primary type in all ethnicities and religions, though has a slightly greater occurrence in white and yellow races

Miscellaneous
1) Medium heart rate (63–73), muscles, bones, height, weight, blood pressure (110/70–120/80)

2) Very symmetrical face and body

3) Can change weight pattern for special needs

Animal Kingdom Examples
A. Not applicable because this is more of a secondary pattern or the most symmetrical of the most symmetrical animals

Celebrity Examples:	Female	Male
	Jane Fonda	Robert Redford
	Mariah Carey	Warren Beatty

Male-Female Comparative
1) Males tend to have a slight adrenal or pituitary constitutional emphasis allowing for a slightly squared facial appearance, as with Robert Redford, or more prominent forehead, as seen in Warren Beatty

2) Females tend to have a slight thyroid or pineal constitutional emphasis allowing for a more V-shaped jaw, as with Jane Fonda, or rounded head, as we find with Mariah Carey

Gonadal Dominant

a.k.a. Type IV or T4
"The Sensually Potent One"

Physical Structure
1) Female: Hourglass shape (very curvaceous) *
   Male: Usually "barrel" chested
2) Female: Usually has naturally large breasts *
   Male: Tends to have male pattern baldness; European, African, and middle Eastern men tend to have heavy beards and profuse body hair
3) Female: Large hips, small waist*
   Male: Generally larger shoulders and smaller hips and legs, although can develop "beer bellies" with age, gaining weight in abdominal area first
4) Female: Very soft skin *
5) Female: Early puberty*

6) Female: Tends to be less than average height

7) Female: General tendency to gain weight

8) Female: Prone to "cellulite appearance" of rear, thighs, and buttocks with progressive weight gain

9) Female: Can have a very "feminine" voice

10) Male: Usually less than average height

11) Male: Can have a very deep voice

Intelligence
1) High social intelligence*

2) Female: Very good mothering ability
   Male: Make good fathers

3) Tends to hold strong views on sexual issues, such as birth control, abortion, pornography, prostitution, etc.—can be either pro or con

Personality
1) Sexually oriented*

2) Sensual

3) Flirtatious

4) Sexually expressive or repressive

5) Can be very moody

Energy
1) Low oxidation rate (allows the body to gain body fat easily) with medium overall oxidation amount (allows for relatively good muscle size although soft)

Blood Type
1) Usually O*

Exercise
1) Does well with group- or team-oriented exercise as opposed to individual activities and sports, unless involves a high degree of human interaction

Ethnicity
1) African, Mediterranean, and Russian dominance, although a strong showing among all races and religions

Miscellaneous
1) Female: May have tendency for low-level rashy appearance of skin at times, mostly in buttock area

2) Generally has exaggerated secondary sexual characteristics: female--very soft skin, small waist with large hips and/or

breasts; male–large shoulders, small hips, and male pattern baldness with masculine voice and some "macho" behavior

3) Nervous system tends to be parasympathetic dominant with a low pulse rate (in the 50s) and blood pressure that is medium normal (110/70 to 125/80)

4) Not always the best digestive patterns

5) Exceedingly high fertility level

6) Need frequent sexual activity

Animal Kingdom Examples

1) Monkey

2) Ape

Celebrity Examples:	Female	Male
	Dolly Parton	Billy Carter
	Sophia Loren	Alec Baldwin
	Monica Lewinsky	Yassir Arafat
	Susan Sarandon	
	Mae West	

Pancreatic Dominant

a.k.a. Type V or T5
"The Chubby Lovable Eater"

Physical Structure
1) Chronically overweight*
2) Very round or "rotund" body and face shape*
3) Thick solid fat layer on body*
4) Double chins and other "chubby" type features*

5)   Muscles appear fatty, soft, and large

6)   Usually medium frame with variable height

Intelligence

1)   Survival intelligence (from effects of famine on genealogy) *

2)   Can be very good at business and food-oriented industries

Personality

1)   Jolly and generally easygoing*

2)   Food-oriented ("live to eat" more than "eat to live")

3)   Can have periods of depression and irritability to extremes

4)   Likes food-centered family structure

Energy

1)   Mid-range to low oxidation rate (allows for dense body fat accumulation)

2)   Highly efficient carbohydrate metabolism (can crave sweets)

3)   Inefficient fat metabolism, which damages cardiovascular system

Blood Type

1)   Usually O but occasionally A

Exercise

1)   Has a special need for extensive aerobic activity combined with a limited carbohydrate intake for best health, fitness, and weight control results

Ethnicity
1) Strong showing among all races and religions, especially Russian, Americanized Europeans, Hispanics, and African groups

Miscellaneous

1) Tendency to have high blood sugar and resultant diabetes

2) Medium pulse rate (60-72 bps); blood pressure 110/70- 115/80

3) Very susceptible to morbid obesity

4) From a genealogical standpoint, supernormal ability to survive famines with a long-term familial trait of overweight tendencies

Animal Kingdom Examples
1) Brown bear

2) Panda

Celebrity Examples:

	Female	Male
	Kathy Bates	Jackie Gleason
	Ella Fitzgerald	John Belushi
	Oprah Winfrey	John Candy
	Roseanne Barr	James Earl Ray
		Rosie Grier

Thymus Dominant

a.k.a. Type VI or T6
"The Tall Creative One"

Physical Structure
1) Tall and "lanky" *
2) Long limbs (arms and legs) *
3) Large rib cage*
4) Knobby joints*

5)   Taller than average: Female--usually 5'7" or more;
        Male–usually 6' or more

6)   Usually wide hips and shoulders

7)   Slightly longer face shape

Intelligence
1)   Creative, artistic*

Personality
1)   Emotionally sensitive*
2)   Generally concerned with love (either very loving and
        extroverted or depressed and withdrawn)

Energy
1)   Mid-range to low-medium rate and amount of oxidation,
        combined with taller size, cause muscle and fat concentrations
        to be low to medium

2)   Susceptible to digestive inefficiency and hyperallergic
        sensitivities, which both resist strong energy production

Blood Type
1)   O, A, or AB, sometimes B

2)   If Rh negative, greater tendency to be hyperallergic to airborne
        and dietary substances

Exercise
1)   Special need for outdoor exercise (pure air) and more negative
        ions

2)   Well suited to high endurance activities like running and
        swimming long distances

Ethnicity

1) Relatively medium incidence in all races with higher concentrations in African and Northern European races and religions (think of tall Swedes and professional basketball players)

Miscellaneous

1) Generally low pulse rate (approximately 50-65, though sometimes as high as 72)

2) Low to medium blood pressure (approximately 100/60-120/80)

3) Can suffer from lymphatic disorders and other immune system imbalances in relation to allergies, although can have a "supernormal" ability to suppress infectious processes especially when there are more Adrenal type characteristics present (Adrenal type characteristics include more squareness in the face, body, and forehead, more muscle on body, curlier hair, coarser hair, etc.); characteristic allergies include mold, pollen, milk, eggs, wheat, corn, shellfish, kelp, acidic plants, nuts, and seeds

Animal Kingdom Examples
1) Giraffe

Celebrity Examples:	Female	Male
	Many supermodels	Wilt Chamberlain
	Carol Burnett	Alan Alda
	Most female pro basketball and volleyball players	Leonard Nimoy

Pituitary Dominant

a.k.a. Type VII or T7
"The Leader" "The Charismatic One"

Physical Structure

1) This is a mind- or personality based type; basic body structure is dependent on the secondary dominance pattern (for example, Golda Meir was a pituitary dominant, gonadal secondary because of her prominent forehead and curvy, overweight stature; another example is Clint Eastwood, who is pituitary dominant, thymic secondary because of his prominent forehead and very tall, long stature) *

2) Large, very prominent forehead in terms of width, depth, and/or height*

Intelligence

1) Leader (loves to be a leader and very effectively leads people)

Personality
1) Extremely charismatic*

2) An energy and thought transmitter

3) Obsessive tendencies

4) Can be depressed without an audience (make good politicians, salespeople, and actors)

5) Strong addictive tendencies to stimulants

6) Highly resistant to personal change

7) Takes control in dreams and creates the world one wants

Energy

1) Generally medium total oxidation allowing for progressive overweight tendencies

2) Maximum energy output requires regular full spectrum sunlight to normalize the neuroendocrine system in relief of depressive tendencies

Blood Type

1) Usually O

Exercise

1) Team or supervised independent activities work well

2) Jogging or hiking outdoors are key exercises

3) Martial arts and Eastern fitness philosophies, such as Tai Chi and meditation, are very helpful for this type

Ethnicity

1) Strong incidence in all races and religions, especially Jews

Miscellaneous

1) Generally smooth skin

2) Low pulse rate (in the 50s) with mid-range blood pressure (110/70-125/80)

3) Female: Slightly recessed hairline during the aging process, adding to the forehead's prominence
Male: May suffer mild balding in time, usually starting at the top and sides of the forehead, adding to its outright prominence

4) Usually soft and medium-sized muscles

5) Can be very allergic to milk and egg whites and tends to have a weaker liver in relation to strong spices and stimulants

Animal Kingdom Examples
1)   Whale

2)   Dolphin

Celebrity Examples

Female

     Golda Meir (Pituitary-Gonadal)
     Margaret Thatcher (Pituitary-Gonadal)
     Jessica Lange (Pituitary-Adrenal)
     Whoopi Goldberg (Pituitary-Pancreatic)
     Meryl Streep (Pituitary-Gonadal)
     Birgitte Nilsen (Pituitary-Thymic)

Male

     Elvis Presley (Pituitary-Adrenal)**
     Bob Hope (Pituitary-Balanced)
     Ted Kennedy (Pituitary-Gonadal)
     Albert Einstein (Pituitary-Thyroid)
     Dolph Lundgren (Pituitary-Thymic)
     Marlon Brando (Pituitary-Pancreatic)
     Rodney Dangerfield (Pituitary-Pancreatic)
     Arnold Schwarzenegger (Pituitary-Adrenal)
     Ed Harris (Pituitary-Balanced) **
     Christopher Reeves (Pituitary-Thymic)
     John Belushi (Pituitary-Pancreatic)
     Charlton Heston (Pituitary-Thymic)

**In the balanced torso pattern, men tend to have an adrenal-type predominance, which keeps the body thinner with slightly more muscle when activity levels are balanced with reasonable food intake. (Elvis Presley could have been lean and "softly muscular" all of his life, if not for the drug overloads, poor eating habits, and reduced activity levels he allowed as he aged.)

COMPLETION COLUMNS—Place the number of +'s you made next to the asterisked (*) descriptors in the following applicable columns. Take the highest number as your primary type, next highest umber as your secondary type:

THYROID	PINEAL	ADRENAL	BALANCED
GONADAL	PANCREATIC	PITUITARY	THYMIC

Extra Guidelines for Accurate Metabolic Typing (For Only The Most Discriminating Typer)

The eight types possess distinctions beyond the general match-up that you can make using Quick Check. If you have some characteristics dispersed throughout the basic types, use them to create a hierarchy of dominance. For example, a male has a barrel-type chest, male pattern baldness, high social intelligence, and blood type O, which are all giveaways for the Gonadal Type. Yet he has an extremely muscular body, very square jaw, strong commitment to athletics, blood pressure of 120/80, and resting pulse rate of 70 bpm. In this case, we have a gonadal primary, adrenal secondary metabolic type.

To help you to clarify your dominant pattern, secondary patterns, and even recessive glands, use following table to pinpoint your metabolic type, pattern, "blend" or genotrophic profile (as Dr. Roger Williams would say) using numerical quantities.

COMPILATION CHART

Physical Data	TI - Thyroid Dominant	TIA - Pineal Dominant	TII - Adrenal Dominant	TIII - Balanced Subclass
Blood Type	A	A	B	AB or A: Male, B: Female
Height	Small to Medium	Any	Short Medium to Tall Medium	Medium
Weight Range	Chronically Low	Low to Frail	Medium Stable	Medium Stable
Resting Pulse	73-86 bpm	65-85 bpm	64-72 bpm	63-73 bpm
Blood Pressure	85/50-105/65	85/60-115/75	120/75-140/85	110/70-120/80
Hair	Usually Profuse	Silky and Straight (Female)	Coarse, Wavy	N/A
Skin	Eruptive	Sensetive	Dry, Thick Warm	N/A
Muscles	Small	N/A	Prominent, Toned	Medium
Bones	Small	N/A	Thick or Dense, Hard	Medium
Body Shape	Thin, Delicate Features	N/A	Compact, Strong Looking	Medium
Head/Face Shape	Delicate Small	N/A	Square (Especially the Jaw)	Very Symetrical
Childhood Dream States	Vivid Dreams	Intuitive Dreams	N/A	N/A
Personality	High-strung, Nervous	Sensitive Aware	Physical	Affable/ Adabtable
Intelligence	Good Technical Ability	Highly Aware	Physical	Flexible
Miscellaneous	Quick Movements	Psychic Intuition	Larger Features	No Overpowering Characteristics
TOTALS				

COMPILATION CHART

Physical Data	TIV - Gonadal Dominant	TV - Pancreatic Dominant	TVI - Thymus Dominant	TVII - Pituitary Subclass
Blood Type	O	O	A, B, O, or AB	O
Height	Short-Medium	Any	Tall: Males 6' +, Females 5'7" +	Any
Weight Range	High or Low	Chronically High	Stable Medium	High or Low
Resting Pulse	40-60 bpm	60-72 bpm	50-72 bpm	40-60 bpm
Blood Pressure	110/70-125/80	110/70-115/80	100/60-120/80	110/70-125/80
Hair	Males: Male Pattern Baldness	N/A	N/A	Balding Over Time, from Front to Back
Skin	Females: Very Soft, Rash Tendency	Fatty, Thick	N/A	Smooth
Muscles	Soft, Medium-sized	Fatty, Soft, Large	Long, Lanky	Soft, Medium
Bones	Medium	Medium	Long	Medium
Body Shape	Females: Curvy Males: Large Upper Torso, Barrel Chest	Round Chubby	Long	Depends on Secondary Type
Head/Face Shape	Females: Curvy Males: Bald Angular	Round Chubby	Long	Large, Prominent Forehead
Childhood Dream States	N/A	N/A	N/A	Transmitting Dreams
Personality	Sensual/Sexual	Jolly	Emotionally Sensetive	Charismatic
Intelligence	Social	Survival	Creative	Leadership
Miscellaneous	Females: Large Hips and/or Breasts Males: Large Shoulders	Round Features	Large Rib Cage	Loves an Audience
TOTALS				

Compute from Compilation Chart:

Primary Metabolic Type Dominance =

Secondary Dominance =

Tertiary Dominance =

Recessive Glands =

In the preceding chart, check off each characteristic that applies to you. Then total up the columns. The one with the highest number of characteristics is your primary, with second highest is secondary, and the third is tertiary; everything beyond this is considered recessive.

NOTE on Dreams:

> **Vivid Dreams**—dreams occurring in a minute detail and easily remembered starting in childhood—can fade as one matures

> **Intuitive Dreams**—constant dreams of future events that often actually come true; can also be the reception of others' thoughts

> **Transmittive Dreams**—dreams where an individual takes control and creates a world he/she wants

Mixed Types

Before we discuss the nutritional ramifications of your non-laboratory mediated metabolic type, we must address a phenomenon that can make typing very difficult: mixed types. A mixed type is a relative rarity but exists when the endocrine dominant pattern doesn't match the appropriate blood type, given that no typing errors were made. These "typing conflicts" result from the suppression of the dominant endocrine pattern in childhood due to physical and/or emotional influences during the formative stages of life. The most common physical factors include traumatic insults such as injuries, invasive or cosmetic surgeries, side effects from heavy medications or strong-acting recreational drugs, too much radiation, infectious disease, and malnutrition before, during, and after the mother's pregnancy. Common emotional factors include overcompensated reactions to misunderstood or traumatic psychological situations. The majority of emotional factors that cause typing conflicts begin in the home, so it is important to recall how your parents treated you and whether you suffered an abusive or over-controlled upbringing. In addition, you can use other information about you and your family to assist in identifying the dominant endocrine pattern, which was suppressed.

If you are having a hard time categorizing yourself or your blood type does not match the type that other characteristics indicate you are, examine these characteristics to see if they help reconcile the discrepancies.

You may be Adrenal Dominant even though your blood type doesn't match if:

- Your family is generally muscular or toned

- You had severe or chronic bacterial diseases in childhood (like chronic strep throat)

- One or both of your parents were exceedingly frightening to you

- You have an innate fear of strength

- You suffered a debilitating spine injury

- You were extremely inactive due to circumstances beyond your control

You may be Gonadal Dominant even if your blood type doesn't match if:

- Your family has pronounced secondary sexual characteristics (large hips, big breasts, male pattern baldness, etc.)

- Both of your parents are blood type O.

- You experienced drug therapy in utero or sometime thereafter

- Your parents are alcoholics

- Your family is very antisexual, very prudish

- You had a competitive parent of the same sex

- The parent of the opposite sex suffered much anxiety about sex or its implications

- You suffered a debilitating injury to the very low back

- You were on a very low fat diet during childhood or early teenage years

- You have a strong fear of obesity.

You may be Pancreatic Dominant if:

- Your family is either obese or diabetic

- You were on extended drug therapy during formative years

- You've suffered liver disorders

- A parent suffered blood type A-O incompatibility jaundice at birth

- You had chronic diarrhea as a child from wheat allergy or tension about obesity

- You suffered a severe mid back injury

You may be Pineal Dominant (as a subclass) if:

- Your family is highly intuitive or psychic

- You have strong precognition or other sensitive abilities

- You've categorically had a fear of psychic ability

- Your parents are very insensitive or against being sensitive

- You experienced a severe injury to the skull

You may be Pituitary Dominant if:

- Both parents have blood type O

- Your family exhibits large or prominent foreheads

- You suffer a severe milk intolerance, which in combination with unbalanced diet has led to a low skull calcium density (determined by frail bones or an x-ray that reveals the condition)

- You suffer a fear of charisma in yourself

- You had an extremely repressive or highly jealous parent or sister/brother

- You suffered a severe head injury

You may be Thyroid Dominant if:

- Your family members are small, thin, and quick (mentally and physically)

- Infectious disease plagued you in childhood

- You suffered excessive radiation as a child

- You have a fear of sensitivity or high intelligence

- One or both of your parents are anxiety prone
- You suffered a severe neck injury

You may be Thymus Dominant if:

- You were plagued by viral disease early on

- Your family is generally tall

- You suffered chronic side effects from drugs

- You were over-irradiated

- You had a liver disorder

- Your parents have differing blood types

- Your tolerance for milk products is low, combined with a low intake of green leafy vegetables, which caused a low overall bone calcium density

- Your parents were chronically depressed and joyless.

The Quick Check has now helped you to better understand your metabolic type, allowing you to take a giant step forward in delineating your biochemical uniqueness. Next we will explore the nutrient "zones" for each type.

Step 2A: Quick Check Zone

As mentioned previously in this section, blood type gives us a theoretical eating pattern while the endocrine dominance profile and its related criteria help us to further refine the basic pattern with more precise information. Just using blood type eating patterns as a guideline is wholly inadequate and may be out of synergy with inherent neuroendocrine factors related to weak and strong glandular function. Merely knowing food's effect on blood fluidity, as in blood typing, while not including the balance of neuroendocrine function (the core pacesetter for metabolism at large) is a severe shortcoming in the overall process of typing. It's similar to knowing how only one software feature in your personal computer functions without being aware of how all the other programs in your computer work, and even worse, the overall capacity of your drive unit which underscores the entire system in the first place. The endocrine and nervous systems drive the metabolic system in all of its ramifications over and above each cell's vital independence while the blood merely functions as a transport system for hormone compounds, buffers, nutrients, and waste material.

For this reason—and for the fact that other typing procedures haven't been implemented—I've had many complaints from patients about "The Blood Type Diet" by D. Adamo as being ineffective. Blood type nutritional programming alone will never completely fulfill an individual's nutritional needs much as only one piece of a complicated puzzle never completes the puzzle. But you still need that piece to complete the puzzle so you must have it at hand! This line of logic applies to each piece of metabolic typing information presented so far!

The Quick Check has now helped you to better understand your non-laboratory mediated metabolic type allowing us to take a giant step forward in delineating your biochemical uniqueness by reflecting your genetic uniqueness. Now we must match back the foods and nutrients which shaped your phenotype through the ancestral tribal line of heredity which created your DNA. In other words, let's feed your genes properly!

Diet Patterns

Simplistically put, Gonadal, Pituitary and Pancreatic Dominant Types are considered Carni-Vegans. They require a diet rich in meats and plants. Even Pancreatic Dominant Blood Type A's will do well in this category.

Pineal Subclass Dominants are generally considered Semi-Lacto-Vegans subsisting best on fermented dairy products like cheese and yogurt, along with a rich diet of plant foods, and with little or no meat.

Thyroid Dominant Blood Type A Europeans and Africans are generally considered Lacto-Vegans thriving on milk products and plants with less meat intake if any. Thyroid Dominant Blood Type A Asians are categorized as Pesca-Vegans, requiring high intakes of fish and plants for maximum health. Thymic Dominant Types also do well with a Pesca-Vegan eating pattern, but require a greater rotational effect in their diet to minimize IgG (a class of antibodies) allergic sensitivities. This is the case for A, B, or O blood types.

Adrenal Dominant and the Balanced Dominant Subtype are categorized as omnivores thriving upon all foods except some fish and especially shellfish. Refer to Appendix C for more details.

The vitamins, minerals, vitamin-like substances, and herbs that optimize metabolism for each of the basic metabolic types in Quick Check are listed in the next chart. Match your type to the charts given for supplement and nutrition zones. Much of what is recommended is based on the special needs of the typically recessive glands, which accompany the dominant ones, along with the vital nutrients and catalysts which optimize the dominant glandular function. The overall goal is to strengthen weak glands while supporting the strong ones to accomplish a more healthful metabolic balance. But, remember, even with this information, as well as the information about diet patterns as applied to you, the typing process is still not complete until profiling is implemented in Workbook Section—Step 3.

TI TYPE—SUPPLEMENTAL AUGMENTATION

*Key Catalysts for Fundamental Metabolism Efficiency
Recessive Glands: Adrenal Glands and Pancreas

Vitamans and Minerals	Daily Male Average	Daily Female Average	Special Notes
A	25,000 iu	15,000 iu	• Vitamin A
*E	600 iu	400 iu	(Use fish oil
*F	Omega 3-200 iu	100 iu	source over
	Omega 6-300 iu	200 iu	Beta Carotene)
*C Complex	3 gm	2 gm	
PABA (Para Amino Benzoic Acid)	300	200	• Vitamin E (D Alpha
*Inositol	300 mg	200 mg	Tocopherol only)
*B's	1,000 mg	500 mg	
*Total B Complex	300mg/mcg	200 mg/mcg	• Vitamin C
Folic Acid	6 mg	3 mg	Taken as whole
Phosphatidyl Choline	300 mg	200 mg	C Comp.
*Potassium	400 mg	200 mg	With
Manganese	60 mg	40 mg	Bioflavonoids
Selenium	100 mcg	75 mcg	
Chromium	100 mcg	75 mcg	
*Zinc	50 mg	30 mg	
*Iodine	150 mcg	100 mcg	
*Magnesium	150 mg	100 mg	
Copper	3 mg	2 mg	
Iron	30 mg	25 mg	

TI Type

Other Helpful Vitamin/Mineral-like Substances:
• HCL (hydrochloric acid) *
• Pepsin (stomach enzyme) *
• Bee Pollen
• Royal Jelly (unless asthmatic)
• Proteases (protein digesting enzymes)
• Acidophilus
• Germ Oils
• Adrenal gland extracts*
• Thyroid gland extracts
• Phenylaniline (an amino acid)
• Tyrosine (an amino acid)
• Tryptophan; males: orchic*
• pituitary and prostate extracts; females: ovary
• pituitary
• uterus extracts
• Pycnogenol*
• SOD (Superoxide Dismutase) *
• DHEA (dehydroepiandosterone)
• broccoli/cauliflower extracts
• all trace minerals (but in particular Vanadium*)
• Molybdenum*
• Germ Anium*
• Lithium Arginate*
• Cobalt*
• Boron*
• Aloe Vera
• Astralagus
• CoEnzyme Q10
• Ginger and Ginseng
• Korean Ginseng for women; Siberian Ginseng for men
• Oat Bran
• the amino acids
• Histidine
• Methionine and Taurine
• Quercitin and Lecithin

Herb Catalysts:
- Yerba Mate
- Gingko Biloba
- Damiana
- Red Beet
- Nutmeg
- Calamus Root
- Oat Straw
- Bean Leaves
- Blueberry Leaves
- Paprika
- Capsacin
- Tumeric
- Bitter Sweet Root
- Anise
- Devil's Claw Root Bark

Detoxification Profile: Tend to easily absorb poisons through the skin and lungs. Yoga breathing is a good detoxifier.

Nervous System Dominance: Sympathetic dominant. Responds well to Yin influences for calming effect.

Primary Digestive Weakness: Difficulty with meat, beans and raw roughage, especially when taken simultaneously. Use smaller more frequent meal pattern.

Cravings: Usually fat, sometimes sugar.

TII TYPE—SUPPLEMENTAL AUGMENTATION

*Key Catalysts for Fundamental Metabolism Efficiency
Recessive Glands: Thyroid and Pineal (Typically)

Vitamans and Minerals	Daily Male Average	Daily Female Average	Special Notes
*A	30,000 iu	20,000 iu	• Trace Minerals = Espec. Boron Cobalt, Lithium Arginate, Molybendum and Vanadium
*D3	800 iu	600 iu	
*E	800 iu 600 iu		
*F	Omega 3-500 iu	400 iu	
	Omega 6-600 iu	500 iu	
*B Complex	150 mg/mcg	100 mg/mcg	
*C Complex	1,500 mg	1,000 mg	
*Calcium	600 mg	500 mg	
*Magnesium	400 mg	250 mg	
*Phosphatidyl Choline (Lecithin)	24 gr	20 gr	
Potassium	200 mg	100 mg	
*Chromium	50 mg	25 mg	
*Selenium	50 mg	25 mg	
*Zinc	50 mg	25 mg	
*Manganese	15 mg	10 mg	
Silica	100 mg	75 mg	
Sulfur	150 mg	35 mg	
Copper	9 mg	6 mg	
*Iodine	50 mcg	25 mcg	
*Vanadium	10 mcg	5 mcg	
*Trace Minerals	.5 mcg	.5 mcg	

TII Type

Other Helpful Vitamin/Mineral-like Substances:
• SOD (Super Oxides Dismutase) *
• Thyroid gland extracts (large amount) *
• Adrenal gland extracts
• Bee Pollen
• Spirulina
• Alfalfa
• all vegetable extracts (except standard mushroom)

- Seaweed and its extracts
- Branched Chain Amino Acids (Leucine, Isoleucine, Valine)
- Cysteine
- Histidine
- Tyrosine—amino acids
- Melatonin; male: (Orchic) extracts; female: (ovarian) extracts
- Pycnogenol
- DHEA (Dichydroepiandosterone)
- Octacosonol
- Smilax
- Yohimbe
- CoEnQ10

Herb Catalysts:
- Siberian Ginseng
- Shiitake Mushroom
- Reishi Mushroom
- Gingko Biloba
- Schizandra
- Kelp
- Chia Seed
- Dulse
- Iceland Moss
- Mustard
- Nettles
- Parsley
- Seawrack
- Calamus
- Chickweed
- Dill
- Licorice Root
- Marigold
- Rhubarb
- Sorrel
- Watercress

Detoxification Profile: Need vigorous exercise to excrete poisons through the skin.

Nervous System Dominance: Sympathetic/parasympathetic balanced. Usually no dominance present.

Primary Digestive Weakness: Usually none present unless meals are nervously/hurriedly rushed.

Cravings: Starches and sometimes certain proteins.

TIII TYPE—SUPPLEMENTAL AUGMENTATION

***Key Catalysts for Fundamental Metabolism Efficiency
Recessive Glands: Normally None**

Vitamans and Minerals	Daily Male Average	Daily Female Average	Special Notes
B Complex	.75 mg/mcg	50 mg/mcg	• All trace minerals are important, but Vanadium, Germanium, Rubidium, Lithium, and Molybendum are a priority
*C Complex	1,000 mg	750 mg	
A	15,000 iu	10,000 iu	
E Complex	200 iu	100 iu	
*Magnesium	100 mg	75 mg	
*Manganese	10 mg	5 mg	
Chromium	20 mg	15 mg	
Selenium	20 mg	15 mg	
*Trace Minerals	Trace	Trace	
Other Minerals: Potassium, Copper, Iron, Phosphorous, Iodine and Calcium	RDA	RDA	

TIII Type

Other Helpful Vitamin/Mineral-like Substances:
• Full Spectrum Glandular Extract (brain, heart, adrenal, kidney, liver, pancreas, pituitary, thymus, spleen, hypothalamus); male: Orchic; female: Ovary
• Spirulina
• Aloe Vera
• CoEnzyme Q10

- Pycnogenol
- Capsicum
- DMG (Dimethyl Glycine)—an amino acid
- Bee Propolis
- Reishi Mushroom Extract
- Shiitake Mushroom Extract
- the aminos
- Carritine
- Glutamic Acid
- Glutamine

Herb Catalysts:

- Yerba Mate
- Siberian Ginseng
- Beet Powder
- MaHuang
- Guarana
- Kola Nut
- Cayenne
- Gymnema Sylvestre
- American Centaury
- Gotu Kola
- Pullulan
- Licorice Root
- Ginger Root
- Kelp
- Ho Shou Wu
- Mallow Leaf
- Hyssop
- Barberries
- Dandelion Root
- Alfalfa Seed
- Yucca
- Mullein Leaf
- Sage Saw Palmetto

Detoxification Profile: Prone to allergic patterns which can lead to liver/thymus stress. Excretes toxins equally through the excretory systems but can have blood impurities (need periodic blood cleansers/builders). Need to avoid standard mushrooms, string beans, corn, black berries and pomegranates unless allergy testing demonstrates compatibility.

Nervous System Dominance: Sympathetic/Parasympathetic Balanced—usually no dominance present.

Primary Digestive Weakness: Usually none present unless overeating occurs or meals are rushed.

Cravings: Usually none unless allergy/addiction syndrome is present as in IgG sensitivities.

TIV TYPE—SUPPLEMENTAL AUGMENTATION

*Key Catalysts for Fundamental Metabolism Efficiency
Recessive Glands: Liver and Pineal

Vitamans and Minerals	Daily Male Average	Daily Female Average	Special Notes
*B Complex	300 mg/mcg	200 mg/mcg	• L-Tryptophan = Amino Acid taken at bedtime
*Niacinamide	750 mg	500 mg	
B6	400 mg	300mg	
B12	500 mcg	400 mcg	
Biotin	1,000 mcg	750 mcg	• Vitamin F as Borage Oil = Essential fatty acid, as Omega 6
*C Complex	600 iu	400 iu	
*Choline	1,000 mg	750 mg	
*Inositol	500 mg	350 mg	
*Magnesium	800 mg	500 mg	
*Calcium	900 mg	600 mg	• Desiccated Liver = Argentine Beef is the best pure" source
*Potassium	300 mg	200 mg	
Vitamin D3	500 iu	400 iu	
*L-Tryptophan	500 mg	400 mg	
*Vitamin F as Borage Oil	750 mg	600 mg	
*Desiccated Liver	1,000 mg	500 mg	
*Zinc	0 mg	30 mg	
Manganese	75 mg	50 mg	
Lysine	500 mg	300 mg	
All Trace Minerals	Trace	Trace	

TIV Type

Other helpful vitamin/mineral-like substances:
- CoEnzyme Q10
- Melatonin
- Silymarin
- Amino Acids—Proline
- Bromelain
- Hydroxyproline
- Serine
- Copper in combination with Selenium as a synergist
- Flaxseed Oil
- L-Carnitine (amino)

Herb Catalysts:
- Oregon Grape Root
- Milk Thistle Seed
- Artichoke Leaf
- Dandelion Root
- Leaf and Flower
- Beet Leaf
- Fennel Seed
- Goldenseal
- Goldenrod
- Cloves
- Mexican Yam
- Calamus
- Chickweed
- Dill
- Licorice Root
- Marigold Flowers
- Rhubarb
- Sorrel
- Watercress
- Pineapple
- Cranberry
- Strawberry
- (Grapefruit extracts are to be avoided)

Detoxification Profile: Prone to excessive toxic elimination. Stress in sexual organs. Special need to avoid nightshade plants like onion, garlic, beets and rhubarb, as well as raw spinach and standard mushrooms. Wise to limit acid fruit intake like lemons, limes, grapefruit, and black berries.

Nervous System Dominance: Parasympathetic dominant

Cravings: Usually fats and candy-like sugars, especially chocolate.

TV TYPE—SUPPLEMENTAL AUGMENTATION

*Key Catalysts for Fundamental Metabolism Efficiency
Recessive Glands: Liver

Vitamans and Minerals	Daily Male Average	Daily Female Average	Special Notes
*B Complex	150 mg/mcg	100 mg/mcg	• Vitamin F = Omega 3/6— 50/50 ratio
*Choline	500 mg	250 mg	
*Inositol	500 mg	250 mg	
*B12	200 mcg	100 mcg	• Vitamin E = Dry or water soluble
*Folic Acid	3 mg	2 mg	
*C Complex	2,000 mg	1,500 mg	
*A	30,000 iu	20,000 iu	
*D3	800 iu	600 iu	•Trace Minerals = Espec. Vanadium, Boron, Silicon, Germanium, and Cobalt
*E	800 iu	600 iu	
Lecithin	60 grain	40 grain	
*Potassium	500 mg	400 mg	
*Chromium	80 mg	60 mg	
*Selenium	40 mg	30 mg	
Calcium	500 mg	400 mg	
Zinc	70 mg	40 mg	
Manganese	75 mg	50 mg	
Vitamin F	600 mg	400 mg	
*Trace Minerals	Trace	Trace	

TV Type

Other helpful vitamin/mineral-like substances:
- Wheat Germ Oil
- Spirulina
- Desiccated Liver
- Pancreatic Extract
- Lipid-Digesting Enzymes
- Proteases
- Bile Salts
- Bromelain; male: Orchic; female: Ovary
- Extracts
- Amino Acids: Methionine
- Arginine*

- Carnitine*
- Taurine*
- Tyrosine*
- Lysine
- Branched Chain Aminos (Leucine, Isoleuchine, Valine)
- Trans Feurlic Acid
- SOD (Super Oxide Dismutase)
- Balanced Spectrum Glandular Extracts

Herb Catalysts:

- Gymnema Sylvestre
- Yerba Mate
- Garcinia Cambogia
- Capsicum
- Ginger
- Green Tea
- Dandelion Root
- Flower and Leaves
- Goldenseal
- Golden Rod
- Silymarin
- Yucca
- Oregon Grape Root
- Artichoke Leaf
- Beet Leaf
- Fennel Seed

Detoxification Profile: Inefficient fat metabolism leading to blood vessel plaquing effect. Need to keep biliary system flowing freely. Tendency to over-produce glucagon and under-produce insulin leading to obesity and diabetes. Limited intake of carbohydrates—a key to keeping the system running efficiently. Special need to avoid all nightshade vegetables, most particularly eggplant, (green) bell pepper, tomato, potato, beets, rhubarb, garlic and onion. Raw spinach and unusual mushrooms require avoidance also.

Nervous System Dominance: Parasympathetic Dominant.

Cravings: Concentrated sugars and "rich" foods (heavy cream, fat and sugar-laden foods).

TVI TYPE—SUPPLEMENTAL AUGMENTATION

*Key Catalysts for Fundamental Metabolism Efficiency
Recessive Glands: Liver

Vitamans and Minerals	Daily Male Average	Daily Female Average	Special Notes
*A	1,5000 iu	10,000 iu	• C Complex = Non-corn base
*B Complex	150 mg/mcg	100 mg/mcy	
*B6	150 mg	100 mg	
B12	150 mcg	100 mcg	• Phosphorous Mostly from diet
Folic Acid	3 mg	2 mg	
Inositol	200 mg	150 mg	
*C Complex	3,000 mg	2,000 mg	• Choline As phosphatidyl/ Choline
*E Complex	200 iu	100 iu	
*Potassium	200 mg	100 mg	
Calcium	500 mg	400 mg	
Magnesium	250 mg	200 mg	
*Selenium	30 mcg	20 mcg	
Phosphorous	200 mg	100 mg	
Manganese	30 mcg	20 mcg	
*Zinc	75 mg	50 mg	
Iron	20 mg	15 mg	
*Trace Minerals	Trace	Trace	
Celtic Sea Salt	200 mg	150 mg	
Choline	200 mg	150 mg	

TVI Type

Other Helpful Vitamin/Mineral-like Substances:

- Pancreatic enzymes
- Spirulina
- Essential Amino Acids (Crystalline)
- Desiccated Liver
- Thymic Extract
- Yakitron
- SOD (Super Oxide Dismutase); male: Lysine 500mg*; female: Lysine 400mg
- Kelp
- Essential Fatty Acids (GLA-EPA) *

Herb Catalysts:
- Comfrey
- Thyme
- Dandelion Root
- Leaf
- Flower
- Oregon Grape Root
- Milk Thistle Seed
- Artichoke Leaf
- Beef Leaf
- Fennel Seeds
- Goldenseal
- Golden Root
- Cloves
- Devil's Club
- Root
- Bark
- Jambul Seed
- Blueberry Leaf
- Bean Pod
- Paprika
- Turmeric
- Bitter Sweet Root

Detoxification Profile: Prone to nutritional and aerial substance sensitivities such as mold, pollen, egg, wheat, corn, milk, some sea animals, grains, acidic plants, nuts and seeds. If Rh negative, there is more of a tendency to be hyperallergic, lymphatic disorders are common, and lymphatic cleansing is in order with age. Special need for more pure air and negative ions. Must be careful to avoid food additives. May be sensitive to supplement ingredients.

Nervous System Dominance: Varies on secondary patterns.

Cravings: Usually fats and oils, but can vary with secondary patterns. Essential fats are helpful across-the-board for all Thymic Types.

TVII TYPE—SUPPLEMENTAL AUGMENTATION

*Key Catalysts for Fundamental Metabolism Efficiency
Recessive Glands: Liver and Pineal

Vitamans and Minerals	Daily Male Average	Daily Female Average	Special Notes
A	10,000 iu	7,500 iu	•Trace Minerals = Espec. Germanium, Silicon, Vanadium, Boron
*B Complex	200 mg	100 mg	
*Niacinamide	750 mg	500 mg	
B6	00 mg	200 mg	
Biotin	250 mg	150 mg	
*B12	500 mcg	400 mcg	
*C Complex	1,000 mg	750 mg	
D3	350 iu	250 iu	
*Magnesium	800 mg	600 mg	
*Calcium	900 mg	800 mg	
*Potassium	300 mg	200 mg	
*Zinc	100 mg	50 mg	
Manganese	50 mg	35 mg	
*Lecithin (Phosphatidyl Choline)	24 grains	20 grains	
*F Essential Fatty *Acids Omega 3 Fish Oils Omega 6 Borage Oil	300 mg 600 mg	250 mg 500 mg	
Trace Minerals*	Trace	Trace	

TVII Type

Other Helpful Vitamin/Mineral-like Substances:
Silicon as Horsetail
- Desiccated Liver
- Amino Acid L-Tryptophan
- 500–1,000 mg
- CoEnzyme Q10
- Melatonin (as a sleep aid)
- Lipase Enzymes
- Proteases
- Amylases

Herb Catalysts:
- Comfrey
- Dandelion Root
- Leaf
- Flower
- Oregon Grape Root
- Milk Thistle Seed
- Artichoke Leaf
- Fennel Seed
- Goldenseal
- Golden Rod
- Cloves
- Mexican Yam
- Calamus
- Chickweed
- Dill
- Licorice Root
- Marigold Flowers
- Sorrel
- Watercress

Detoxification Profile: Sensitive to Nightshade Plants (eggplant, bell pepper, tomato, potato, beets, rhubarb, onion, garlic, raw spinach, usually mushrooms, acid fruits, such as lemon, lime, pineapple, cranberry, strawberry, grapefruit and blackberry can stimulate either allergic T-cell sensitivity or other sensitivity rebound—of course the lab-mediated component of Metabolic Typing will verify this clearly). Very susceptible to stimulant addictions and should be wary of excessive coffee (caffeine), nicotine and amphetamine intake. Can easily become addicted to cocaine. Special need for full spectrum sunlight to help balance overall endocrine system and counteract depressive tendencies. Strong spices should be avoided, along with sugar, salt and alcohol. Liver and colon cleansing periodically is advisable when the system gets off balance from stress.

Nervous System Dominance: Parasympathetic Dominant.

Cravings: Usually stimulants, such as sugar, salt and alcohol.

TIA TYPE—SUPPLEMENTAL AUGMENTATION

***Key Catalysts for Fundamental Metabolism Efficiency
Recessive Glands: Adrenal Glands and Pancreas**

Vitamans and Minerals	Daily Male Average	Daily Female Average	Special Notes
A	30,000 iu	20,000 iu	• C Mineral Complex Buffered Form (Ester C)
*C (Mineral Complex)	3,500 mg	2,500 mg	
*B Complex	150 mg	100 mg	
*Bioflavanoids	500 mg	350 mg	
*B5	1,000 mg	800 mg	• Bioflavanoids Full Spectrum
Folic Acid	10 mg	8 mg	
*E Complex	800 iu	600 iu	
*F Essential Fatty Acids			
Omega 3	400 mg	300 mg	
Omega 6	400 mg	300 mg	
*Inositol	500 mg	400 mg	
Phosphatidyl Choline (Lecithin)	20 grain	16 grain	
*Potassium	400 mg	300 mg	
PABA (Paraminobenzoic Acid)	500 mg	400 mg	
*Calcium	600 mg	400 mg	
*Zinc	100 mg	75 mg	
Magnesium	300 mg	200 mg	
*Chromium	150 mg	100 mg	
Manganese	100 mg	75 mg	
Selenium	75 mg	50 mg	
Iodine	150 mcg	125 mcg	
Copper	400 mcg	200 mcg	
Niacinamide	100 mg	75 mg	

TIA Type

Other Helpful Vitamin/Mineral-like Substances:
- Silicon as Horsetail*
- Sulfur as MSM (methylsulfanylmethane)*
- Pancreatic Enzymes*
- Pepsin*

- Pepsin*
- Betaine HCL (Hydrochloric Acid)
- Bee Pollen
- Royal Jelly (unless asthmatic)
- Acidophilus
- Wheat Germ Oil
  (unless allergic to wheat/gluten)

- Adrenal Gland Extracts
- Thyroid Gland Extracts
- Pituitary Gland Extracts
- L-Phenylaniline—L-Tyrosine
- L-Tryptophan (amino acids)
- L-Methionine

Herb Catalysts:
- Wild Cherry Bark
- Cherry Juice Extract
- Yucca
- Saw Palmetto
- Sage*
- Siberian Ginseng Root
- Licorice Root
- Oat "Milky Seed," Jamaican
  Sarsaparilla Root
- Prickly Ash Bark; men: extra
  Jamaican Sarsaparilla Root
- American Ginseng Root
- Saw Palmetto Berry

- Damiana Leaf and Powder
- Cardamom Pod with Seed;
  women: Hebonias Rhizome
- Squaw Vine Herb
- Cramp Bark
- Blue Cohosh
  (Rhizome and Root)
- Ginger Rhizome
- Calendula
- Yarrow
- Nettle

Detoxification Profile: Sensitive to corn, most beans, blackberries, snow-white mushrooms. Generally have weak digestive systems, are prone to nervous exhaustion and require calm environments and deep relaxation to keep system clear and balanced. Yoga and Yoga breathing techniques are very helpful for detoxification and balanced energetics. Strenuous exercise is generally not helpful.

Nervous System Dominance: Sympathetic Dominant.

Cravings: Usually starches and sometimes sugar.

METABOLIC TYPES:
CONNECTING "THE DOTS"

Dominant Glands	Characteristics	Blood Type	Food Pattern
Thyroid (European Genealogy)	Slender, delicate features, Small-boned	A	Lacto-Vegan (milk and plants primarily)
Thyroid (Asian)	High-strung, quick mentally	A	Pesca-Vegan (fish and plants primarily)
Thyroid (African Persian)	Quick movements, good technical ability	A	Modified-Vegan (milk, especially non-cow), plants, fish and some red meat
Pineal	Small-medium stature, delayed puberty, extremely sensitive/intuitive, psychic, vivid dreams, large rear skull	A	Semi-Lacto-Vegan (Yogurt and plants primarily)
Adrenal	Square jaw, lean, hard muscles (women are less muscular) very athletic, physically practical	B	Omnivore (All foods except some fish and shellfish)
Balanced	Medium frame, medium muscles medium fat, flexible, affable, no overpowering characteristics	A B	Omnivore (All foods except some fish and shellfish)
Thymus	Tall and lanky, sensitive, creative	A or B or O	Pesca-Vegan Rotation Diet
Gonad	Male: Pattern baldness usually with hairy bodies, Female: Hourglass figure, soft skin. Both male and female go through early puberty	A	Carni-Vegan (Primarily meat and plants)
Pancreas	Chronic obesity, jolly/easygoing, food oriented	O or A	Carni-Vegan (Primarily meat and plants)
Pituitary	Large, wide or prominent forehead, extremely charismatic, very outgoing, with leadership qualities, good focus and memory	O	Carni-Vegan (Primarily meat and plants)

THE ZONES OF TYPING

ZONE I: Interproportion of 3 Food Categories

Endocrine Dominance and Blood Type	Carbs as % of Calories	Proteins as % of Calories	Fats as % of Calories
Thyroid, Bl. Type A1 (T1)	50	25	25
Pineal, Bl. Type A2 (T1A)	50	25	25
Adrenal, Bl. Type B (T2)	40	40	20
Balanced, Bl. Type B, AB or O (T3)	45	35	20
Gonad, Bl. Type O (T4)	40	45	15
Pancreas Bl. Type O (T5)	40	45	15
Thymus, Bl. Type A (T6)	50	30	20
B (T6)	40	30	30
O (T6)	45	35	20
AB (T6)	45	25	30
Pituitary, Bl. Type O (T7)	40	45	15

THE ZONES OF TYPING

ZONE II: Interproportion of Each Protein Type

Endocrine Dominance and Blood Type	Fish	Veg. & Grain	Dairy & Eggs	Red Meat	Light Meat
Thyroid, Bl. Type (T1)					
A1, European	25	15	30	5	25
A2 Other (Asian, etc.)	30	25	10 (as eggs only)	5	30
Pineal, Bl. Type A2 (T1A)	15	25	40	15	15
Adrenal, Bl. Type B (T2)	20	20	20 (milk variable)	20	20
Balanced, Bl. Type AB, A, B, O (T3	20	20	20	20	20
Gonad, Bl. Type O (T4)	25	10	10	30	25
Pancreas Bl. Type O (T5)	20	10	10	30	30
Thymus, Bl. Type A (T6)	20	40	20	5	15
B (T6)	20	35	10	10	25
O (T6)	25	20	10	20	25
AB (T6)	15	40	15	15	15
Pituitary, Bl. Type O (T7)	15	15	15	25	30

THE ZONES OF TYPING

ZONE III: Interproportion of Each Carbohydrate Type

Endocrine Dominance and Blood Type	Dilute Cal. Complex Carb (High Fiber)	Dense Cal. Starchy Carb (Varied Fiber)	Natural Simple Sugar (Fruits & Some Veg.)	*Man-Made Simple Sugars
Thyroid, Bl. (T1)				
Type A1, European	30	40-42.5	25	5 or less
Type A2 Other (Asian, etc.)	30	45-47.5	20	5 or less
Pineal, Bl. Type A (T1A)	25	35-37.5	27.5	2.5 or less
Adrenal, Bl. Type B (T2)	32.5-35.0	35-37.5	25-27.5	7.5 or less
Balanced, Bl. Type AB, AB, A, B, O (T3)	32.5	32.5-35	30	5 or less
Gonad, Bl. Type O (T4	40-42.5	30	25-27.5	5 or less
Pancreas, Bl. Type O (T5)	45-47.5	30	25	2.5 or less
Thymus, Bl. Type A, AB, B, O (T6)	40	30-35	25	5.0 or less
Pituitary, Bl. Type O	42.5-45	35	20	2.5 or less

*Manmade sugars are generally very concentrated, causing dramatic blood-sugar "spikes," resultant pancreatic stress and powerful neuropeptide fluctuations, which alter brain function noticeably. So it's better to keep their intake to a bare minimum. Your tooth enamel and digestive linings will also benefit from lowered (manmade) sugar intake.

THE ZONES OF TYPING

ZONE IV: Interproportion of Each Fatty Acid Type

Endocrine Dominance and Blood Type	P.U.F. as Polyunsaturated Fats	M.U.F. as Monounsaturated Fats	S.A.F. as Saturated Fats
Thyroid, Bl. Type A, European (T1)	50	35	15
Type A, Other (Asian, etc.) (T1)	45	35	20
Pineal, Bl. Type A (T1 A)	40	40	20
Adrenal, Bl. Type B (T2)	30	30	30
Balanced, Bl. Type AB, A, B, O (T3)	40	35	25
Gonad, Bl. Type O (T4)	40	40	20
Pancreas, Bl. Type O (T5)	50	40	10
Thymus, Bl. Type A, AB, B, O (T6)	45	35	20
Pituitary, Bl. Type O (T7)	45	40	15

THE ZONES OF TYPING

ZONE V: Interproportion of Acid/Alkaline Foods

Note: Saliva and Urine pH has to be taken in order to modify your foods and/or intraproportions of nutrients. More on this after Zone VI A.

ZONE VI: Interproportion of Micronutrients

Note: Micronutrient ranges have been given for each Metabolic Type previously in Quick Check under "Supplemental Augmentation." Further lab-mediated Typing and Profiling is required to refine these ratios into more precise proportions, which can be variable over time depending on one's lab-measured metabolic status up-to-the-moment. A simple pH test using the differential measurement between saliva and urine can, however, demonstrate which type of calcium and in what amounts the body requires before proceeding into further testing. (Remember, just deriving one's pH ranges and adjusting diet and calcium accordingly can have a profoundly positive effect on metabolic balance, most poignantly when done in conjunction with Quantification/ Qualification and Quick Check.)

ZONE VI A: Interproportion of Micronutrients

According to biological ionization principles, our good health begins with mineral availability to the basic structures chemically formed by the liver. PH is considered the major indicator of the cumulative direction of molecular resistance within the entire body chemistry. More simply stated, when one's pH levels are higher or lower than a narrow range, the relationships the mineral content of the body is not optimum, which undermines the entire metabolic function of the body starting with the liver and proceeding throughout all aspects of body function. This degenerates the entire system, depriving it of usable energy to fight fatigue and disease, and the overall aging process. In essence, pH is very important to the body's vitality and should be measured in each person.

One's pH can be taken using "pH paper" obtainable at almost any pharmacy (or in the pH lab kit in the back section of this book). The pH paper is placed on the tongue for a few seconds for a saliva evaluation. The pH paper will give you a number that your will use in a simple mathematical formula. Another fresh strip of pH paper is dipped in a cup of midstream urine ("midstream" means that urine flow is initiated for a few brief moments before it is collected and collection is halted a few seconds before the bladder is completely empty). Again, the pH number is taken from the used strip and written down. For best results, both urine and saliva test is performed together in the morning before eating breakfast, as this is the best time for unfettered results. (The ingestion of food just prior to this test will alter results unfavorably.)

pH Test

The pH numbers from this test are written into the following formula:

$$\frac{2\ (\text{Saliva pH}) + 1\ (\text{Urine pH})}{3} = \quad \text{Test Average (Weighted Average)}$$

$$\text{Example:}\ \frac{2\ (5) + 1\ (8)}{3} = \quad 6\ \text{pH}$$

Once you've calculated your pH test average (known as a weighted average), you can understand which type of calcium is best for your unique body chemistry. (Keep in mind that as calcium increases in proportion to other minerals within a particular tissue, there will be a subsequent decrease in the other minerals and vice versa to a certain degree depending on each type of tissue's properties.)

This pH test is the most sensitive indicator of calcium changes and since calcium is the most important mineral relative to all of the other minerals in the body, a change in calcium content alters basic molecular structure and subsequent body function. There is more to this in relation to all biologic life, from soil to humans, and in relation to Phosphorus and Potassium (which exist in a life-sustaining proportion of approximately 2:1), but for the purposes of Quick Check, it's important to simply match your weighted average to the calciums that match in the following chart:

TYPE OF CALCIUM REQUIRED

Saliva	Average	Urine	Range	Type of Calcium Req.	Synergist (Sups)	Synergist (Foods)
4.70 4.80 4.90 5.00 5.10 5.20 5.30 5.40	4.70 4.80 4.90 5.00 5.10 5.20 5.30 5.40	4.70 4.80 4.90 5.00 5.10 5.20 5.30 5.40	E	Calcium Hydroxide Calcium Orotate Calcium Citrate Calcium Carbonate (Tums) Calcium Gluconate Bicarbonates Lime Water (Liq. Oxide)	Vitamin D D3 50,000 iu 1/Day D3 5,000 iu 2/Day	Organic milk, broccoli, green leafy veg., white cheeses, barley, green parsley
5.50 5.60 5.70 5.80 5.90 6.00 6.10	5.50 5.60 5.70 5.80 5.90 6.00 6.10	5.50 5.60 5.70 5.80 5.90 6.00 6.10	D	Calcium Orotate Calcium Hydroxide Calcium Citrate Calcium Carbonate (Tums) Calcium Gluconate Lime Water	Vitamin D 1,000 iu 2/Day	Organic milk, broccoli, green leafy veg., white cheeses, barley, green parsley
6.20 6.30 6.40 6.50 6.60	6.20 6.30 6.40 6.50 6.60	6.20 6.30 6.40 6.50 6.60	A	Calcium Hydroxide Calcium Gluconate/ Orotate 1/4 of each type daily Calcium Lactate Calcium Gluconate/ Orotate	Vitamin C Males: 1,000 mg 2/Day Females: 745 mg 2/Day	Organic milk, broccoli, green leafy veg., white cheeses, barley, green parsley
6.70 6.80 6.90 7.00 7.10	6.70 6.80 6.90 7.00 7.10	6.70 6.80 6.90 7.00 7.10	B	Calcium Lactate Calcium Gluconate Calcium Orotate	Vitamin C Males: 1,500 mg 2/Day Female: 1,000 mg 2/Day	Almonds, brazil nuts, buttermilk, sour cream, molasses, beans (legumes)
7.20 7.30 7.40 7.50 7.60 7.70 7.80 7.90 8.00 8.10	7.20 7.30 7.40 7.50 7.60 7.70 7.80 7.90 8.00 8.10	7.20 7.30 7.40 7.50 7.60 7.70 7.80 7.90 8.00 8.10	C	Calcium Lactate Calcium Gluconate Calcium Orotate	Vitamin C Males: 3,000 mg 2/Day Female:2,000 mg 2/Day Vitamin C Males: 3,000 mg 2/Day Female:2,000 mg 2/Day	Almonds, brazil nuts, buttermilk, sour cream, molasses, beans (legumes)

Amount of Calcium taken for E, D, A, B, C ranges appear in the above chart. (Calcium Aspartate, Calcium/Hydroxyapatite, and Calcium in multiple amino chelations can substitute for Calcium Orotate/Carbonate.)

Note: Cod Liver Oil can be used as an extra synergist to improve Vitamin D metabolism in ranges D and E:
    1. Tablespoon with Vitamin D supplement taken in Range D
    2. Tablespoons with Vitamin D supplement taken in Range E

Rates of Calcium Intake

(Based on 4 pH Patterns from Urine and Saliva)
Pattern I:
- Urine is considered alkaline (pH is more than 6.40)
- Saliva is considered to be alkaline (over 6.40)
- *Weighted* average to be alkaline

Pattern II:
- Urine is alkaline (pH over 6.40)
- Saliva is alkaline (pH over 6.40)
- *Weighted* average is alkaline (pH over 6.40)

Pattern III:
- Urine is acid (pH under 6.40)
- Saliva is acid (pH under 6.40)
- *Weighted* average is acid (pH under 6.40)

Pattern IV:
- Urine is alkaline (pH over 6.40
- Saliva is acid (pH under 6.40)
- *Weighted* average is acid (pH under 6.40)

Note: Match your pH urine/saliva pattern to either Pattern I, II, III, or IV. Next, write down your pH result for urine and saliva as follows, using Pattern I–IV and Ranges A, B, C, D, D:

Example: Saliva pH = 8.0 = Range "C" = Alkaline
Urine pH = 6.0 = Range "D" = Acid

[Weighted Average = 7.3 = Alkaline (range is not important for Weighted Average other than if alkaline or acid in value.]

Next: Place urine and saliva pH values side by side (as in above), urine range value first:

Urine (6.0) = Range C   Urine/ Saliva
Saliva (8.0) = Range D or C/D   = CD

To simplify again from your home pH tests:

Urine pH_____ Saliva pH_____
Match to range and combine letters for *Combined Range*. Now we can compute your calcium daily dosage using the next chart.

Note: In the Calcium Dosage Rates Chart on the next page, 6.40 is considered "neutral" or "balanced" as a combined average, whereas 7.00 is considered neutral on a standard pH scale. For all intents and purposes, 6.40 is considered neutral in Biological Ionization and overall optimum for good health. A person with a 6.40/6.40/6.40 (Urine pH/Combined Average/Saliva pH) uses his Metabolic Type's Supplemental Range as 1/2 Calcium Lactate and 1/2 Calcium Gluconate. PH evaluation should be accompanied once every 60 days and dosages adjusted according to the previous formula and charts. Once 6.40 pH is achieved, you are considered "pH balanced" and should recheck urine/saliva pH once every four (4) months to double-check your progress.

CALCIUM DOSAGE RATES

Pattern	Ph Urine	Combined Ave. Ph	Ph Saliva	Combined Range	Calcium Type	Daily Calcium Dosage
I	*6.40	+6.40	+6.40	AA	Lactate	800 mg
				BB	Lactate	1,200 mg
				CC	Lactate	1,800 mg
				AB	Lactate	800 mg
				AC	Lactate	1,200 mg
				BC	Lactate	1,800 mg
II	*-6.40	+6.40	+6.40	AA, AB	Lactate	400 mg
					Hydroxide	800 mg
					or Citrate	800 mg
				AC, BC	Lactate	800 mg
					Hydroxide or	400 mg
					Citrate	400 mg
				DB, DC	Lactate	400 mg
					Hydroxide and	800 mg
					Citrate	400 mg
					Lime Water	2 TBSP
				EB, EC	Lactate	400 mg
					Hydroxide	1,200 mg
					Citrate	800 mg
					Lime Water	2 TBSP
II	-6.40	-6.40	-6.40	DA, EA	Hydroxide	1200 mg
					Citrate	800 mg
					Carbonate	100 mg
					Lime Water	4 TBSP
					Vitamin B12	2,000 mcg
				DD, ED, EE	Hydroxide	1,800 mg
					Citrate	800 mg
					Carbonate	200 mg
					Lime Water	2 TBSP
					Vitamin B12	3,000 mcg
					1,200 mg	
II	+6.40	-6.40	-6.40	BA, BD, BE, CA, CD, CE	Hydroxide	800 mg
					Citrate	200 mg
					Lactate	800 mg
					Vitamin B12 (Sublingual)	2,000 mcg

* + = Above 6.40,   - = Below 6.40

Zone V (Revisited)

Now that you know your pH levels, you can proceed to proportion foods into your diet to help balance your metabolic system. These foods serve to logically integrate with your respective Metabolic Type diet pattern as a temporary priority, but, not in conflict with your specific pattern. In other words, if your Metabolic Type requires a Carni-Vegan Diet, and your pH levels (urine and salvia) are −6.40 when calculated as a weighted average, you are considered *too acidic*, but you will not add in alkaline foods that are incompatible with your Type. Therefore, increasing the consumption of milk is *not* an option. (Carni-Vegans have milk as a "Least Healthy Food" in their diet pattern.)

A general rule of thumb is to add: 8 to 10 ounces more alkaline foods per day for pH Range E. (You can use food synergists listed in the previous Type of Calcium chart.)

- 6 to 8 ounces or more alkaline foods per day for Range D
- 6 to 8 ounces or more acid foods per day for Range B
- 8 to 10 or more acidic foods per day for Range C
- For Range A, follow Metabolic Type Diet Patterns

Alkaline/acid food changes are superimposed on to Zoned Diet Patterns, and are considered priority foods within any Type until pH is more neutral.

If you are too acidic, consumption of the following foods will help rebalance your system, provided they are *not* "Least Healthy" for your type.

Fruits/Sugars	Vegetables	Proteins	Nuts and Grains
Apricots Apples Bananas Berries (All Types) Cherries Currants Dates Fits Grapes Honey Pumpkin Persimmons Rhubarb Syrup (Maple)	Avocados Alfalfa Artichokes Beans (String) Beans (Wax) Carrots Cucumbers Corn Cauliflower Celery Knobs Greens (All Types) Kohlrabi Leeks Lettuce Okra Parsley Spinach Squash Sweet Potatoes White Potatoes Yams	Cottage Cheese Cheese (White) Dairy Products Milk	All Types of Nuts No Grains except for Chestnuts and Peanuts

If you are too alkaline, eat more of the following foods that are not incompatible with your type.

Fruits/Sugars	Vegetables	Proteins	Nuts and Grains

Grapefruit
Lemons
Oranges
Peaches
Plums
Prunes
Raisins
Tangerines
	Asparagus
	Beans
	  (Brown or White)
	Cabbage
	Chickpeas
	Eggplant
	Lentils
	Olives
	Sauerkraut
	Sprouts (Brussels)
	Tomatoes
		All Meat, Fish
		and Fowl
			Chestnuts
			Barley
			Grains (Almost all
			Grains, including
			  Wheat, Rye,
			  Oats Etc.)
			Pasta
			Rice
			Tapioca

The general rules of thumb to either "acidify" or "alkalize" your body chemistry to achieve a more optimum pH balance are:

1. Have 60-70% of your calories consumed daily from the appropriate acid or alkaline food categories until your next pH test (30 to 60 days). Chances are that simply adhering to your Quick Check Metabolic Typed Diet Pattern will automatically rebalance your system if it tested too acid or alkaline. But, using this rule of thumb guarantees faster results. For fastest results (especially if you are extremely acid/alkaline) is to consume 80-90% of your daily food calories from the appropriate acid/alkaline food category and retest your pH every 1 to 2 weeks until it is close to optimum and then switch back to your Typed Diet Pattern in its normal balance.

2. Follow the calcium and associated synergists in conjunction with the food recommendations above. These calcium recommendations take the place of the calcium ranges noted under the "Supplemental Augmentation" profile for each Metabolic Type.

Summation of Quick Check

You have now traveled through several steps deep into the final frontier of nutritional healing. At this time, you have uncovered your Metabolic Type using non-laboratory mediated Typing in conjunction with you first lab-mediated Typing procedure (pH testing). (Thanks to pH paper, you do not need a lab—if you don't know your blood type, home kits using a mere pinprick are available.) Nutritional Patterns, Supplemental Augmentation and Zones of Typing are now superimposed onto Appendix A in order to tighten up your specific program. It's simply a matter of basic mathematics and a "ruling in" and "ruling out" of your foods and supplemental ranges to match the information Quick Check has provided.

Going back to Robin's diet plan or your own, of course:

1. Recompute Step V using your Quick Check macronutrient ratios (carbohydrates/proteins/fats) In Robin's case, as Pituitary Dominant/Adrenal Secondary O Blood Metabolic Type, her best macro ratios are:

   - Protein: 45%   20%
   - Carbs: 40%   Instead of   60%
   - Fat: 15%   20%
                                        (According to NAS RDAs)

   - 1,424 multiplied by .45 = 641 Kcals   - Proteins
   - 1,424 multiplied by .40 = 597 Kcals   - Carbs
   - 1,424 multiplied by .15 = 214 Kcals   - Fat

1. Recompute Step VI (using 4.35 and 4.1 substitutions)

   - Protein: 641 Kcals divide by 4.3 Kcals/gm = 147 gm
   - Carbs: 597 Kcals divide by 4.1 Kcals/gm = 146 gm
   - Fat: 214 Kcals divide by 9.0 Kcals/gm =   24 gm

1. Rule in and rule out your "Typed" food sources in Step VII. In Robin's case, she's a Carni-Vegan. She must choose foods from that pattern in the proper protein, carbohydrate and fat intraproportions (Zone II, III, IV) For the purposes of this book, fatty acid ratios need not be computed because Zones I, II, III will suffice to balance Zone IV without creating confusion.

In effect, Robin's Zone II and III should correspond to the Pituitary Dominant category:

Zone II =	Fish	25 % of protein gms (147)
	Vegetable & Grain	15% of protein gms
	Dairy/Eggs	5% of protein gms
	Red Meat	30% of protein gms
	Light/White Meats	25% of protein gms

Zone III = Complex Carbs   45 % of carb gms (146)
(Low Calorie/High Fiber)

Complex Carbs   35% of carb gms
(Starches)

Simple Sugars   20% of carb gms
(Natural)

Simple Sugars   0% of carb gms
(Manmade)

Let the fats fall where they may according to the Metabolic Typing Food Patterns/List for now (Zone IV).

The information from the pH test is superimposed over the remainder of Appendix A, along with the Supplemental Ranges given per your personal Metabolic Type. If no pH test is taken, simply follow the supplemental/food recommendations per your type as you customize your final nutrition plan (Steps VIII through XIII). In Step XI, one more zone can be computed based on raw/cooked food intake known as Zone IA or raw/cooked interproportion.

Step 3A: How to Use This Workbook

This book is designed to empower you with the ability to take precise control of your health and to understand the severe shortcomings of conventional wellness wisdom. This book reveals the only provable way nutrition can effectively be used as "the most powerful weapon against disease on earth"! It's designed to save you thousands of dollars, wasted time and much confusion about *one-size-fits-all* diet plans and ineffective nutritional products. Follow through with the testing procedures in this section in addition to the Ph test and you will be fully Typed and Profiled.

There are two parts to Step 3: Part I answers the question, "What's wrong with my body?" Part II demonstrates how to repair your body with perfect nutrition.

Nutritional Stereotyping is Out— Biochemical Individuality is In

One-size-fits-all nutrition is the basic philosophy of choosing foods and nutrition supplements on the premise of "what's good for you must be good for me, too." We see it every day in doctors' offices, health food stores, supermarkets, on television, at fitness centers, at home and in most nutrition and wellness books. A commercial touts a certain drug. There is a news story about the benefits of a particular herb. Your friends extol the virtues of a particular diet plan or supplement and insist that you must try it too. The underlying message of each example is "this worked for me so it will work for you, too."

It is this errant philosophy that we must fight to correct. But first we have to understand the reasons why this philosophy has become so ingrained in our society today. They are political, economic, cultural, and due to just plain ignorance of the facts. As previously mentioned, there are endless dangers in this narrow-minded thinking. It has already been scientifically demonstrated that no two people are alike. Logic, science, and startling research contradictions fully validate this "everyone is unique" approach to understanding the essence of wellness.

Part 1
What's Wrong With My Body?

Metabolic Typing Theory vs. Metabolic Profiling Science

The theories of *Metabolic Typing* developed over a period from 5000 years ago to the present have been reviewed and condensed in this book. To summarize, typing is the process of categorizing certain genetically predetermined constitutional elements into subclasses of physical, psychological and physiological distinction. Blood type, vital statistics, glandular balance, ethnicity, personality, body and face shape, fat distribution pattern, and other human distinctions can add up to as many as 37 metabolic types with corresponding food patterns. This all makes for interesting reading in the pursuit of discovering our metabolic and biochemical individuality, but, it has the most dire shortcoming that virtually renders it useless.

These issues simply have nothing to do with what nutritional state the body is in at this very moment! Only specialized testing featured in the process of *Metabolic Profiling* can provide this information precisely. How much vitamin C, calcium, or copper is present in my body? What are my hidden allergies, toxic accumulations, and glandular stresses? Without this up-to-the-moment information derived from direct metabolic chemistry measurement, (such as hair, saliva, urine, blood, etc.), you cannot know exactly what nutrition your body needs to be put back into perfect balance. Metabolic Profiling consists of all the tests, which precisely determine every discernible mineral, vitamin, amino acid, fatty acid, toxin, sensitivity, and diet-related hormone pattern present, and whether in or out of balance. These insights allow us to customize diet and supplements exactly to body specifications with no guesswork whatsoever. And, best of all, you can measure your personal wellness success with retests in the future for comparison to ensure that the personalized nutrition program is working properly.

Metabolic Typing by itself is a process of grouping genetic subclasses in order to distinguish one's metabolic identity, but without testing direct metabolic need as accomplished in Metabolic Profiling you cannot determine your true biochemical individuality.

Subject 1:
Pretesting Metabolic Genetics With Quick Check

In 1956 Dr. Roger Williams published *Biochemical Individuality*, presenting his theory that each person is biochemically unique in their anatomy and chemical composition. Dr. Williams' research showed wide variations among healthy, "normal" humans. He related these differences to genetic inheritance and revealed unique needs for particular nutrients due to inherited digestive, absorptive, enzymatic concentrations, and abilities to transport nutrients and to excrete the by-products of metabolism. Thousands of years before Dr. Williams the Chinese, Ayurvedics (espoused by Deepak Chopra), Greeks (Hippocrates), Egyptians, and many more developed Typing systems to uncover individuality (as discussed in Section III).

Years later, my Quick Check System serves to streamline these theories and the landslide of modern Typing research, to bring forth the best of what Metabolic Typing theory has to offer. It's organized into a simplified system of self-application which allows us to quickly categorize our genetic set in preparation for moving on to the essence of biochemical individuality—Metabolic Profiling—where tests scientifically reveal our innermost uniqueness. Light years beyond mere Typing theory, Profiling eliminates doubts, involves no guesswork, leaves "no stone left unturned," and requires no doctor.

Subject 2:
The Nutrition Testing/Profiling Procedures

The smallest particles of visible matter in the universe are minerals. They are categorized in chemistry and physics books as the elements on the Periodic Table. These atoms are the building blocks of all matter and all life in the universe (including our bodies, of course). Their presence in varying degrees and proportions specifies the nature of each life (and non-life) form in all properties and characteristics. Humans are composed of 4% minerals by weight. The rest of our bodyweight is matter derived from minerals including water, protein, tissue enzymes, hormones etc. There are 76 minerals identified in humans. They each exert varying electromagnetic force and inertia upon each other (as degrees of attraction, repulsion, and displacement), and their presence relative to one another not only defines "humanoid" within the universe, but defines the wellness state of each individual human within itself. They are involved in every process within the body and their exact proportion to one another, either as synergy or antagonism, **affects** the efficiency of the total organism.

One's lifespan, state of wellness or sickness, fatness, energy level, and all other factors of one's life process is directly or indirectly related to the ratio of one mineral to the next. This is the most important nutrient factor to test and where we always begin the testing process. Hair, urine, saliva, and one particular blood test are introduced and discussed as the most reliable indicators of mineral presence and function as deficiency, excess, or imbalance within the body. And, as with all the following tests, doctors are optional.

List of Primary Tests:
1. TMA (Hair Analysis)*
2. Metabolic Urine Analysis*
3. Organic Acid Analysis (Urine)*
4. Saliva*
5. Blood/Mineral Profile

* Indicates that no blood specimen is required.

Vitamins, or "vital minerals," are our bodies' molecular minerals. This means that structurally they are slightly larger groups of atoms, or molecules, made from mineral combinations. These eighteen biochemicals have less to do the actual support substance of the body than minerals, like calcium which gives bone its hardness and strength or copper which gives muscle elasticity, but are involved with every life process much as minerals.

In fact, collectively, vitamins and minerals are the spark plugs of life. Much as spark plugs ignite gas in autos, vitamins and minerals provide the spark of life to enzymatically create and process energy from air, water, and food for all aspects of our existence. Their internal presence, properly proportioned, effects wellness from life to death. Vitamins are both synergistic and antagonistic to each other and to minerals as well. **The nature of this attraction-repulsion pattern renders all A–Z multiple vitamin-mineral supplements functionally useless.** The exact relationships are well understood and proportions within the body must be precisely measured and then synergistically remediated where necessary to effect perfect balance. Urine, hair and a blood test reveal all one needs to know to get this right.

List of Primary Tests:
1. TMA (Hair Analysis) *
2. Metabolic Urine Analysis*
3. Antioxidant Profile (Blood)
4. Organic Acid Analysis (Urine) *

Amino Acids are the smallest constituents of proteins for wellness. They organize the 70%+ of your body's water into the matter that you see, feel, and refer to as the body. Created from minerals, vitamins, air, water, and sunshine, 40 amino acids combine to form enzymes, hormones, immunoglobulins, neurotransmitters, cellular and tissue proteins. Collectively, they provide all body structure and many of its functions. From the way you're built physically and the way you think, to the way your body moves and fights disease, all of these behaviors are related to your amino pattern. Specific patterns within the body as measured in urine, blood, hair, and feces give us dramatic insights into the body's current state of metabolic efficiency (in conjunction with the vitamins and minerals evaluated previously).

List of Primary Tests:
1. Blood and blood "spots"
2. Organic Acid Analysis*
3. Comprehensive Digestive Function (Stool/Urine) *

Fatty Acids are considered the body's homeostatic equalizers providing many functions ranging from nerve and body insulation to immune system fortification to hormonal synergy. Their combined effect is to provide a template from which other biochemicals can work in harmony. They also provide a slow release energy source to help fill in the body's energy needs. Excessive storage of fat on the body is the #1 problem facing the U.S. today, over and above all other nutrition issues. Fatty acid imbalances create a large amount of metabolic "short circuits" which can severely undermine good health and prevent a lean physique. A special (very inexpensive) blood test reveals which of 38 fatty acids is in or out of balance and why.

List of Primary Tests:
1. Blood Plasma
2. Organic Acid Analysis (Urine) *
3. Comprehensive Digestive Function (Stool/Urine) *

Nutritional Sensitivities: These hidden killers, when left undetected, lead to 25 major disease states and can make daily living downright miserable. This class of sensitivities does not cause the typical, easily identified allergic reaction we are used to seeing. The effects are very subdued and therefore hard to detect. In fact, the majority of hidden sensitivities when triggered cause an immediate release of adrenaline which in turn gives us a lift. This stimulating response can actually lead to an addiction cycle where we crave foods that we're actually allergic to—a very dangerous problem.

Within 72 hours of eating an offending food, concentrated vitamin/mineral, sugar or spice, the body becomes deadlocked in a biochemical war that literally tears up the body. This problem has emerged from the constant interbreeding of genetically different populations in combination with the increasing rejection of traditional ethnic diets in favor of "modern" generic diets which have little connection to our individual genetic digestive, absorptive, assimilation, and excretory capabilities. A huge array of problems results, ranging from heart disease and headaches, to premature death. There is a special blood test to identify the offenders and customized food rotations treat the problem naturally.

List of Primary Tests:
1. TMA (Hair Analysis) *
2. IgE/IgG Sensitivity Test and Glucose Tolerance (Blood)
3. Comprehensive Digestive Analysis (Stool) *

Toxic Accumulation brings on slow death, the result of bodily infusion of heavy metals such as mercury and aluminum; anti-corrosives like chromium 6, and strong carcinogens such as formaldehyde (FMA), trimellitic and phthalic anhydrides, isocyanates, TDI, benzene, and a host of others. Excessive minerals and vitamins (hyper-mineralosis and hyper-vitaminosis), free radicals and other easily detectable poisons all combine to severely deteriorate body functions. Special hair, urine, blood and feces tests reveal these chemical killers so that the proper detoxification can be instituted long before serious disease takes hold.

List of Primary Tests:
1. TMA (Hair Analysis) *
2. Antioxidant Profile (Blood)
3. Organic Acid Analysis (Urine) *
4. Toxic Challenge (Blood/Urine)

Hormone Patterns provide your own personal glandular profile, as revealed in saliva and hair tests. Any imbalances found are nutritionally correctable. Hormones are the chemical messengers of the body connecting the brain to each cell as complement to nerve connections. When synchronized properly, the life force is maximized.

List of Primary Tests:
1. Saliva*
2. TMA (Hair Analysis) *
3. Blood Plasma

Test information is available from Dragon Door or the ASAP. The ASAP is strongly dedicated to providing effective alternatives and adjuncts to conventional medicine and nutrition that defeat the cause of disease and our fatness at the level of the nutrition-toxin disease connection.

Membership entitles you to the ASAP Newsletter (Dr. Tefft is the executive editor) and the chance to purchase Dr. Tefft's expanded self-help workbook, *The Tefft System For My Body Only*. Although Dr. Tefft's name is truly his name, it also stands for "*Today's Evaluation For a Finer Tomorrow*." This book is one of many from the For Your Body Only audio visual library series. The expanded workbook is signed by Dr. Tefft and will have your name embossed on the front cover.

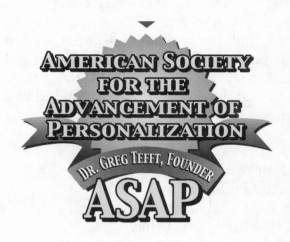

Part II:
Let's Repair My Body With Perfect Nutririon!

Now that your biochemical uniqueness from the preceding testing is understood, we must customize diet and supplements into a perfect nutrition program For Your Body Only.

Subject 1:
Food Patterns and Nutrient Zones

There are seven basic food patterns which have shaped our metabolic genetics over thousands of years. We are each designed to be either carnivores, carni-vegans, vego-vegans, semilacto-vegans, pescalacto-vegans, pesca-vegans, or omnivores. Your basic genetic pattern is identified in Quick Check and its corresponding food pattern outlined here. The seven nutrient zones are then used to divide foods and supplements into the proper ratios and ranges for each Metabolic Type. Next, test results as revealed in your Metabolic Profile from Part I are used to refine these ratios perfectly.

Subject 2:
Balance Mineral Ratios

Balancing mineral proportions is the most overlooked aspect of conventional nutrition yet is the most important variable of all. The relationship of one mineral to the next as synergism or antagonism, sedation or stimulation, yin or yang, acid or alkaline, has to be taken into account. Too much calcium in your system? Excess calcium depresses the absorption of iron, which in turn increases the body's need for copper and so on. If one's heavy metal accumulation is found to be high, then increasing other mineral intake such as calcium, zinc, and iron can rid these killers from the body in combination with proper prevention measures. Once the intake of minerals as food and supplements is corrected to actual body needs the other variables of a perfect nutrition program can be fit into place harmoniously.

Subject 3:
Synergize Vitamin Proportions

Strategizing vitamin intake is based on a simplified system of do's and don'ts specific to your test findings and in relation to vitamin-to-vitamin-and-vitamin to mineral synergies and antagonisms. If a test shows that you have a vitamin A deficiency then vitamins C, E, B1, B2, B3, and B6 must be increased in order to increase vitamin A absorption, as well as increasing A intake from foods and supplements. Add too much E into the mix and you'll antagonize A utilization and depress the other vitamins synergistic with A. Your A deficiency may be caused by deficiencies of zinc, potassium, phosphorous, selenium, magnesium, and manganese which showed up in your mineral tests. Balancing these nutrient chemicals and all others according to test results "bulletproofs" your body against metabolic breakdown.

Subject 4:
Equalize Protein Intake

Having tested amino acid profiles, it's time to proportion protein food and supplements in order to correct any imbalances found. Perhaps a test reveals that your personal biochemistry is low in the amino acid methionine, which is **typical of overweight people.** Simply consume more methionine-rich foods such as chicken and fish to compensate for the metabolic imbalance and to stimulate weight-loss. Sulfur-rich aminos such as cysteine can be taken individually to draw heavy metals such as mercury out of the body when necessary. Other aminos "layer into" the nutrient customization process for total biochemical synergy.

Subject 5:
Proportion Fats

If your test results reveal any fatty acid disorders specific foods and supplements can rectify the problem directly. A good example of this is deficiencies of Omega 6 fats, as discussed in "The Zone. This problem is remedied by a greater consumption of sunflower seeds, vegetable oils, and borage oil supplements in conjunction with balancing the minerals, vitamins, proteins, sugar, and glands you've tested.

Subject 6:
The Sugar Equation

Setting the ratio of one sugar to the next within the "carbohydrate interzone" is critical. Sugar intolerance reveals itself in nutritional sensitivity and mineral tests. Knowing this biochemical criteria allows us to balance metabolism precisely by using sugar as high energy fuel instead of as a metabolic irritant. Easy-to-follow do's and don'ts simplify this process.

Subject 7:
Food Rotation and Detoxification

Profiling tests reveal your hidden nutrition sensitivities and toxic accumulation. Applying the test findings to a strategic sequence of alternating food consumption allows us to clean the body out of this chemical stress so that it can function at peak efficiency. Most hidden allergies can be reduced significantly and in some cases eliminated altogether using the 1-4-7-alternation process. Toxic accumulations may require special supplements in addition to modified food intake depending on their nature. For example, if you were found to have a mild sensitivity to spinach and an abnormal mercury level in your body then you would avoid all spinach six out of seven days per week for the next 90 days, then you would have spinach once every four days for the next 120 days at which time a retest should reveal a major sensitivity reduction to spinach. Mercury detox requires an increase in sulfur-rich foods, like garlic, in conjunction with increased intake of supplemental zinc, selenium, iron, sulfur and the herb, "Captomer." A 10-dollar mail order hair analysis confirms results in 120 days. Your personalized process of rotation and detox is exceedingly important to extend life, promote healthy DNA, and minimize disease potential.

NOTE: When you take any/or all of the tests described in Part I, the information explained in Part II will automatically be included in your test results, based precisely on your needs. You can apply this information on your own or use my self-help profiling workbook (*For My Body Only*) to help yourself in your quest for the perfect nutrition plan.

Subject 8:
Hormone Maximization

Hormone Pattern Evaluation quickly reveals disturbances within the glandular system which can be eliminated and/or diminished using nutritional customization. Merely adding a hormone or pro-hormone into this delicate system either indiscriminately or based upon purely static conventional reference range tests only serves to increase stress to the hormonal system at large. The above practice usually leads to drug hormone dependence because nutrient-deprived under-functioning glands are further shut down when hormones and some prohormones are given to make up for any deficits. Ultimately the normal stimuli which activate glands are taken away and the target glands will cease to function properly ever again even with proper nutrient customization. Using hormone profiling "functional tests" on top of nutrient customization can help us to strategically implement prohormones, adaptogens, natural hormones, and even drug hormones to gently revive the endocrine system. This will expedite a more efficient metabolism and help the body to wake up to a higher energy yield. The end result is: faster results, less (if any) stress to the body, and minimal (if any) long term drug dependencies.

Summation

For Your Body Only is the last self-help nutrition book you will ever need to read. Readers can finally create the perfect nutrition program for their one-of-a-kind body and mind with the utmost precision and confidence. No other philosophy, fad, or one-size-fits-all "latest finding" can upstage the **scientific solidarity** found in these pages. Standing out from its thoroughly historical backdrop, this work fully encapsulates the entire phenomenon of nutritional individualization, from crude theory to the cutting edge of scientific testing to enhance reader perspective. The self-help format has been designed to allow readers to rediscover themselves in all of their nutrition-related uniqueness and then attain the perfect wellness they've always dreamt of. We can each take final control over our personal wellness destiny as we're guided to greater longevity, a leaner physique, a clearer mind, and so much more out of life. It's simply a matter of follow-through. Take the tests to be your best! There simply is no other way to get it right.

Call **1-888-899-5111** to obtain more information.

APPENDIX A

Psychological Typing
Combined with Bodytyping

William Sheldon, Ph.D., developed a three-body type system previously mentioned in Chapters 3 and 4, which is based on the amount of "derm" present in the body. His work is based on Jung's categories of people derived from the particular psychological characteristics they possessed.

In his research, Dr. Sheldon studied 4,000 photographs of college-age men, showing front, back, and side views of the whole body. After careful examination of these photographs, he found that there were three primary elements that, in combination, made up "physiques" or "somatotypes" (i.e., body types). With further persistence in his research he was able to work out methods to directly measure these three elements and to express them in numerical terms, so that any human body could be described in terms of three characteristic numbers.

Dr. Sheldon was able to standardize his system so that two independent observers could arrive at very similar conclusions about each body type. These primary characteristic elements were named "ectomorphy," "mesomorphy," and "endomorphy." They were each derived from the three cellular layers of the human embryo known as the ectoderm, the mesoderm, and the endoderm (sometimes called the entoderm).

Ectomorphy—	Related to the tissue components of the brain and nervous system
Mesomorphy—	Related to the muscles and circulatory system
Endomorphy—	Related to the abdomen and the entire digestive system

Our bodies contain all three elements in varying degrees. We all possess digestive, circulatory, and nervous systems, but in different proportions as part of our human uniqueness. No one is simply an ectomorph without having at the same time some mesomorphic and endomorphic characteristics in varying degrees.

Dr. Sheldon's work reflected the degree to which a derm component was present using a scale ranging from 1 to 7, with 1 as the minimum and 7 as the maximum number. An example of this would be a rating of 711, where 7 represents endomorphic characteristics, the first 1 represents mesomorphic characteristics, and the second 1 represents ectomorphic characteristics. A 711 rating is the most extreme endomorphic body type, with only a trace of mesomorphy and ectomorphy.

Temperament

Dr. Sheldon looked into the basic components of temperament. He interviewed several hundred people, searching for traits that would describe the basic elements of their behavior. He eventually came up with three components that he termed "ectotonia," "mesotonia," and "endotonia."

Ectotonia—	Centered on privacy, self-restraint, and a highly developed self-awareness
Mesotonia—	Focuses on being assertive and a love of action
Endotonia—	Demonstrated by the love of relaxation, comfort, food, and people

Dr. Sheldon developed a way of numerically rating the occurrence of each of the three categories, based on a checklist of 60 characteristics that describe the three basic components of behavior. Again, as with the derm-based body types, the number 711 reflected extreme endotonia, 117 extreme ectotonia, and 171 extreme mesotonia. Dr. Sheldon was able to correlate similarities between the endomorphic body type and the endotonic temperament, the mesomorphic body type and the mesotonic temperament, and the ectomorphic body type and the ectotonic temperament.

When you combine the methodologies of Dr. Sheldon and Dr. Jung there is a correlation between the two typologies:

Sheldon	Jung
Endotototonics	Dominant Extroverted Sensing Types (ESTP and ESFP)
Mesotototonics	Dominant Extroverted Thinking Types (EST and ENTJ)
Ectotonics	Dominant Introverted Intuitive Types (INTJ and INFJ)

When it comes to other psychological types discovered by Jung, some questions arise as to how they fit into Dr. Sheldon's systems. Dr. Sheldon did not provide detailed descriptions of the mixed temperaments from which other psychological types could be extracted.

The following descriptions cover the three types that are categorizable.

Type 1
Personality Type: Dominant Extroverted Sensing Types (ESTP and ESFP)
Body Type: Extreme Endomorph (fatty roundness)

Physical Description:
- Skin is soft and smooth
- Roundness and softness characterize the body (some development of the breast is present in males)

- Most mass is concentrated in the abdominal area
- Body has smooth contours without projecting bones and a high waist
- Hair is fine
- Whole head is spherical, tendency towards premature baldness beginning at the top of the head spreading in a circle
- Fullness of the buttocks
- Arms and legs are short and tapering
- Upper arms and thighs have more mass development than lower arms and legs
- Hands and feet are comparatively small

Temperament:
- Very friendly
- Love to eat, socialize; good food digesters
- Enjoys sitting around after a good meal
- Don't have nervous stomachs often
- Readily falls asleep
- Frequently snores
- Relaxed and slow moving
- Breathes deep and regular, and from the abdomen
- Speech is unhurried
- Limbs are usually limp
- Has slow reactions
- Slow pulse, slow breathing rate, and low body temperature
- Poor extremity circulation

According to Dr. Sheldon, this type is a biologically introverted organism with all of its energy focused on the abdominal area, leaving less for the limbs and face, all of which gives the impression of a lack of intensity. He also felt that biological introversion predisposed psychological extroversion. Since the bodies of endotonics are so focused on the digestive system, they need and crave social stimulation in order to feel more complete socially. Social contact stimulates them when focus on food is switched to a social focus. Endotonics love to socialize while they eat and meal sharing is very important. This type makes excellent hosts; they love company, desire to be liked and approved of, and are "non-controversial" in their choices, so that they avoid the disapproval of others.

Endotonics are "open" even when it comes to emotions that can flow out of them spontaneously with little inhibition. During happiness or sadness they enjoy having people around them for empathy; they are very sympathetic to others as well. Drinking alcohol stimulates endotonics to become even more jovial and demonstrate an even greater love of people. This type is family-oriented; they love babies and young children, and have a highly developed maternal and paternal instinct. This type is particularly nonjudgmental and quick to accept people as they are.

Type 2

Personality Type:	Dominant Extroverted Thinking Types (ESTJ and ENTJ)
Body Type:	Extreme Mesomorph (muscular)

Physical Description:
- Hair is coarse, balding starts at the front of head
- Face is wide and long
- Head tends toward a cubicle shape
- Cheekbones are well-defined
- Jaw is square and heavy
- Head and face bones and muscles are prominent
- Neck muscles on sides create triangular shape
- Chest area dominates over abdominal area
- Torso tapers to a narrow and low waist
- Wrist and fingers are thick and heavy
- Skin is thick and coarse, holding tan well, but can develop a leathery appearance with many wrinkles
- Overall body is square and hard-looking due to thick bones and high muscle tone
- Lower and upper arms and legs are well developed

Women show less sharp angularity than men, have less prominent bone structure, less pronounced muscularity, but can still look muscular. Contours are smoother in women, chest area dominates over the abdomen, and both upper and lower arms are well muscled. Skin is finer than in males, though women can also exhibit the same characteristics of tanning and wrinkling.

Temperament:
- A "person of action"
- Muscles seem to have a "mind of their own"
- Good posture, energy abundance, and fatigue doesn't come easily
- Can labor for long periods, evincing an overall need to exercise and an enjoyment of physical activity
- Inactivity causes restlessness and dejection
- Risk-taking and physical fearlessness
- Difficult and argumentative
- Slow to anger, acting out rage physically on occasion
- Highly competitive
- Craving forward motion
- Psychologically callous
- Practical tendencies
- Not overly sentimental
- Walks forcefully over obstacles (and people) who stand in their way
- Eats food rapidly and randomly, often neglecting set meal-times
- Sleeps less than the other types, often thrashing about
- Shows insensitivity to pain
- Tendency for high blood pressure, with large blood vessels prominent on exposed skin
- Generally noisy, with a voice that carries
- Very active when speaking, with a tendency to glorify younger days (that's when physical powers were optimum)
- Early maturation patterns, possibly looking older than one's age
- Quick decision-making
- May be unaware of other aspects of personality
- Tendency to be disassociated with dream life
- Enjoys wide open spaces, as well as freedom from the restraints of clothes
- Can convey exceptional calmness and amenability
- May expect special treatment
- When provoked can easily show true colors

Women's mesotonic traits are similar but are toned down to "more acceptable feminine levels" and channels acceptable within social limits.

Type 3
Personality Type: EDominant Introverted Intuitive Types (INTJ and INFJ)
Body Type: Extreme Ectotonic (linear)

Physical Description:
- Physique is fragile and delicate
- Light bones and small muscles
- Hair is fine and fast growing, with baldness being rare
- Facial features are fragile and sharp
- Face shape is triangular
- Chin is point of triangle
- Teeth are often crowded on lower jaw, which may seem to be receded
- Drooping shoulders
- Ribs clearly visible and delicate
- Upper arms and thighs are weak
- Overall body appearance is linear and extended
- Rrelatively long limbs
- Long fingers and toes, long neck
- Dry skin, which tends to burn and peel easily; poor tan retention

Temperament:
- Highly tuned receptive system and tends to be reflective
- Proficient at picking up all stimuli or may think in terms of strategies that can be narrowed down to details
- Very aware of sudden loud noises, which may interfere with attention to delicate sounds
- Doesn't like to make or be subjected to noise
- Likes to cross legs when sitting
- Tends to curl up to minimize exposure to the exterior world
- Avoids crowds and large groups of people, preferring small, protected places
- Suffers from extreme heat or cold due to greater surface area of skin in relation to body mass
- Quick to hunger and quick to satiate, favoring a high-protein and high-calorie diet
- Tends to snack frequently due to small digestive systems

- Tendency to have a nervous stomach and bowels
- Light and quiet sleeper, often plagued by insomnia and tending to sleep on one side with legs drawn up
- Finds sleep hard to shake off in morning
- Possesses low energy levels with fast reactions
- Suffers from marginal chronic fatigue and must avoid too much heavy exercise
- Blood pressure is low, respiration shallow and rapid, with a rapid but weak pulse
- Body temperature is elevated slightly above normal and can rise rapidly when illness strikes
- Resistant to many major diseases
- Suffers excessively from insect bites and skin rashes
- Susceptible to pharyngeal streptococcal infections, which can cause swelling and strangulation effects

APPENDIX B

Blood Type Diet Categories (5 Examples)

1. OMNIVORE DIET FOR BLOOD TYPES B AND AB

Usually in combination with **Adrenal Dominance**, also seen in the **Balanced Types** and sometimes in strong **Thymic Types**.

Note: According to scientists, Blood Type B occurred about 10,000 years ago with a genetic mutation allowing for better milk digestion. This new strain of Blood Type B is the newest and rarest of the blood types, appearing about 1,000 years ago.

Food Type	Healthy Foods	Least Healthy Foods
Dairy Products	European Descent: butter, yogurt, kefir, cottage cheese, cheeses, no Homo/pasteurized milk (cow)	Oriental Descent or Other Ethnicity: No cow's milk products, ice cream
Eggs, Fats	Eggs, unprocessed seed oils (olive, flaxseed), avocado	Margarine, sesame oil, corn oil, cottonseed oil, peanut oil
Meats, Poultry, Fish	Most meats including: some beef, lamb, liver, fowl, light colored deep water cold fish (including white albacore tuna	Some fish: opaleye, trout, salmon, dark tuna goose, snail, pork, tuna, turtle, salmon caviar, caviar in general, some shellfish, snake meat
Vegetables	Leafy green vegetables: all greens including lettuce, cabbage, spinach, seaweeds (kelp), spirulina, snow peas, bamboo shoots, celery, water chestnuts, tomatoes, alkaline vegetables including squashes, cucumbers, carrots, starchy vegetables: Including yams, sweet potato, white potato, jicama, cruciferous vegetables Including broccoli, cauliflower, asparagus, brussels sprouts, etc.	Unusual mushrooms, artichokes, corn, tomatoes, radishes, lima beans, mung sprouts, peppers

Grains	Almost all grains, including wheat, corn, rye, barley, millet, oats, rice, pumpernickel	Buckwheat, kasha, couscous, bulgar wheat
Beans	Some beans including green beans, peas, tofu, soybean & alfalfa sprouts lima beans, pinto beans, peas, lentils, tofu, soybean sprouts, alfalfa sprouts, navy beans, black beans	Black-eyed peas, castor beans, field beans, soybeans, beans, fava beans
Nuts, Seeds	Almonds, cashews, brazil nuts, sunflower seeds, pecans	Peanuts, sesame seeds, filberts, pignolas
Fruit	All fruits including most citrus, peaches, apricots, apples, dates, nectarines, all berries, cherries, pineapple, pears	Pomegranates, coconuts, persimmons, rhubarb
Beverages	Herb tea, vegetable and fruit juices, pure water, vegetable broths	Carbonated soft drinks, coffee, black tea, hard liquor, cocoa
Misc.	Carob, raw honey, maple syrup, malt, onions, herbs, spices	Chocolate, sugar, salt, junk foods, artificial sweeteners

2. CARNI-VEGAN DIET FOR BLOOD TYPE O

Usually seen in combination with **Gonad** and **Pituitary Dominance** and sometimes with **Pancreatic** and **Thymic Dominance**.   **Note:** Blood Type O is the human race's oldest blood type. Gluten intolerance and celiac sprue is very common in Type O's, which is why they need to avoid wheat in the diet. Step 3 (**Tefft System**) Lab Typing can determine if there truly is an incompatibility.

Food Type	Healthy Foods	Least Healthy Foods
Dairy Products	None except butter, mozzarella, goat cheese	Milk, cream, cheese, cottage cheese, Yogurt, cream cheese, kefir, ice cream
Eggs, Fats	Egg yolks, unprocessed seed oils, cottonseed & safflower okay, olive oil, avocado	Raw egg whites, margarine, sunflower oil, corn oil
Meats, Poultry, Fish	Most meats including beef, lamb, liver, fish, fowl, shellfish, game meats	Pork, fatty meats, , catfish, goose, veal, eel, halibut, opaleye fish, caviar, conch
Vegetables	Leafy greens vegetables: lettuce, cabbage, parsley, cooked spinach, most greens., bean sprouts, alkaline vegetables: squashes, cucumber, vegetable marrow, okra, starchy vegetables: sweet potato, yams, jicama, plantains, carrots, cruciferous vegetables: broccoli, cauliflower, asparagus, Brussels sprouts, etc.	Night shade vegetables: Bell peppers, eggplant, potato, tomato, other: beets, garlic, onion, raw spinach, rhubarb, unusual mushrooms, corn, black olives
Grains	Certain grains: barley, corn, millet, oats, rye, brown rice , buckwheat	All wheat as found in bread, cake, cookies, cereals, crackers, pasta
Beans	Green beans, lentils, peas, pinto, aduke, azuki, black eye, soy	Kidney, copper, navy, soybeans
Nuts, Seeds	Almond, filbert, walnuts, chestnut, pecan, sesame, macadamia, pumpkin	Sunflower seeds brazil nuts, litchi, peanuts
Fruit	Alkaline fruits: apples, blueberries, bananas, cherries, dates, grapes, mango, peach, persimmon, plum, apricot, nectarine, fig, pear, prunes	Acid fruits:(to be limited): lime, pineapple, cranberry, grapefruit, orange, kiwi, tangerine, blackberry, coconut, plantains
Beverages	Herb tea, vegetable & fruit juices, pure water, vegetable broths tea,	Carbonated soft drinks, coffee, black hard liquor, cocoa
Misc.	Carob, raw honey, maple syrup, herbs, date sugar	Chocolate, sugar, salt, vinegar, spices, junk foods, artificial sweetener

2. PESCA-VEGAN DIET FOR BLOOD TYPE A1
(Asian Descent)

Usually seen in combination with **Thyroid Dominance.**

Food Type	Healthy Foods	Least Healthy Foods
Dairy Products	Butter, soya dairy substitutes,	Fresh milk, cream, cheese, cottage cheese, kefir, yogurt, ice cream,
Eggs, Fats	Eggs, avocado, olive & flaxseed oils	Margarine, corn oil, most seed oils
Meats, Poultry, Fish	Fish, fowl, liver, shellfish, some tender beef occasionally	Escargot, garfish, halibut, brown trout, pork, goose, rabbit, lox, caviar, Fish clams, turtle, tough red meats, snake meat, anchovy, conch
Vegetables	Leafy green vegetables: all greens, lettuce, cabbage, seaweed (kelp, nori), water chestnuts, snow peas, spinach, celery, bamboo shoots, onion, starchy vegetables: yams, potatoes, jicama,, artichokes cooked carrots, cruciferous vegetables: broccoli, cauliflower, asparagus	Alkaline vegetables: cucumber, squash, other: horse gram, string beans, snow white mushrooms, Raw roots, raw tubers
Grains	Rice, wheat, oats, barley, millet, rye, most grains	Corn products
Beans	Alfalfa sprouts, peas, lentil soup, tofu, soybeans (cooked), green beans, blackeye peas	Copper, navy, lima beans, field beans, tora beans, uncooked soybeans, garbanzo
Nuts, Seeds	Majority of nuts and seeds: almonds, brazil, cashews, filberts, pecans, sesame, sunflower	Raw coconut
Fruit	Oranges, grapefruit, kiwi, tangerines, apricots, berries, dates, figs, apples, peaches, pears, plums, prunes, pineapple, pomegranate, persimmon, nectarines, raisins	Blackberries, rhubarb
Beverages	Herb tea (green tea), vegetable and fruit juices, pure water, vegetable Broth	Carbonated soft drinks, coffee, black hard liquor, cocoa
Misc.	Carob, raw honey, maple syrup, onions, herbs, spices	Chocolate, sugar, salt, vinegar, spices, junk foods, artificial sweeteners, yeast

PESCA-LACTO-VEGAN DIET FOR BLOOD TYPE A1
(European Descent)

Usually seen in combination with **Thyroid Dominance.**

Food Type	Healthy Foods	Least Healthy Foods
Dairy Products	Raw milk, butter, most cheeses, cream, cottage cheese, kefir, yogurt	Highly aged hard cheeses
Eggs, Fats	Eggs, avocado, unprocessed seed oils	Margarine, corn, oil
Meats, Poultry, Fish	Fish, fowl, liver, shellfish	Brown trout, clams, escargot, garfish, turtle, snake meat, halibut, red meat in general
Vegetables	Leafy green vegetables: lettuce, cabbage, seaweeds, all greens, snow peas, celery, spinach , tomato, starchy vegetables: potato, artichoke, yams, cooked carrots, jicama, cruciferous vegetables: broccoli, cauliflower, asparagus, Brussels sprouts, etc.	Reduce alkaline vegetables: squash, cucumber, other: horse gram, string beans, raw tubers and roots, snow white mushrooms
Grains	Rice, barley, oats, wheat, rye, millet	Corn products
Beans	Alfalfa sprouts, lentils, peas, tofu	Soybeans sprouts, lima beans, field beans, tora beans
Nuts, Seeds	Almonds, brazil, cashews, filbert, pecans, sesame, sunflower	Raw coconut
Fruit	All citrus fruits, apricots, berries, dates, apples, figs, peaches, pears, plums, pineapple, persimmon, Pomegranates, prunes, nectarines	Blackberries
Beverages	Herb tea, vegetable and fruit juices, pure water, vegetable broths	Carbonated soft drinks, coffee, black tea, hard liquor, cocoa
Misc.	Carob, raw honey, maple syrup, malt, onions, herbs, spices	Chocolate, sugar, salt, junk foods, yeast, bleached flour

SEMI LACTO-VEGAN DIET FOR BLOOD TYPE A2

Usually in combination with **Pineal Dominance.**
Note: In theory Blood Type A's are better suited to vegetarian types of diets than any
other blood type. Type A is considered to be the second blood type to evolve on earth.

Food Type	Healthy Foods	Least Healthy Foods
Dairy Products	Butter, cottage cheese, yogurt, kefir	Milk, cream, ice cream, highly aged cheeses
Eggs, Fats	Eggs, avocado, unprocessed seed oils	Margarine, corn oil
Meats, Poultry, Fish	Fish, fowl, shellfish, some lean red meat	Brown trout, escargot, halibut, garfish, turtle, snake meat, fatty meats
Vegetables	Leafy green vegetables: lettuce, cabbage, all greens, spinach, seaweed, celery, snow peas, bamboo shoots, starchy vegetables: potatoes, sweet potatoes, yams, artichokes, carrots, jicama, cruciferous vegetables: broccoli, cauliflower, asparagus, Brussels sprouts, etc.	Horse gram, string beans, snow white mushrooms
Grains	Rice, oats, barley, wheat, millet, rye	Corn products
Beans	Alfalfa sprouts, tofu, peas, lentils	Soybeans sprouts, lima beans, field beans, tora beans
Nuts, Seeds	Almonds, brazil, cashew, filberts, pecans, sesame, sunflower	Raw coconut
Fruit	Citrus, apricots, berries, apples, figs, peaches, pears, plums, pineapple, persimmon, pomegranate, prunes, Nectarines	Blackberries
Beverages	Herb tea, vegetable and fruit juices, pure water, vegetable broths	Carbonated soft drinks, coffee, black tea, hard liquor, cocoa
Misc.	Carob, raw honey, maple syrup, malt, onions, herbs, spices	Chocolate, sugar, salt, junk foods, artificial sweeteners

APPENDIX C

Food Groups

Complex Carbohydrates		
Low Calorie / Calorie Dilute	**Starchy / Calorie Dense**	
Non-Leafy Vegetables	**Grains**	
Alfalfa Sprouts String Beans Artichokes Olives Bean Sprouts Onions Beets Peppers (all colors) Carrots Pumpkin Celery Radish Cabbage Squash (see cabbage below) Tomatoes Cucumber Turnips Eggplant Water Chestnuts	Cold Cereal Brown Rice Bread White Rice* Hot Cereal Tapioca Pasta (all types)	
	Legumes	
	Lima Beans Peas Peanuts All beans Soybeans Pinto Beans Lentils	
Cabbage Family and Cruciferous Group	**Other Starchy Vegetables**	
Asparagus Broccoflower Broccoli Cauliflower Brussels Sprouts Cabbage (all types)	Corn Carrots (some clinica Potatoes (all types) nutritionists consider Yams carrots as a starchy Sweet potatoes vegetable) Jicama	
Leafy Vegetable		
Lettuce (all types) Swiss Chard Kale All "greens" Spinach		

*White rice naturally increases blood sugar faster than most complex carbohydrates. Consequently, many nutritionists consider it a simple sugar instead of a complex dense starch.

Simple Carbohydrates

Apricots	Coconut	All grapes	Mangoes	Papaya	Plums
Bananas	Dates	Guava	All melons	Peaches	Prunes
All berries	Figs	Lemons	Nectarines	Pears	Raisins
Cherries	Grapefruit	Limes	Oranges	Pineapple	Tangerines

OTHER GROUPINGS

Proteins	Fats	Spices/Condiments	
Egg Whites	Flaxseed Oil	Basil	Dill
Whole Eggs**	Olive Oil	Bay leaf	Fennel Seed
Fish	Peanut Oil	Caraway	Garlic
Poultry	Canola Oil	Olives	Ginger
Shellfish	Safflower Oil	Cinnamon	Mace
Cheese**	Sunflower Oil	Clove	Mustard
Beef	Butter	Cocoa	Oregano
Pork	Seeds	Coffee	Paprika
Lamb	Nuts	Cumin	Pepper
Organ Meats	"Light" Mayonnaise	Curry	Rosemary
Yogurt*	Egg Yolk	Parsley	Sage
Milk*	Avocado	Tarragon	Butter Buds
	Vinegar		

Fungi	Special Amino Seasoning
Mushrooms (all kinds) Yeast (Baker's or Brewer's)	Bragg's Liquid Amino Acids

**There are substantial amounts of fat in these proteins, which can be sidestepped by using low fat or non-fat versions or simply by reducing intake.

FOOD IRRITANTS & ALLERGENS: (generalized) chocolate, yeast, salt, sugar, junk foods, coffee, alcohol, preservatives, artificial dyes, bleached flour, fried foods, processed deli meats (hot dogs, salami, etc.). (See also Appendix E "Harmful Food Additives.")

APPENDIX D

Common Food Families
Used Through The Centuries

Food Families	Foods
Plum	Plum, cherry, peach, apricot, nectarine, almond, wild cherry
Papaw	Papaw, papaya, papain
Blueberry	Blueberry, huckleberry, cranberry, wintergreen
Mustard	Mustard, turnip, radish, horse-radish, watercress, cabbage, kraut, Chinese cabbage, broccoli, cauliflower, Brussels sprouts, collards, kale, kohlrabi, rutabaga
Laurel	Avocado, cinnamon, bay leaf, sassafras, cassia buds or bark
Sweet Potato or Yam	Wheat, corn, rice, oats, barley, rye, wild rice, cane, millet, sorghum, bamboo sprouts
Grass	Parsley, aster, corn, tomato
Orchid	Vanilla
Protea	Macadamia nut
Birch	Filberts, hazel nuts
Conifer	Pine nut
Fungus	Mushrooms and yeast (Brewer's yeast, etc.)
Bovid	Milk products—butter, cheese, yogurt, beef and milk products, Oleomargarine, lamb
Tea	Sassafras, papaya leaf, mate, lemon verbena, comfrey, fennel, Kaffir, alfalfa, fenugreek
Oil	Corn oil, butter, fats from any bird on this list, soybean, Peanut, cottonseed, safflower
Sweetener	Cane sugar, sorghum, molasses, corn syrup, glucose, dextrose, Date sugar, orange honey, beet sugar, carob syrup, clover Honey, buckwheat honey, safflower honey or sage honey
Citrus	Lemon, orange, grapefruit, lime, tangerine, kumquat, citron
Banana	Banana, plantain, arrowroot (Musa)
Palm	Coconut, date, date sugar
Parsley	Carrots, parsnips, celery, celery seed, celeriac, anise, dill, Fennel, cumin, parsley, coriander, caraway

Food Families	Foods
Beet	Beets, spinach, Swiss chard, lamb's quarters (greens)
Pepper	Black and white pepper, peppercorn
Herbs	Nutmeg, mace
Cashew	Cashew, pistachio, mango
Bird	All fowl and game birds including chicken, turkey, duck, Goose, guinea, pigeon, quail, pheasant, eggs
Grape	All varieties of grapes and raisins
Pineapple	Juice pack, water pack or fresh
Rose	Strawberry, raspberry, blackberry, dewberry, loganberry, Youngberry, boysenberry, rose hips
Melon (gourd)	Watermelon, cucumber, cantaloupe, pumpkin, squash, other Melons, zucchini, acorn, pumpkin or squash seeds
Pea (legume)	Pea, black-eyed pea, dry beans, green beans, carob, soybeans, Lentils, licorice, peanut, alfalfa
Mallow	Okra, cottonseed
Subucaya	Brazil nuts
Flaxseed	Flaxseed
Swine	All pork products
Mollusks	Abalone, snail, squid, clam, mussel, oyster, scallop
Crustaceans	Crab, crayfish, lobster, prawn, shrimp
Apple	Apple, pear, quince
Mulberry	Mulberry, figs, breadfruit
Olive	Black, green or stuffed with pimento
Gooseberry	Currant, gooseberry
Buckwheat	Buckwheat
Aster	Lettuce, chicory, endive, escarole, artichoke, dandelion, Sunflower seeds, tarragon
Potato	Potato, tomato, eggplant, peppers (red & green), chili pepper, Paprika, cayenne, ground cherries
Lilly (onion)	Onion, garlic, asparagus, chives, leeks
Spurge	Tapioca
Herb	Basil, savory, sage, oregano, horehound, catnip, thyme, Spearmint, peppermint, marjoram, lemon balm
Walnut	English walnut, black walnut, pecan, hickory nut, butternut
Pedalium	Sesame
Beech	Chestnut
Saltwater Fish	Sea herring, anchovy, cod, sea bass, sea trout, mackerel, Tuna, swordfish, flounder, sole
Freshwater Fish	Sturgeon, herring, salmon, whitefish, bass, perch

APPENDIX E

Harmful Food Additives

Chemical	Description	Potential Damage
Blue No. 1, Citrus Red No. 2	Artificial coloring	Cancer risk
Blue No. 2	Artificial coloring	Brain tumors (FDA unsure)
Green No. 3	Artificial coloring	Bladder cancer (FDA unsure)
Red No. 3	Artificial coloring	Thyroid tumors
Red No. 40	Artificial coloring	Final verdict not in
Yellow No. 5	Artificial coloring	Allergic response
Yellow No. 6	Artificial coloring	Strong cancer risk
All "Artificial Flavoring" (hundreds of compounds, mostly in junk foods)	Artificial flavoring	Hyperactivity
Aspartame	An artificial sweetener	Cancer risk, behavioral effects, PKU
Brominated Vegetable Oil (BVO)	Emulsifier, clouding agent	Controversial
Butylated Hydroxy Anisole (BHA)	Antioxidant	Cancer risk (Japanese study)
Butylated Hydroxy Toluene (BHT)	Antioxidant	Cancer risk (controversial)
Concentrated Caffeine	Stimulant	Increase fibrosystic breast disease, miscarriages, birth defects
Carrageenan	Thickening and stabilizing agent	Colon damage
Corn Syrup	Sweetener, thickener	Tooth decay, high glycemic index
Dextrose (Corn Sugar, Glucose)	Coloring agent, sweetener	Tooth decay, high glycemic index
Heptyl Paraben	Preservative	Controversial
Hydrogenated Vegetable Oil	Oil, fat source	Potential immunity impairment
Hydrolyzed Vegetable Protein (HVP)	Flavor enhancer	Contains MSG—allergic responses

Chemical	Description	Potential Damage
Invert sugar	Sweetener	Cavities, high glycemic index
Monosodium Glutamate (MSG)	Flavor enhancer	Nerve damage, burning sensation, headache
Phosphoric Acid, Phosphates	Acidulant, buffer, chelating agent, emulsifier, discoloration inhibitor	Osteoporosis risk
Propyl Gallate	Antioxidant	Cancer risk
Quinine	Flavoring	Birth defects
Saccharin	Synthetic sweetener	Cancer risk
Sodium Chloride (salt)	Flavoring	Heart disease
Sodium Nitrite, Sodium Nitrate	Preservative, coloring, flavoring	Cancer risk
Sucrose (sugar)	Sweetener	Cavities, high glycemic index
Sulfur Dioxide, Sodium Bisulfide	Preservative, bleach	Allergy, B1 deficiency

APPENDIX F

Gland Composition And Relationships

Glands	Related Organ Systems	Minerals	Vitamins	Amino Acids
1 Adrenal	Kidney, Stomach Muscles, Heart, Colon	Sulfur Phosphorus Potassium Chloride Copper, Iron Manganese Selenium	A, D, E, F, C, B5, Paba	Methionine Cysteine Carnitine Phenylanine
2 Gonad	Reproductive	Phosphorus Iodine, Zinc Manganese	Paba, E, F	Leucine Isoleucine Valine
3 Pancreas	Small Intestine	Phosphorus Sodium, Zinc Chromium Manganese	B Complex, Folic Acid B12	Tryptophan
4 Pineal	Brain, 5 Senses Sympathetic Nerves	Phosphorus Zinc, Silica Manganese	B Complex Paba, B6	Tryptophan
5 Pituitary	Brain, Eye, Other Glands	Phosphorus Zinc Manganese Magnesium	B, E, F	Glutamine Arginine Carnitine
6 Thymus	Lymph, Spleen	Phosphorus Sulfur/Magnesium Calcium Copper Iron, Zinc	B12, A, C, K	Lysine Arginine

Glands	Related Organ Systems	Minerals	Vitamins	Amino Acids
7 Thyroid	Skin, Membranes, Hair, Bones, Teeth	Calcium Potassium Magnesium Phosphorus Sulfur Iodine, Silica Zinc, Copper	A, D, B6, B1	Tyrosine Methionine
8 Liver	Gall Bladder, Intestines Master Chemist	Sodium Potassium Magnesium Trace minerals Calcium	B Complex Folic Acid	All Amino Acids Methionine

APPENDIX G

Master List of
Essential Nutrients Used in Typing

I. Minerals

Minerals are atomic elements found in the earth's crust; they are constituents of human tissue and human food. Many are considered essential to human life, while others are thought to be harmful. About 70 of the 100 known elements have been isolated in human body tissues. There are two types of minerals: macro (major) and micro (trace) minerals. **Macro-minerals** are required in 100 milligrams (mgs) or greater amounts every day. **Trace minerals** are required in less than 100 mg-per-day amounts and out of these many are required in only microgram (mcg) amounts daily. Minerals occur as:

- Components of certain essential organic molecules such as metalloenzymes (or iron containing cytochromes), amino acids (the sulfur in cysteine and methionine), and others such as iron in hemoglobin, and iodine in thyroid hormones.
- Structural components of various tissues such as calcium, phosphorus, and fluorine in teeth, bones, hair, nails, etc.
- Free ions (sodium, calcium, and potassium) in blood and all other body fluids and which assist in acid/base balance, nerve impulse transmission, muscle contraction, and as catalysts for enzymatic reactions.
- Toxins when taken in excessive amounts or in unbalanced ratios.

Major Minerals		Trace Minerals			
Calcium	Sulfur	Iron	Bismuth	Copper	Gold
Magnesium	Chlorine	Chromium	Lithium	Zinc	Nickel
Potassium	Sodium	Selenium	Platinum	Vanadium	Ruthenium
Phosphorus		Manganese	Scandium	Molybdenum	Silver
		Boron	Strontium	Cobalt	Tin
		Germanium	Tungsten	Silicon	Zirconium
		Antimony	Fluorine	Berilium	

Trace Minerals—Rare Earth

Lanthanum	Cerium	Praseodymium	Terbium	Dysprosium	Holmium
Lutetium	Neodymium	Promethium	Erbium	Thulium	Ytterbium
Samarium	Europium	Gadolinium			

Trace Minerals—Miscellaneous

Curium	Rubidium	Erbium	Tellurium	Gallium	Thallium
Gadolinium	Thorium	Iridium	Titanium	Neodymium	Yttrium
Neptunium	Palladium	Niobium			

Trace Minerals—Highly Toxic

Arsenic	Plutonium	Beryllium	Radon	Aluminum	Chlorine
Cadmium	Uranium	Lead	Mercury	Radium	

Signifigant Minerals Ratios Used in Typing

Calcium / Phosphorus	Sodium / Potassium	Zinc / Copper
Sodium / Magnesium	Calcium / Magnesium	Iron / Copper
Copper / Molybdenum	Selenium / Silver	Chromium / Vanadium
Selenium / Tin	Potassium / Lithium	Potassium / Cobalt
Magnesium / Boron	Sulfur / Copper	Calcium / Potassium
Zinc / Tin	Iron / Cobalt	Calcium / Strontium

Toxic Mineral Ratios Used in Typing

Calcium / Lead	Selenium / Mercury	Sulfur / Mercury
Iron / Lead	Zinc / Cadmium	Sulfur / Cadmium
Iron / Mercury	Zinc / Mercury	Sulfur / Lead

II. Vitamins

Vitamins are organic compounds:

- Required in trace amounts by the body.
- That perform specific metabolic functions like stimulating enzyme action. Also known as coenzymes or cofactors because of this property.
- Are not synthesized by the body (except for A,D,and K to some extent) and are considered "molecular minerals"
- Do not produce energy in and of themselves. They require enzymes to work with for energy production.
- In excess can be toxic to the body—a condition known as clinical or subclinical hypervitaminosis. Are either synergistic or antagonistic to each other and minerals.
- Come in two forms: fat soluble and water soluble.

Vitamin Names

- **Vitamin A**—fat soluble—3 forms:
  - A1 a.k.a. retinol
  - A2 a.k.a. dehydroretinol
  - A3 a.k.a. pro vitamin A a.k.a. beta carotene (precursor substance for vitamin A)

- **Vitamin B Complex**—water soluble—multiple forms:
  - B1 a.k.a. thiamin
  - B2 a.k.a. vitamin G a.k.a. riboflavin
  - B3 a.k.a. niacin in 2 forms:
    - nicotinic acid
    - niacinamide a.k.a. P.P. factor (pellegra preventing factor, a.k.a. antipellegra factor)
  - B5 a.k.a. pantothenic acid
  - B6 group a.k.a.
    - pyridoxine
    - pyridoxal
    - pyridoxamine
  - B7 a.k.a. Bc, vitamin M, folic acid, Bc conjugate

B10 a.k.a. vitamin H, biotin

B12, a.k.a. anti-pernicious anemia factor, comes in 2 forms:
>   cyanocobalamin a.k.a. B12
>   hydroxocobalamin a.k.a. B12b

B15 a.k.a. Pangamic Acid

B17 a.k.a. Laetril

- **Vitamin C Complex**—water soluble—2 forms:
  > C a.k.a. ascorbic acid, anti-scurvy factor, anti-scorbutic factor
  > Bioflavonoid Complex—multiple forms:

flavones	flavanones	flavanonals
eriocitrin	hesperedin	naringen
naringenin	rutin	turmeric
quercitin		

- **Vitamin D**—fat soluble—3 forms
  D1 a.k.a. D, calciferol
  D2 a.k.a. cholecalciferol
  D3 a.k.a. ergocalciferol

- **Vitamin E Complex**—fat soluble—3 forms:
  E1—d'alpha tocopherol (most active form)
  E2—d'beta tocopherol
  E3—d'gamma tocopherol

- **Vitamin F (a.k.a. essential fatty acids)**—fat soluble—4 forms:
  Omega 6 a.k.a. cis linoleic acid (LA)
  Omega 3 a.k.a. alpha linolenic acid (ALA)
  GLA* a.k.a. gamma linolenic acid
  EPA* a.k.a. eicosopentanoic acid

* These two forms of fatty acids (i.e., activated fatty acids) can be manufactured by the body. I have observed severe metabolic disturbances in regard to their efficient production, so I consider them essential. Therefore, it is necessary to derive them from exogenous sources (food and supplements) through the "typing and profiling" process. Proper TPing minimizes the inhibition of these two fatty acids in metabolism by keeping resistance factors like insulin and vitamin deficiencies to a minimum.

- **Vitamin K**—fat soluble—3 forms:
    K1 a.k.a. phytonadione
    K2 a.k.a. menaquinone
    K3 a.k.a. menadione

- **Vitamin L**—water soluble—2 forms:
    L1 isolated from beef liver extract
    L2 isolated from yeast

Vitamin-Like Factors

Chlorophyll	Ubiquinone (coenzyme Q10)
Choline	PABA (para-aminobenzoic acid)
Inositol	Pangamic Acid (vitamin B15)
Octacosanol	All bioactive non-toxic compounds
Lipoic Acid	and herbs
Pycnogenol	Glandular extracts
Colostrum	

Enzymes

- Metabolic (produced in body from amino acids—endogenous)
- Digestive (proteases, amylases, lipases, cellulases—**endogenous** and **exogenous**)
- Exogenous (naturally occurring enzymes in all foods)

Phytonutrients

Phytonutrients (a.k.a. phytochemicals) are known (and unknown) nutritive compounds found in all plant life, including but not limited to vitamins, minerals, and other pre-classified nutrients. Some phytonutrients are known to prevent certain diseases, such as cancer, but their full metabolic functions are still not well understood; there are thousands more to be discovered.

Alkaloids	Kavalactones	Allium
Glycosides	Allyl Sulfides	Chlorogenic Acid
Caffeic Acid	Polyphenolcatechins	Ellagic Acid
Genistein	Sulfonamides	Daidzein
Sulforaphane	Ginsenosides	Limonene
Disogenin	Dithiolthiones	Schisandrins
Protease	Inhibitors	Salicin
Phytosterols	Ligustilides	Isoflavones
Anthocyanosides	Saponins	Ginkolides
Phytic Acid	Indoles	Isothiocyanates
Polyphenols	Hippuric Acid	Proanthocyanadins
Parthenolides	Eleutherocides	

III. Amino Acids

These are the smallest component parts of protein and represent the building blocks of the body, from which all tissues are synthesized. Many metabolic control factors are derived from amino acids, in the form of hormones, enzymes, neurotransmitters, and immunoglobulins.

I. Neutral Aliphatic	I. Neutral Aliphatic
Threonine* Isolucine (a.k.a. branch chain amino)* Lucine (a.k.a. branch chain amino)* Valine (a.k.a. branch chain amino)*	Gycine Alanine Serine Norleucine
II. Neutral Cyclic aka Aromatic aka Heterocyclic	**II. Neutral Cyclic aka Aromatic aka Heterocyclic**
Phenylanaline* Tryptophan*	Tyrosine** Proline (loosely classified) Hydroxyproline (loosely classified)
III. Neutral Sulphur Containing	**III. Neutral Sulphur Containing**
Cysteine Methionine*	Taurine Homocysteine Cystathionine
IV. Basic	**IIIA. Acidic**
Histidine* Lysine* Arginine	Aspartic Acid Asparagine Glutamic Acid Hydroxyglutamic Acid GABA—(Gamma Glutamine Amino Butyric Acid)
	V. Miscellaneous
	Citrulline (from urea cycle) Phosphoserine Ammonia (from urea cycle) Sarcosine Alpha Amino Adipic Acid Ethanolamne Alpha Amino-n-butyric acid Anserine Phosphoethanolamine Carnosine, Methionine Sulfoxide Carnitine Methylhistidine

*Basic eight essential amino acids
**Can replace the need for some phenylalanine in metabolism

IV. Fatty Acids

Omega 3:
1. Alpha Linolenic
2. Eicosapentaenoic (EPA)
3. Docosapentaenoic
4. Docosahexaenoic

Omega 6:
1. Linoleic
2. Gamma linolenic
3. Eicosadienoic
4. Dihomogamma linolenic (DGLA)
5. Arachidonic.
6. Docosadienoic
7. Docosatetraenoic

Monounsaturated :
1. Vaccenic
2. Myristoleic
3. Palmitoleic
4. Oleic
5. 11-Eicosenoic
6. Erucic
7. Nervonic

Saturated:

1. Capric	6. Arachidic
2. Lauric	7. Behenic
3. Myristic	8. Lignoceric
4. Palmitic	9. Hexacosanoic
5. Stearic	

Odd Chain:
1. Pentadecanoic
2. Heptadecanoic
3. Nonadecanoic
4. Heneicosanoic
5. Tricosanoic

Trans Fat:
1. Palmitelaidic
2. Elaidic

Ratios:
1. Polyunsaturated/Saturated
2. Stearic/Oleic
3. Linoleic Acid/DGLA
4. Eicosapentaenoic/DGLA
5. Arachidonic Acid/EPA

All of the above nutrients, vitamins, minerals, amino acids, and fatty acids are accounted for through TPing procedures and are synergistically proportioned within the individualized nutrition programs, according to biochemical uniqueness.

APPENDIX H

Antagonism and Synergy Between Minerals and Vitamins

Nutrients can either work together or against each other. This occurs at the atomic and molecular level. The process of nutrients working together to metabolize more efficiently is known as "synergy"; it is known as "antagonism" when nutrients counteract each other. This phenomenon exists both outside of the body—as in making a supplement mixture—and inside the body, spanning from the digestive tract through to each cell's ability to absorb and utilize nutrients.

An example of nutrient synergy within the digestive tract can be seen when we consider vitamin C and iron relationships. The presence of vitamin C within food enhances or "synergizes" the absorption of iron by intestinal cells. Vitamin D enhances calcium absorption in a similar fashion. Within each cell, potassium retention is increased by the presence of magnesium. Hence, a "cellular" potassium deficiency can be treated by the addition of more magnesium from the diet. This works in relation to iron and copper balance when hemoglobin (blood cell protoplasm) is formed by the body. Too little copper sabotages the use of iron in forming blood cells. Therefore, a copper deficiency can cause anemia just as much as a deficiency of iron. It's important to note here that over 50% of American women who suffer from slight to full-blown anemia are actually suffering from copper deficiency as well as iron deficiency because the two are so closely related.

Nutrient antagonism occurs between calcium and zinc. Excessive calcium in our food, or supplements for that matter, reduces the absorption of zinc, iron, phosphorus, and magnesium by the intestine; excessive iron impairs copper absorption. Likewise, cellular metabolism is adversely affected by calcium-iron-phosphorus-magnesium copper imbalances. The phenomenon of antagonism and synergism between atoms and molecules continues throughout all constituents of the human body, including the hormones.

Due to the antagonistic/synergistic relationships between vitamins, minerals, and other nutrients "one-a-day, all-in-one" vitamin/mineral supplements are functionally useless. You simply cannot put all of these very potent nutrients into the same pill at the same time and expect optimum results. First of all, the nutrients literally oxidize or in some cases "go up in smoke" as they interact within the pill without "gobs" of extenders, fillers, buffers, antioxidants, neutralizers, and other material present. Secondly, the body won't accept pills which have a high degree of internal antagonism. This antagonism causes nutrient cancellation and properties of high ionicity, which resist the digestive, absorptive, and assimilation processes. This is why so many deficiency studies using "one a day" takers as subjects reveal a predominant pattern of nutrient imbalances not significantly better than non supplement takers. In order to create a functionally effective vitamin/mineral supplement nutrient ratios must be balanced for maximum synergism and in accordance with what the body really needs as determined through testing.

A brief list of primary nutritional mineral antagonists includes:

1. **Calcium and**
   a. Phosphorus
   b. Potassium
   c. Magnesium
   d. Lead
   e. Strontium

2. Phosphorous and
   a. Calcium
   b. Iron
   c. Manganese
   d. Magnesium
   e. Zinc
   f. Copper

3. Magnesium and
   a. Calcium
   b. Phosphorous
   c. Sodium
   d. Lead
   e. Manganese

4. Sodium and
   a. Potassium
   b. Calcium
   c. Magnesium

5. Potassium and
   a. Sodium
   b. Lithium
   c. Cobalt
   d. Calcium

6. Copper and
   a. Iron
   b. Zinc

A brief list of secondary nutritional mineral antagonists includes:
   Ca/Sr, Cr/V, Cu/Mo, Fe/Co, K/Co, K/Li, Mg/B, S/Cu,
   Se/Ag, Se/Sn, Zn/Sn

A brief list of nutritional versus toxic minerals as antagonists includes:
   Ca/Pb, Fe/Pb, Fe/Hg, Se/Hg, Zn/Cd, Zn/Hg, S/Hg,
   S/Cd, S/Pb

Mineral	Synergistic Minerals
Calcium	Magnesium-Phosphorus-Copper-Sodium-Potassium-Selenium
Magnesium	Calcium-Potassium-Zinc, Manganese-Phosphorus-Chromium
Sodium	Potassium-Selenium-Cobalt-Calcium-Copper, Phosphorus-Iron
Potassium	Sodium-Magnesium-Cobalt-Manganese-Zinc-Phosphorus-Iron
Copper	Iron-Cobalt-Calcium-Sodium-Selenium
Zinc	Potassium-Magnesium-Manganese-Chromium-Phosphorus
Phosphorus	Calcium-Magnesium-Sodium-Zinc-Potassium-Iron
Iron	Copper-Manganese-Potassium-Sodium-Chromium-Phosphorus-Selenium
Chromium	Magnesium-Zinc-Potassium
Manganese	Potassium-Zinc-Magnesium-Iron-Phosphorus
Selenium	Sodium-Potassium-Copper-Iron-Manganese-Calcium

Vitamin Antagonisms include:

B_1/B_2, B_1/B_6, B_1/B_{12}, B_2/B_3, B_6/B_3, B_2/B_6, A/D, A/E, A/B_3, B_{12}/C, A/B_6

Vitamin Synergisms include:

A	$C-E-B_1-B_2-B_3-B_6$
D	$E-B_{12}$
E	$A-C-B_1-B_3-B_5-B_6-B_{10}-B_{12}$
B_1	$A-E-C-B_2-B_3-B_5-B_6-B_{10}-B_{12}$
B_2	$A-B_3-B_{10}$
B_6	$A-E-B_1-B_3-B_5-B_{10}-B_{12}$
B_{12}	$C-D-E-B_1-B_3-B_5-B_6-B_{10}$
C	$A-E-B_3-B_5-B_6$
B_3	$A-E-B_1-B_2-B_5-B_6-B_{10}$
B_5	$A-C-E-B-B_3-B_6-B_{10}$

Vitamin and Mineral Antagonisms include:

A/Cu, A/I, A/Ca, A/Na, B_1/Mn, B_1/Ca, B_1/Zn

B_2/Se, B_2/B, B_2/Na

B_3/Cu, B_3/Ca, B_3/Zn

B_5/Cu

B_{10}/Mg, B_{10}/K, B_{10}/Zn

B_{12}/Mn, B_{12}/Zn, B_{12}/K, B_{12}/Mg, B_{12}/Cr

D/P, D/K, D/Zn

E/Ca, E/Zn, E/Fe, E/Ag, E/Mg

Vitamin and Mineral Synergisms include:

Vitamin	Synergistic Mineral
A	Zinc-Potassium-Phosphorus-Selenium-Magnesium
B_1	Selenium-Cobalt-Sodium-Potassium-Iron-Manganese-Phosphorus Magnesium-Copper-Zinc
B_2	Iron-Phosphorus-Magnesium-Zinc-Potassium-Chromium
B_3	Zinc-Potassium-Iron-Phosphorus-Magnesium-Manganese-Sodium-Chromium-Selenium
B_5	Chromium-Sodium-Potassium-Zinc-Phosphorus
B_6	Zinc-Chromium-Magnesium-Sodium-Potassium-Phosphorus
B_{12}	Selenium-Copper-Calcium-Cobalt-Sodium
C	Iron-Copper-Manganese-Zinc-Selenium-Phosphorus-Magnesium
D	Calcium-Magnesium-Sodium-Copper-Selenium
E	Sodium-Potassium-Calcium-Iron-Manganese-Zinc-Phosphorus-Selenium

NOTE: As you may have observed in the above sometimes vitamins and minerals which are synergistic can also be antagonistic in certain proportions. It is in these cases that ratios are critical to achieve balance because a slightly higher or lower atomic proportion can cause antagonism when synergism is desired.

Thanks to the work of Drs. Albert Einstein, David L. Watts, Roy Dittman, and many, many others, we now understand mineral and vitamin relationships better than ever before. We can use these nutrient relationships and many others very precisely to both measure and correct our metabolic function for a longer, more energetic, fat- and disease-free life.

APPENDIX I

Common Fallacies and Myths Among Non Typers

MYTH 1   Obesity and overweight tendencies are purely genetic
conditions.

Reality: There are far too many variables involved in becoming overweight to simply blame it all on genetics. Genetics always plays **some** role in the process of weight gain, but fat can easily be controlled using the TPing process to maximize one's body type and allow one to live up to his/her full health and fitness potential chemistry.

Social Pitfall: Far too many irresponsible advertising campaigns attempt to draw you into drug-mediated medical weight loss programs on the basis of your inability to control your own weight, because it's not your fault that you're fat in the first place (according to them)— they say it's the fault of your genes! And of course these programs have that magic silver bullet (another fallacy), which is usually a side-effect laden drug (or two) meant to get you hooked on their product for as long as possible.

Suggestion: Use TPing to lose weight healthfully. (Consider the terrible consequences Phen-Fen consumers suffered prior to that product being removed from the market.) If you are so desperate and impatient that you just have to go on weight loss drugs to get started, choose only those clinics who custom make your nutrition and exercise program using scientific procedures like those found in Personalized Nutrition, *The Tefft System*, or its other adjunctive programs. In this way, you can be typed and profiled properly to optimize weight loss and health gain results while taking any drugs on the program and beyond the program for the rest of your life.

MYTH 2   **Vitamin and mineral supplementation is controversial.**

Reality: The fact is that modern-day foods have less essential nutrient density than ever before. The result is that the average person (most often in industrialized nations) has far greater nutrient deficiencies and imbalances than in the past. The research consensus confirms that it is increasingly more difficult to find all of the necessary nutrients you require from your food. Given this, the logical deduction is that we need nutrient supplements to compensate for losses in our foods— hence, the titanic growth of the supplement industry. The problem is that our conventional mainstream drug and *one-size-fits-all* traditional research bodies are at least 30 years behind in their supplement research, due to a unanimous preoccupation with "magic bullet" drug research. (After all, drugs are patentable, right? Vitamin and minerals are not!) Even so, there is a mammoth research body proving the values and need for nutrient supplementation, which is finally receiving some attention from research traditionalists and getting published in the mainstream.

The dilemma here is that many health authorities haven't caught up with all of the available research. Especially that research having to do with proving the importance of individualized supplementation over one-size-fits-all supplementation. In scientific actuality there is no controversy over the need for nutrient supplementation once you've passed through the preliminary *one-size-fits-all* research body and on into the final frontier of individualized nutrition research. This is where the magic bullet of health really resides.

The problem is that the average health authority who still sees supplementation as controversial has barely entered into the realm of one-size-fits-all supplementation information, let alone learned about TPing. Given this, what can you expect? Their ignorance of the facts (in particular, about TPing) is what keeps the idea of supplementation (of any kind) controversial, at least in their minds. The only real supplement controversy revolves around the use of *one-size-fits-all* techniques instead of individualized, properly synergized supplementation. But even this should begin to fade away as the true benefits of TPing are revealed to all.

Social Pitfall: People are constantly confused by certain health authorities who condemn or diminish the virtues of nutrient supplementation. Even though these authorities are fast being replaced by more responsible scientists and doctors, some of their ideas have swayed people from taking supplements or even valuing them in the process of attaining well-being. This phenomenon has only resulted in more people suffering from nutritional disorders which lead to more serious dis-ease states, which otherwise are highly preventable (especially with TPing). The controversy over which *one-size-fits-all* entity is best for you is capitalized upon by supplement retailers, in order to sell you more products—many of which are not right for you. This way, you end up spending more money and receiving far less benefit than you may think while retailers make higher profits.

Suggestion: Use TPing to free yourself of controversies and misconceptions others less insightful than you may have. Realize that it will take some time for research- ignorant health authorities to catch up with you and the many thousands of health authorities who are already typers or those who are starting to finally catch on. Don't sacrifice your health for a moment longer: you need not wait for the most backward authorities to concede that the controversy isn't really over supplementation, but *one-size-fits-all*.

MYTH 3   Diets don't work (especially for fat loss).

Reality: *One-size-fits-all* diets don't work properly. But a diet custom made according to specific TPing considerations will always work.

Social Pitfall: Serious health consequences result when "magic bullets"—such as drugs and hormones—take precedence over real nutrition in the quest for wellness and fat loss.

Suggestion: Get into TPing and a specific nutrition program, and get away from artificial diet aids and gimmicks.

MYTH 4   Processed food has close to or the same nutrient value as garden fresh foods.

Reality: No matter what the label says, processed foods cannot even come close to the nutritional value of fresh foods. Processed food represents a violation of natural food chemistry beyond the plethora of chemical additives (including artificial vitamins and minerals), genetic alterations, toxins, and nutrient scarcity already present in garden fresh food. Over the course of their production, processed foods may even undergo inversion of the natural electrolyte relationships in food, like sodium and potassium, which has the far-reaching and widely recognized effect of inducing disease in people. In most cases, food processors have to actually put back ("enrich"?) some obvious artificial vitamins and minerals to meagerly make up for those lost during processing, containment, and storage, so that at least there's something left in the way of nutrients to put on the label so you'll buy it.

Social Pitfall: A prevalent attitude that these processed foods can stand in place nutritionally for fresh foods, thanks to their widespread use for reasons of extra taste and convenience. Truly, they cannot.

Suggestion: Minimize the use of highly processed foods in favor of increasing the consumption of fresh, unmodified foods as much as possible. Use only TP'd supplementation in conjunction with a customized fresh food nutrient plan.

MYTH 5   The FDA (Food and Drug Administration) has full knowledge of and control over the field of nutrition.

Reality: You and I have access to the same nutrition research that the FDA relies on for developing nutritional insights. The problem is that, due to the FDA's finite size and funding limitations, it has historically been caught up in a battle to keep up with the latest revelations in the science of nutrition.

Philosophically, the FDA has been more focused on pharmacological developments due to the inherent dangers that most drugs pose to humans and has kept a better pace in that area. It has, however, compiled and controlled an extensive list of dangerous nutritional practices, including most aspects of society's *one-size-fits-all* pursuits. In fact, much TPing research ends up under FDA scrutiny and is actually one of the motivating reasons why the FDA expends time and money trying to protect people from *one-size-fits-all* nutritional abuses. This is also the reason why some foods and vitamin/mineral supplementation at one time were being legislatively considered for consumer use by prescription only. What would the nutrient prescriptions be based on? Patient-specific criteria revealed from TPing, of course! So you could say that TPing is FDA user-friendly because it is inherently highly individualized. This eliminates any excesses, bad proportions, or other dangerous *one-size-fits-all* nutrition practices the FDA is supposed to fight against in the first place!

Someday in the near(we hope) future, the law of the land may require every citizen to be completely typed and given a full lifetime prescription of nutrition and exercise, effectively putting an end to *one-size-fits-all*, once and for all! Agricultural retailing of foodstuffs and nutrients will be strategized specific to the measure of the needs of each person in the most efficient food and lifestyle market ever seen. One day, wasted food will be unheard-of and planned surpluses will be more extensively used for worldwide peace and harmony. Seventy to eighty percent of all disease will disappear from the human race and retirement ages will reach toward the hundred-year mark.

Social Pitfall: The FDA can't keep pace with all developments in nutrition, especially when it comes to new scientific knowledge and legislative control. The result of this lagging behind is only more *one-size-fits-all* legislation and related confusion about what's best for our health.

Suggestion: Get into the process of TPing now and become healthier than ever before as you wait for the rest of the world of non-typers to catch up with you and for the FDA and other agencies to eventually legislate what you're already putting healthfully into practice.

MYTH 6   Food politics has little effect on your (nutrition-related) health.

Reality: Food politics can either work for you or against you according to the prevailing forces of the consumer market and that which controls it—commonly held knowledge and beliefs. Of course, common knowledge is controlled by governmental and non-governmental health authorities, which may be controlled by the ulterior capitalistic interest of special interest industries: they buy up the most media air time and typically receive the greatest attention from the masses. A good example of the occurrence of food politics can be seen in the plight of Dr. Harvey Wiley, the founder and first director of the FDA in 1906. He was a physician, chemist, and U.S. Department of Agriculture administrator, who quit his post in disgust in 1912. His resignation came about because his vain attempts to ensure the safe processing of foodstuffs were consistently resisted and negated by high-level politicians. As Thomas Riddick stated, "since then (1912), the names, faces, and political parties have changed many times, but not the politics."

The point Dr. Wiley stated in regard to certain food and agricultural additives (from his 1929 book "*The History of a Crime Against The Food Law*"):

> "From the earliest days of food regulations the use of alum (aluminum sulphate) has been condemned. It is universally acknowledged as a poison and deleterious substance in all countries. The United States is the only country that permits, of course illegally, the addition of alum to our food supply. If the Bureau of Chemistry had been permitted to enforce the law as it was written and as it tried to do—no food produced in our country would have any trace of benzoic acid, sulfurous acid or sulphites or any alum or saccharin, save for medical purposes. Our food and drugs would be wholly without any form of adulteration or misbranding. The health of our people would be vastly improved and their life greatly extended."

According to Riddick and many others, the addition of alum to dramatically increased and not diminished compounding our health problems from heart disease to Alzheimer's. At least they finally took aluminum out of antacids a couple of years ago, right? But that's only the microtip of the "food politics iceberg." When there are hundreds of billions of dollars at stake in maintaining the status quo, our individual health levels are always of last and least consideration.

Social Pitfall: Widespread sickness has the consequence of fueling prevailing profit oriented special interests like the drug and medical industries. These special interest groups considered to be health authorities in turn actually help to shape our beliefs in order to favor their profit attainments.

Suggestion: Become a TPer and help to change the prevailing nutrition consciousness of society into one that demands only the healthiest user-friendly nutrition from its industrial suppliers and their political counterparts.

MYTH 7   Drugs are more important than nutrition.

Reality: Drugs have nothing to do with the life sustaining needs of the body. They are in existence only because many people do not meet the specific nutrient needs of their particular body and mind. Progressively depriving the body of its exact nutritional needs causes people to become sick and then have to resort to "quick fix" symptom relief drugs in order to reduce their suffering. Hence, drugs were created to cover up the root cause of problems to relieve crises quickly. The cost, though, comes in the form of many side effects that degenerate the body's wellness. And unfortunately we tend to be dependent on drugs in the long term because the nutrient related root cause is not found and repaired naturally.

Social Pitfall: Today, more drug-dependent sick people artificially sustain their **low quality lifestyles** than ever before in the world's history. Plus, more people are being hurt by the same drugs they take to reduce symptoms to the point where the AMA has classified the side effect complications from conventional prescription medications as the fourth leading cause of death in the U.S. As times goes on, more drugs are being added to "the mix" in order to control further complications because true healing cannot be achieved by an artificial drug—only essential nutrient chemicals.

Suggestions: Don't let anyone talk you out of the importance of nutrition over drugs. You must become aware of all nutrient-drug interactions so that you can successfully protect yourself from a drug's side effects, thus nutritionally minimizing their negative effects on your body.

MYTH 8   **There can't be such a thing as TPing—it sounds too good to be true.**

Reality: TPing is real and it is truly good.

Societal Pitfall: The perpetuation of *one-size-fits-all* by those people that don't know any better.

Suggestion: Become a typer and join the **ASAP**, reap the benefits, and spread the word about the existence of metabolic typing and profiling.

Variations of Mineral Content in Vegetables

The following charts show the average phosphorus and minor nutrient content of snapbeans and tomatoes, and lowest individual values for these and three other vegetables, through several states in the U.S. (P) is the percentage and minor elements in parts per million dry matter.

	P	B	Mn	Fe	Mo	Cu	Co
Snapbeans							
Georgia	0.27	14	24	83	0.5	12	0.02
S. Carolina	0.27	17	9	110	0.4	13	0.05
Virginia	0.28	12	21	68	0.1	17	0.05
Maryland	0.22	12	30	75	0.2	11	0.12
New Jersey	0.25	25	7	88	0.6	14	0.03
New York	0.23	16	20	74	0.5	9	0.06
Ohio	0.27	15	14	77	3.0	16	0.06
Indiana	0.24	20	7	130	5.0	14	0.03
Illinois	0.25	19	7	129	3.4	30	0.05
Colorado	0.26	16	4	130	4.3	24	0.06
Highest	0.36	73	60	227	8.1	69	0.26
Lowest	0.22	10	2	10	0.1	3	0.00

	P	B	Mn	Fe	Mo	Cu	Co
Tomatoes							
Georgia	0.25	8	6	107	0.1	10	0.03
S. Carolina	0.27	10	4	119	0.1	11	0.06
Virginia	0.27	7	3	59	0.2	21	0.01
Maryland	0.19	10	5	97	0.1	16	0.04
New Jersey	0.24	9	7	113	0.2	20	0.08
New York	0.23	11	2	87	0.1	26	0.04
Ohio	0.27	20	3	96	0.3	12	0.02
Indiana	0.29	12	4	52	0.5	14	0.06
Illinois	0.30	12	2	179	2.0	27	0.03
Colorado	0.25	13	4	265	0.5	24	0.11
Highest	0.35	36	68	1,938	1.3	53	0.63
Lowest	0.16	5	1	1	0.0	0	0.00
Cabbage							
Highest	0.38	42	13	94	24.1	48	0.15
Lowest	0.22	10	2	20	0.0	0.4	0.00
Spinach							
Highest	0.52	88	117	1.584	5.6	32	0.25
Lowest	0.27	12	1	19	0.0	0.5	0.20
Lettuce							
Highest	0.43	37	169	516	4.5	60	0.19
Lowest	0.22	6	1	9	0.0	3	0.00

Other extrapolations from this extensive study showed highest and lowest nutrient densities as follows:

	Ash	Calcium	Magnesium	Potassium	Sodium
Cabbage					
Highest	10.38	60.0	43.6	148.3	20.4
Lowest	6.12	17.5	15.6	53.7	0.8
Spinach					
Highest	28.56	96.0	203.9	257	69.5
Lowest	12.38	47.5	46.9	84.6	0.8
Lettuce					
Highest	24.28	71.0	49.3	176.5	12.2
Lowest	7.01	16.0	13.1	53.7	0.0

Ash values are given in percentages and other mineral cations (positively charged minerals) in milli-equivalents per 100 grams dry water. Source: Firman E. Bear Report from Rutgers University. Contributing researchers include Steven J. Toth, Arthur L. Prince, and Arthur Wallace.

APPENDIX K

Diseases And Dis-eases That Respond To Metabolic Typing/Profiling

Achiness
Acclimitization
Acne (All Types)
Acute Pain
Addiction (All Types)
Adrenergic
  Hypersensitivity
Aging
AIDS
Alcoholism
Allergies (Airborne,
  Environmental,
  Atopic, Nutritional)
Alopecia
Alzheimer's
Amino Acid
  Imbalance
Amoebic Infestation
Anaphylaxis
Anemia
Anger
Angina Pectoris
Ankylosing
  Spondylitis

Anorexia
Anxiety
Arrythmia
Arteriosclerosis
Arthritis
Asthma
Atherosclerosis
Atopic Dermatitis
Autoimmune
  Disorders
Back Pain
Bacterial Infection
Bad Breath
  (Halitosis)
Bed Wetting
Bell's Palsey
Birth Defects
Bloating
Blood Clotting
  (Abnormal)
Blood Pressure
  (High/Low)
Blood Sugar
  (High/Diabetes)

(Low
  Hypoglycemia)
Body Fat
  Abnormalities
  (High/Low)
Brain Allergies
Brain Disorders
Burkitts Disease
Burns
Calcium Oxalate
  Kidney Stones
Cancer (All Types)
Candidiasis (Yeast
  Infection)
Canker Sores
Carbuncles
Cardiovascular
  Disease (All Types)
Carpal Tunnel
  Syndrome
Cataracts
Celiac Disease
Cellulite
Cervical Dysplasia

Charley Horse
Chemical Sensitivities
Circulating Immune
  Complexes
Chest Pain
Child Birth
  Difficulties
Chronic Fatigue
  Syndrome
Coated Tongue
Chlamydia
Cholecystitis
Cholelithiasis
Colitis (Spastic)
Collagen Disease
Constipation
Cramps
Crohn's Disease
Dandruff
Deficiencies
  (Nutritional)
Degenerative Joint
  Disease
Dementia
Depression
Dermatitis
Diabetes Insipidus
Diabetes Mellitus
Digestive Disorders
  (Diarrhea, Hypo-
  chlorhydria,
  Hyperchlorhydria,
  Irritable Bowel
  Syndrome, etc.)
Diverticulitis/
  Diverticulosis
Dumping Syndrome
Duodenal Ulcer

Dysentery
Dysmenorrhea
Dyspepsia
Ear Ringing
Eczema
Edema/Water
  Retention
Endocrine
  Dysfunction
  (Glandular
  Enteritic
  Imbalance)
Excessive Skin
  Dryness (Scaling)
Excessive Thirst
Eyesight
  Dysfunction/Loss
Fatigue
Fatty Liver
Fever
Fibrocystic Disease
Fibromyalgia
Food Allergies
Fractures
Frozen Shoulder
Gall Bladder Disease
Gas
Gastric Ulcer
Gastritis
Gastroenteritis
Genetic Disease
Glaucoma
Gluten Sensitivity
Gouty Arthritis
Hair Loss
Halitosis (Bad
  Breath)
Hangovers

Hay Fever
Hearing Loss
Headaches
Heart Disease
Heartburn
Hemorrhoids
Hepatitis
Herpes
Hiatal Hernia
Hives
Hormonal
  Imbalances
Hot Flashes
Hyperactivity
Hyperchlorhydria
Hypermobile Joints
Hyperpigmentation
Hypertension
Hypervitaminosis
Hypochlorhydria
Hypoglycemia
Hypometabolism
Hypotension
Hypothyroidism
Hypovitaminosis
  Immune System
  Dysfunction
Infections (Chronic)
Infertility
Inflammatory Bowel
  Disease
Influenza
Insomnia
Intestinal Parasites
Irritable Bowel
  Syndrome
Jaundice
Joint Swelling

Juvenile Delinquency
Kidney Failure
Kidney Stones
Lactation
Lactose Intolerance
Leaky Gut Syndrome
Learning Impairment
Leg Cramping
Ligament Laxity
Loss of
    Concentration
Low Birth Weight
Low Self-Esteem
Lumbalgia
Malabsorption
Malnutrition
Manic Depression
Marasmus
Memopause
Memory Loss
Menstrual Disorder
Metabolic
    Dysfunction
    (Including
    Acidosis/Alkalosis)
Metabolic Rate
    Slowdown
Migraine Headaches
Miscarriage
Moods Swings
Mucus Accumulation
Multiple Sclerosis
Muscle Cramps
Muscle Spasms
Muscular
    Dystrophies
Myalgia
Myofascitis

Nephritic Syndrome
Nervous Disorders
Neuralgia
Neuritis
Neuropathy
Neuroses
Nutrient Deficiencies
Osteoarthritis
Obesity
Osteoporosis
Otitis Media
Overeating
    Syndromes
Pain (All Types)
Pancreatitis
Panic Disorder
Parkinson's Disease
Parasites
Pellagra
Pelvic Inflammatory
    Disease
Periodontal Disease
Personality Disorders
Phenyl Ketouria
Phlebitis
Phobias
Pleurisy
Pneumonia
Poisoning
Polymyositis
Polyneuritis
Polyneuropathy
Post-Partum
    Depression
Pregnancy
Discomfort
Premature Birth
Premenstrual

Syndrome
Prenatal Health
Prostanoid Imbalance
Prostatic
Hypertrophy
Prostatitis
Pruritis
Psoriasis
Psychosomatic
Disorders
Regional Enteritis
Restless Leg
Syndrome
Reyes Syndrome
Rheumatoid Arthritis
Rhinitis
Rickets
Schizophrenia
Senility
Sensitivities
    (Chemical,
    Nutritional)
Silicosis
Sjogren's Syndrome
Smoking Dependence
Spinocerbellar
    Degeneration
Spontaneous
    Abortive
    Tendencies
Sports Injuries
Steatorrhea
Stiffness
Stress Management
Stretch Marks
Systemic Lupus
    Erythematosus
Tendonitis

Tension Disorders
Thrush
Thyroid Disorders
Tinnitis (Ear ringing)
TMJ Syndrome
Tooth Decay
Tropical Sprue
Ulcerative Colitis

Ulcerative Cystitis
Ulcers (Gastric,
    Duodenal)
Undereating (Loss of
    Appetite)
Urate Stones
Urticaria
Vascular Disease

Vasospasm
Viral Infection
Weight Loss/Gain
Wheezing
Worms
Zollinger–Ellison
    Syndrome

GLOSSARY

A Typers Vocabulary

absorption—the physiological process by which the body takes in through the digestive mucosa the smallest individual components left after the digestive process is completed.

Actual Daily Calorie Consumption (ADCC)—the actual amount of calories that you're taking in per day. When this figure is higher than your TCND figure, you'll gain weight. If it is lower, then you'll lose weight; if they are both the same, you'll stay the same weight.

anabolism—the building-up phase of metabolism.

Ancestral (or Tribal) Typing—using the science of genealogy to trace one's phenotypic origins during the process of determining biochemical individuality.

assimilation—the process by which the body utilizes the nutrient compounds provided by digestion and absorption for metabolism.

Autonomic Nervous System—controls your overall response to stress; that part of the nervous system concerned with regulating the activity of cardiac muscle, smooth, muscle, glands, and other involuntary functions.

balascopy—patented perceptual technology with a cascade of 15 methodologies devised for the detection, extraction, quantification, assessment, and mapping of multiple relationships within a given system (in this case, human metabolism).

Basal Metabolic Rate (BMR; expressed as calories)—the daily rate at which your body consumes calories in a resting state to sustain life (as if you were to lie in bed all day—24 hours). Males burn 24 Kcal/Kg of bodyweight per day. Females burn 21.9 Kcal/Kg of bodyweight per day.

biochemical—any chemical compound found within the body which is involved with the vital processes and physiological chemistry of life.

biochemical individuality—a phenomenon of personal uniqueness where "no two people are exactly alike" in the way their bodies and minds are structured and function and therefore in the precise needs of their bodies and minds for overall wellness.

Blood Typing—using the chemical groupings and sub-groupings of blood to help delineate metabolic types to further distinguish individual biochemical identity.

Calorie Deficit (Negative Calorie Balance)—a lower calorie intake or fewer calories than the body needs to maintain itself at its present weight. The body is forced to come up with missing food calories from fat storage because its not receiving enough calories form the diet to maintain its current weight level.

calorimetry—specific scientific procedures which measure the amount of heat given off as measured in calories by a living individual or for measuring the potential energy in food. All heat measures are given in calories or their equivalent.

carni-vegan—person with a type of diet containing red and white meats and mostly low starch alkaline vegetables and fruits.

carnivorous—referring to a pure meat-eater (over 70% of calories in diet from animal and fish sources). Traditional Eskimos are considered pure carnivores.

catabolism—the breaking down phase of metabolism.

catalyst—any substance that increases the velocity of a chemical reaction or process which in itself is not consumed in the net chemical reaction or process.

clinical nutritionist—a highly trained professional nutritionist with degrees in nutrition, biology or physiology with thousands of hours of professional school in the basic and clinical sciences including every basic and clinical knowledge parameter from cadaver dissection to treating diet-related illnesses in the clinical environment. Addressed as "Doctor" and uses physical examination and laboratory procedures in nutritional work-ups.

Coefficient of Activity—the measurable level of the sum total of all biochemical processes in relation to the process of ionization which forms the nature of one's metabolism.

coenzymes—also known as cofactors, vitamins, and minerals all of which stimulate enzyme action.

Daily Physical Activity Need (DPAN—also known as the Energy Level of Physical Activity)—the caloric energy needs of your body as a "result" of getting out of bed, moving around, and exercising.

Deductive Reasoning—reasoning from the general to the specific.

desaturase—any enzyme that catalyzes the desaturation of a fatty acid.

desaturation—chemical process of introducing a double bond between the carbon atoms of a fatty acid.

detoxification—process of removing the health damaging effects of a toxic substance.

digestion—chemical process by which the body breaks apart all of food's nutrients into their smallest individual components.

drug—Any chemical which can create symptomatic relief, but that is not already part of or derived from the body's chemical structure or essential needs; i.e., Vitamin C is not a drug because the body becomes sick without it. Prozac is a drug because it doesn't occur naturally within the body nor is it essential to the body's life processes.

ectoderm—the outermost of the three primary embryonic germ layers which forms the skin and nervous system, the predominance of which in a given body relates to the high strung, highly intelligent, lean or seemingly underweight Ectomorph Type.

ectomorph—an individual having a type of body in which tissues derived from the ectoderm predominate: preponderance of linearity and fragility, with large surface area, thin muscles and subcutaneous tissue, low body fat, and slightly developed digestive viscera (digestive systems).

ectotonia—psychological state of being centered on privacy, self-restraint, and a highly developed self awareness.

eicosanoids—"super hormones" manufactured by every living cell of the human body as derived from essential fatty acids within the diet.

elimination—the process by which the body rids itself of residual chemical waste products produced by the body as a result of metabolism.

elongation—the chemical process of increasing the length of a molecule.

endocrine glands—organs that secrete hormones directly into the circulatory system influencing metabolism and other bodily processes including behavior.

Endocrine Typing—using the strength and weakness hierarchy of the body's endocrine glands to group people into body types, metabolic types or constitutional types to help delineate individual biochemical identity.

endoderm (a.k.a. entoderm)—the innermost of the three primary germ layers of the embryo from which is derived the digestive tract and linings of the pharynx, respiratory tract, bladder, and urethra.

endogenous—referring to substances produced within the body.

endomorph—an individual who has a body build predominately composed of tissues from the "endo" or entoderm. Possesses a preponderance of soft roundness throughout the body with large digestive viscera and fat accumulation, large trunk and thighs, and tapering extremities.

endotonia—psychological state of being demonstrated by the love of relaxation, comfort, food, and people.

energy (human)—the electrochemical force that sustains life released through the biochemical processing of nutrients, air, and water.

enzyme—a cellular protein capable of accelerating the chemical reaction of a substance into a product without being destroyed or altered during the process.

exogenous—referring to substances from outside the body.

food assay—qualitative and quantitative analysis of the nutrient and non-nutrient composition of food.

Forced Feeding Incompatibility Syndrome (FFIS)—a phenomenon where-one-size-fits-all symptom relief marketing promoters encourage unsuspecting consumers to risk their health by eating foods, which are either generically unhealthy or specifically incompatible with an individual; meanwhile they promise to relieve the symptomatic consequences that one will suffer from eating these foods with their special symptom-blocking wonder drug.

free energy—the life force available to the body above and beyond that being consumed to counteract resistance within the body and mind.

genotype—reflection of the entire genetic constitution of a person that distinguishes his or her physical appearance.

Health Index—the degree of metabolic balance reflected by the mathematical ratio of energy to resistance expressed as a factor of probability.

homeostasis—the mechanism of the body that keeps it in life sustaining balance; a tendency toward stability in the normal body states (internal environment) of an individual achieved by a system of control mechanisms activated by negative feedback.

Inductive Reasoning—reasoning from the specific to the general.

ionization—the metabolic process by which nutrients are moved from one place to another by ions or dispersed as ions internally.

ions—positively or negatively charged particles. Elemental minerals are all ions with either positive or negative charges until neutralized as salt or chelation compound.

Laboratory Typing—a.k.a. Profiling--that component of the overall Typing process which utilizes human specimens (blood, urine, feces, saliva, hair, etc.) to help determine biochemical identity by measuring nutrient and toxin states in the body.

macronutrients—basic nutrients which we need to consume as humans on a daily basis in "larger than gram" amounts. They consist of proteins, fat, carbohydrates, water and air and each have their own caloric and metabolic value. Ethanol is considered a non-essential macronutrient.

megadoser—someone who takes in too much of anything (usually foods, drink, supplements, drugs or exercise).

mesoderm—the middle layer of the three primary embryonic germ layers which forms the connective tissue and muscles and is therefore associated with the typically muscular Mesomorph Type.

mesomorph—an individual whose body build is characteristic of mesodermal predominance: possesses a preponderance of muscle, bone, and connective tissue usually with a hard, heavy physique and with rectangular or squarish appearance.

mesotonia—psychological state of being which focuses on being assertive and on a love of action.

metabolic balance—when the chemistry of the body is working at peak efficiency and follows the relative path of least resistance for energy production.

metabolic map—a graphic representation of both balanced and imbalanced metabolic relationships between body chemicals as demonstrated through the phenomenon of metabolic networks. Metabolic maps can also be considered metabolic patterns.

metabolic network—a network of metabolic relationships which reflect metabolic function as an integrated whole and not as a list of isolated variables.

Metabolic Typing (patterning)—process of categorizing certain constitutional elements of the body into their own unique subgroups to help determine biochemical identity. Includes all aspects of typing short of Profiling.

metabolism—the total profile of all biochemical activity required to maintain life.

micronutrients—essential nutrients your body needs in "less than gram" amounts, e.g. vitamins, minerals, and vitamin-like substances.

MUFA (Monounsaturated Fatty Acids)—nutritional fats with a characteristic single open molecular bond per carbon chain.

negative feedback—an inhibitory (resistive) controlling effect on the output of a system. Example: the build-up of acids in the blood from anaerobic exercise triggers an increase in bicarbonate output by the kidneys to buffer the acids and restore pH balance.

Nerve Typing—using the sympathetic/parasympathetic dominance hierarchy to help delineate metabolic types and to further distinguish individual biochemical identity.

novice nutritionist—self proclaimed nutritionist who does not have years of study nor the necessary degrees to fully understand the body's inner workings and the clinical application of precise nutritional science to optimize body function. May possess a correspondence degree or some minor degree of schooling.

nutrient—any naturally occurring essential substance that provides or catalyzes energy production for the functional growth and maintenance of the human organism.

nutrition—the process by which nutrients maintain the life of the body and mind.

omnivore—person who can eat all types of foods.

omnivorous—able to eat all types of foods for efficient metabolism.

overfat—a specific amount of body fat accumulation which when reached creates resistance to overall metabolic balance and is characteristically different for each body type and each individual as measured by the science of Typing and Profiling.

oxidation (biological)—the enzymatic processing of oxygen by which food is metabolized resulting in the release of energy.

Oxidation Typing—using oxidation rates and amounts as the basis to delineate metabolic types in the quest to distinguish biochemical identity. Used in conjunction with Nerve Typing and Endocrine Typing as a secondary distinguishing feature of metabolism.

Parasympathetic Nervous System—controls the alkaline cells or basophils which is that part of the nervous system which has a calming effect on the body including digestion.

phenotype—body classification which reflects the entire physical, biochemical, and physiological make-up of an individual as determined both environmentally and genetically.

phytonutrients (a.k.a. phytochemicals)—nutrient compounds found in vegetables and fruits including vitamins, minerals, enzymes, and other compounds.

piecemealer—someone who takes a little bit of this and a little bit of that of food and supplements (not knowing if they really need them or not) to try to make a complete diet and supplement plan.

Profiling—see Laboratory Typing.

Psychological Typing—using patterns of personality in the quest to determine biochemical identity.

Pseudonutritionist—self-proclaimed nutritionist with absolutely no formal training in nutritional sciences whatsoever.

PUFA (Polyunsaturated Fatty Acids)—nutritional fats with characteristic open molecular bonds throughout the carbon chain mostly from plant sources particularly grains, seeds, and vegetables. Includes the body's essential fatty acids: cis linoleic and alpha linolenic acids.

Pure Typing—using only those typing procedures not directly involving laboratory procedures of specimen evaluation.

purine—by-product of nucleic acid (genetic material) breakdown in red meat which forms uric acid; found in high concentrations in red meats. Can cause gout in people who are biochemically susceptible or have certain mineral deficiencies.

ratio—proportion of one nutrient to the next construed as either synergistic or antagonistic in terms of physiologic response.

resistance—(overall) the electro-chemical inhibition of "free energy" production within the body due to the presence of inadequate nutrition, pathological (disease) states, physical degeneration (including premature aging), and/or the spiritual condition of the individual. Electrochemical resistance—the effect produced when atomic particles of varying energy potentials encounter one another and release energy.

SAFA (Saturated Fatty Acids)—nutritional fats with characteristic closed molecular bonds predominantly from animal sources.

shotgunner—someone who takes a huge variety of nutrients and supplements thinking that they are going to cover all of their metabolic needs.

Single Nucleotide Polymorphism—single point mutations in the genetic code which impair certain protein and enzyme production in cells and are associated with many chronic diseases.

Somatyping—using the predominate pattern of primal derm distribution when categorizing metabolic types.

Specific Dynamic Activity (SDA)—the calorie energy required for the process of digestion and reflexive fat thermogenesis after eating.

State of Health—the continuing variable adaptation of the biochemistry of metabolism between the internal environment and the external environment of a living organism relative to its coefficient of activity.

submetabolic—a small profile of biochemical activity which contributes in some part to the total profile of metabolism.

substrate—a substance upon which an enzyme acts.

Sympathetic Nervous System—the part of the Autonomic Nervous System, which controls acid cells known as acidophilus and which is the part of the nervous system that prepares our bodies for "fight or flight."

thermogenesis—heat production by the body. About 75% of the energy created by the human body is given off as heat.

Total Caloric Need Per Day (TCND)—the amount of calories your body needs to maintain itself at a constant weight without a net gain or loss of weight.

toxic overload—when the presence of toxins internally stresses the process of metabolism beyond its capacity to neutralize the deteriorative effects of the toxins.

toxin—any substance present internally or externally that increases resistance or stress to the metabolic process.

TPing—the science and art of determining a person's unique biochemical identity utilizing all aspects of metabolic typing (endocrine, blood, psychological, body shape and features, nerve, oxidation, laboratory assessment, quantification and qualification).

YoYo Diet—a dietary syndrome of rapid weight loss followed by rapid weight gain which can repeat itself many times over.

Zeta Potential—mathematical basis for the physical chemistry governing the stability of liquid-solid systems. In more biological terms, the maintenance of fluidity within the aqueous (water-based) systems of both plant and animal life based upon inherent ionization properties.

INDEX

BIBLIOGRAPHY

Abravanel, Elliot, D., M.D. *Dr. Abravanel's Bodytype Diet*. New York: Bantam Books, 1983.

Bajusz, E., M.D. *Nutritional Aspects of Cardiovascular Disease*. London: Crosby, Lockwood, and Son, 1965.

Balch, James F., M.D. and Balch, Phyllis A., C.N.C. *Prescription For Nutritional Healing*. New York: Avery Publishing Group, 1990.

Beach, Rex. "Modern Miracle Men," United States Government Printing Office Washington, 264 (1936).

Beasley, J. D., M.D. and Swift, Jerry, M.A. *The Kellogg Report: The Impact of Nutrition & Lifestyle on the Health of Americans*. New York: Annandale-On-Hudson, 1989.

Beddoe, A. F. *Biologic Ionization As Applied To Human Nutrition*. Grass Valley, CA: Agro-Bio Systems 1990.

Bieler, Henry G. and Block, Maxine. *Food Is Your Best Medicine*. New York: Random House, 1965.

Bland, Jeffrey, Ph.D. *Trace Elements in Human Health and Disease*. Bellvue: Washington: Northwest Diagnostic Services, 1979.

Braly, James, M.D. *Dr. Braly's Food Allergy & Nutrition Revolution*. New Canaan, Connecticut: Keats Pubishing, 1992.

Brody, Jane. *Jane Brody's Nutrition Book*. New York: Bantam Books, 1981

Bucci, Luke R., Ph.D., C.C.N., C(ASCP). "Role of Individualized Convenient Assessment," *CCA Journal*, 19:3 (March, 1994).

Cheraskin, E., M.D., D.M.D., et al. *Diet and Disease*. New Canaan, Connecticut: Keats Publishing, 1977.

Colgan, Michael, Ph.D. *Your Personal Vitamin Profile*. New York: William Morrow & Company, 1982.

Collin, Jonathan, M.D. "Food and Drug Insider Report," *Townsend Letter For Doctors*, 108 (July, 1992).

Colt, George Howe. "Heal Me," *Life Magazine*, (September, 1996).

Communications Research Machines, Inc. *Biology Today*. Del Mar, California: CRM Books, 1972.

Crawford, Michael, Ph.D. and Marsh, David, Ph.D. *The Driving Force—Food, Evolution and The Future*. New York: Harper & Row, 1989.

D'Adamo, James, N.D. "ABO Bias May Signal Innate Differences In Natural Immunity," *Journal of Naturopathic Medicine*, 2:1 (1991).

D'Adamo, James, N.D. *One Man's Food*. Madrid, Spain: Everest, 1980.

D'Adamo, Peter, N.D. *Eat Right For Your Bodytype*. New York, New York: G.P. Putnam's Sons, 1996.

Deepak, Chopra, M.D. *Perfect Health*. New York: Harmony Books, 1991.

Deepak, Chopra, M.D. *Quantum Healing: Exploring The Frontiers of Mind-Body Medicine*. New York: Bantan Books, 1989.

DeGowin, Elmer L., M.D. and DeGowin, Richard L., M.D. *Bedside Diagnostic Examination*. New York: Macmillan Publishing Cmpany, 1981.

DeRoeck, Richard E., D.C. *The Confusion About Chiropractors*. Danbury, Connecticut: Impulse Publishing, 1989.

Eaton, S. Boyd. M.D. *The Paleolithic Prescription*. New York: Harper & Row, 1988.

Erasmus, Udo, Ph.D. *Facts That Can Heal Facts That Can Kill*. B.C., Canada: Alive Books, 1996.

Feuer, Elaine. *Innocent Casualties: The FDA's War Against Humanity*. Pittsburgh: Dorrance Publishing Co., 1996.

Galsey, Alan R., M.D. "Literature Review and Commentary," *Townsend Letter For Doctors*, 108 (July, 1992).

Gelb, Barbara Levine. *The Dictionary of Food and What's In It For You*. New York: Ballantine Books, 1978.

Gittleman, Ann Louise, M.S., C.N.S. "A New Year, A New You," *Healthy Talk*, Premier Issue (1996).

Goldfinger, Steven E., M.D., ed. "By The Way, Doctor," *Harvard Health Letter*, 19:10 (August, 1994).

Goldfinger, Steven E., M.D.,"Food Allergies That Stretch To Latex," *Harvard Health Letter*, 19:5 (March, 1994).

Goldfinger, Steven E., M.D., "Unkind Milk," *Harvard Health Letter*, 18:12 (October, 1993).

Goodhart, Robert S., M.D., D.M.S. and Shils, Maurice E., M.D. Sc.D. *Modern Nutrition in Health and Disease*. Philadelphia: Lea & Febiger, 1980.

Guthrie, Helen Andrews. *Introductory Nutrition*. Saint Louis: C.V. Mosby Company, 1971.

Guyton, Arthur C., M..D. *Textbook of Medical Physiology*. Phildelphia: W. B. Saunders Company, 1981.

Hausman, Patricia and Hurley, Judith Benn. *The Healing Foods*. Emmans, Pennsylvania: Rodale Press, 1989.

Herbert, Victor, M.D. "What You Should Know About Vitamins— The Case Against Supplements," *Bottom Line*, 15:23 (December, 1994).

Horrrobin, David, M.D., Ph.D. *Clinical Uses of Essential Fatty Acids*. Montreal—London: Eden Press, 1982.

Jacobsen, Michael, Ph.D., ed. "Pumping Immunity," *Nutrition Action Health Letter*, 20:3 (April, 1993).

Jacobsen, Michael, Ph.D., "Short Takes," *Nutrition Action Health Letter*, 20:10 (December, 1993).

Jacobsen, Michael, Ph.D., "Viva La Difference: Aspirin," *Nutrition Action Health Letter*, 22:2 (March, 1995).

Jung, Carl. *Psychological Types or The Psychology of Individuation*. New York: Pantheon Books, 1923.

Jung, Carl. *Psychological Types*. California: Princeton University, 1976.

Kennedy, Charles C., M.D., ed. "Beta Carotene Supplements—Do They Prevent Or Promote Lung Cancer?" *Update Mayo Clinic Health Letter*, April 14, 1994).

Kennedy, Charles C., M.D., "Breakfast Cereal," *Mayo Clinic Health Letter*, 12:9 (September, 1994).

Kennedy, Charles C., M.D., "Herbal Supplements," *Mayo Clinic Health Letter*, 12:6 (June, 1994)

Kennedy, Charles C., M.D.,"Second Opinion," *Mayo Clinic Health Letter*, 12:8 (August, 1994).

Klafs, Carl E., Ph.D., F.A.C.S.M. and Arnheim, Daniel D., D.P.E., F.A.C.S.M., F.A.C.T.A. *Modern Principles of Athletic Training*. Saint Louis: C.V. Mosby Company, 1973.

Kreutler, Patricia A., Ph.D. *Nutrition In Perspective*. New Jersey: Prentice-Hall, Inc., 1980.

Langman, Jan, M.D., Ph.D. *Medical Embryology*. Baltimore: Maryland, 1981:

Liebman, Bonnie, M.S. "Antioxidants: Surprise, Surprise," *Nutrition Action Health Letter*, 21:5 (June, 1994).

Liebman, Bonnie, M.S. "Coffee Lovers," *Nutrition Action Health Letter*, 21:3 (April, 1994).

Liebman, Bonnie, M.S. "Fish Oil Flops," *Nutriton Action Health Letter*, 20:6 (July/August, 1993).

Liebman, Bonnie, M.S. "Just The Calcium Facts," *Nutrition Action Health Letter*, 22:4 (May, 1995).

Liebman, Bonnie, M.S. "M.D. = Mediocre Diet?" *Nutrition Action Health Letter*, 21:3 (April, 1993).

Liebman, Bonnie, M.S. "Non-Trivial Pursuits: Playing The Research Game," *Nutrition Action Health Letter*, 21:8 (October, 1994).

Liebman, Bonnie, M.S. "Quick Studies: Trans Wreck," *Nutrition Action Health Letter*, 22:4 (May, 1995).

Liebman, Bonnie, M.S. "Short Takes," *Nutrition Action Health Letter*, 21:3 (April, 1994).

Liebman, Bonnie, M.S. "Sneak Previews," *Nutrition Action Health Letter*, 20:1 (January/February, 1993).

Liebman, Bonnie, M.S. "Tea For 250 Million?" *Nutrition Action Health Letter*, 21:9 (November, 1994).

Luciano, Dorothy S.; Vander, Arthur J. and Sherman. James H. *Human Function and Structure*. New York: MacGraw-Hill Book Company, 1978.

Malter, Rick, Ph.D. "Trace Mineral Analysis and Psychoneuro-immunology," *Journal of Orthomolecular Medicine*, 9:2 (1994).

Margolis, Simeon, M.D., ed. "Drugstore Aisle," *Johns Hopkins Health After 50 Medical Letter*, 6:6 (August, 1994).

Margolis, Simeon, M.D., ed. "Our Readers Ask," *Johns Hopkins Health After 50 Medical Letter*, 6:8 (October, 1994).

Margolis, Simeon, M.D., ed. "Tamoxifen: Cancer Cause or Cure," *Johns Hopkins Health After 50 Medical Letter*, 6:8 (October, 1994).

Margolis, Simeon, M.D., ed. "Weighing The Latest Cancer Risks," *Johns Hopkins After 50 Medical Letter*, 6:10 (December, 1994).

Mathews, Donald K. and Fox, Edward L. *The Physiological Basis of Physical Education and Athletics*. Philadelphia: W. B. Saunders Company, 1976.

Mendelsohn, Robert, M.D. *Confessions of a Medical Heretic*. New York: Warner Books, 1979.

Metropolitan Life Insurance Company Statistical Bulletin, July–September 1992

Monte, Tom. *World Medicine*. New York: Perigee Books, 1993.

Napier, Christine, K. "What Is A Good Checkup?" *Harvard Health Letter*, 20:3 (January, 1995).

National Center for Health Statistics, Data from the National Health Survey, Series II, No. 231, Department of Health & Human Services, 1984 .

National Center for Health Statistics, First Health & Nutrition Examination Survey, DHEW Pub No. (PHS) , U.S. Public Health Services, 1984.

National Academy of Sciences Recommended Dietary Allowances, 9th Edition, National Academy of Press, Washington, D.C., 1980.

Nussbaum, Bruce. *Good Intentions*. New York: Penguin Books, 1990.

Oppenheim, Michael, M.D. *The Complete Book of Better Digestion*. Emmaus, Pennsylvania: Rodale Press, 1990.

Page, Melvin E., M.D. *Your Body Is Your Best Doctor*. New Canaan, Connecticut, Keats Publishing, 1972.

Pataki, Ladislov, Ph.D. and Holden, L. *Winning Secrets*. U.S.: Pataki and Holden, 1989.

Pennington, J. A. and Young, B. E. "Nutritonal Elements in U.S. Diets: Results From The Total Diet Study, 1982–1986," *Journal of the American Dietary Association*, 89:659 (1989).

Personal Health Response, "*The Metabolic Health Map— Professional's Guide*." San Francisco, California, The Human Technologies Group, Inc. and Personal, 1996.

Power, Richard T., Ph.D. and Power, Laura, B.A. *Metabolic Typing: Old and New Systems*. Maryland: self-published, 1982.

Rath, Matthias, M.D. *Eradicating Heart Disease*. San Francisco, California: Health Now, 1993.

Reams, C. A., Ph.D. and Dudley, Cliff. *Choose Life or Death*. Tampa, Florida: Holistic Laboratories, 1990.

Rector-Page, Linda G., N.D., Ph.D. *Healthy Healing: An Alternative Healing Reference*. 9th edition, California: Healthy Healing Publications, 1992.

Riddick, Thomas. *Control of Colloidal Stability Through Zeta Potential*. New York: Zeta Meter, Inc. 1968.

Riddick, Thomas. *Heart Disease: A New Approach To Prevention and Control*. Vermont: International Study Group For Research In Cardiac Metabolism, 1970.

Robbins, Stanley, M.D. and Cotran, Ramzi S., M.D. *Pathologic Basis of Disease*. Philadelphia: W.B. Saunders, 1979.

Sanders, T. A. B. "Essential and Trans-Fatty Acids In Nutrition," *Nutrition Research Reviews*, 1 (1988).

Schardt, David. "Phytochemicals: Plants Against Cancer," *Nutrition Action Health Letter*, 21:3 (April, 1994).

Schardt, David. "Pumping Immunity," *Nutrition Action Health Letter*, 21:3 (April, 1993).

Schwartz, Bob, Ph.D. *Diets Don't Work*. Houston, Texas, 1996.

Sears, Barry, Ph.D. *The Zone*. New York: HarperCollins, 1995.

Segarnick, David, Ph.D. and Rotrosen, John, M.D. "Essential Fatty Acids, Prostaglandins, and Nonsteroidal Antiinflammatory Agents: Physiological and Behavioral Interactions," *Alcoholism: Clinical and Experimental Research*, 11:1 (January/February 1987).

Selye, Hans, M.D. The Stress of Life. New York: McGraw-Hill, 1956.

Sheldon, William H., Ph.D. *Varieties of Human Physique*. New York: Harper, 1940.

Sica-Cohen, Robban, M.D. "What You Should Know About Vitamins," *Bottom Line*, 15:22 (November 15, 1994).

Silver, Helene. *The Body-Smart System*. Sonora, California: Bantam Books, 1994.

Solomon, T. W. Graham. *Organic Chemistry*, Second Edition. New York: John Wiley & Sons, 1980.

Stern, Mark, M.D. "Clinical Applications of the Metabolic Urine Study," *A Report compiled by the Utilization Review Associates for Personalized Nutrition.*

VINIS: Vitamin Nutrition Information Service (2:2). New Jersey: Hoffman-LaRoche, Inc., 1981.

Wallach, Joel D., B.S., D.V.M., N.D. "Exercise: Without Supplementation is Suicide," *Health Consciousness*, 15:3 (February, 1995).

Walker, N. W., Sc.D. *Fresh Vegetable and Fruit Juices: What's Missing In Your Body*. Prescott, Arizona: Norwalk Press, 1970.

Watson, George, Ph.D. *Nutrition and Your Mind*. New York: Harper & Row, 1972.

Watts, David, D.C., Ph.D. *Trace Elements*, Texas: Watts, 1995.

Weil, Andrew, M.D. *Spontaneous Healing*. New York: Alfred A. Knopf, 1995.

Weir, Edith C., Ph.D., et al. *An Evaluation of Research in the United States on Human Nutriton: Report No. 2: Benefits from Nutrition Research*. Washington D.C.: U.S. Department of Agriculture, 1971.

Wilson, George, Ph.D. *Nutrition and Your Mind: The Psychochemical Response*. New York: Harper, 1972.

Wilson, George, Ph.D. *Personality, Strength, Psychochemical Energy*. New York: Harper, 1979.

Williams, Roger J., Ph.D. *Alcoholism: The Nutritional Approach*. University of Texas Press, 1959.

Wilson, George, Ph.D. *Biochemical Individuality*. New York: Wiley & Sons, 1956.

Wilson, George, Ph.D. *Nutrition Against Disease*. New York: Bantam Books, 1971.

Wilson, George, Ph.D. *A Physician's Handbook on Orthomolecular Medicine*. Keats, 1979

Wilson, George, Ph.D. *The Wonderful World Within You: Your Inner Nutritional Environment*. Bio-Comm. Press, 1987.

Wilson, George, Ph.D. *You're Extraordinary*. New York: Random House, 1967.

Williams, Roger John, Ph.D. and Lansford, Edwin M. *The Encyclopedia of Biochemistry*. New York: Reinhold, 1967.

ABOUT THE AUTHOR

Dr. Gregory Tefft is a Chiropractic Doctor and a Board Certified Naturopathic Physician treating patients since 1984. On an accelerated Ph.D. program he's surpassed his M.S. requirements in Exercise Physiology and is completing the remainder of this third doctorate in holistic nutrition. His two B.S. degrees are based upon three majors in Physical Education, Health Science, and Biology.

Dr. Tefft's accomplishments include being a 3 time Natural America, a Master's Class powerlifter, a fifth placing in track and field at the Jr. Olympics, and Olympic Team alternate classification in swimming.

Dr. Tefft has been a drugless physician, personal training and nutritional consultant for numerous celebrities including Dolph Lundgren and Larry Wilcox.

TESTING RESOURCES

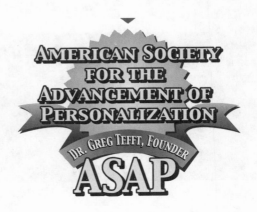

ASAP, in conjunction with Dragon Door Publications, will be offering the following testing services to help you better determine the diet you were born to eat.

- Saliva—Calcium Typing Test
- Detoxification Capacity Test
- Urine—Original Precision Metabolic Stress Profile (short form)
- Total Precision Panel a.k.a. Cellular Energy Profile (short and long forms)
- pH/Calcium Type Test
- Protein Digestion Efficiency
- Hair—Trace Mineral Analysis
- Blood—Typing,
- Cholesterol

For complete information on these testing services, including pricing, call **1-800-899-5111** or visit the Dragon Door website www.dragondoor.com.

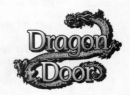

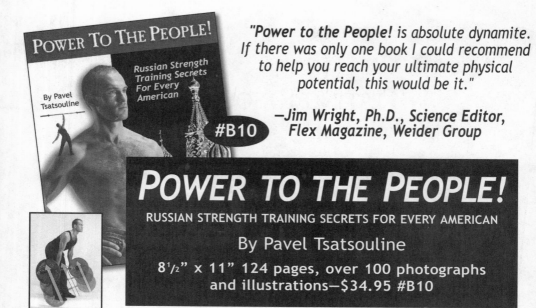
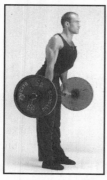

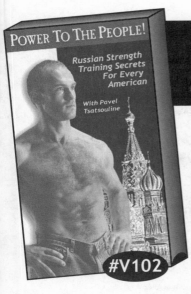
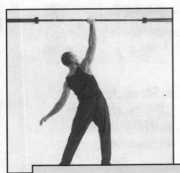
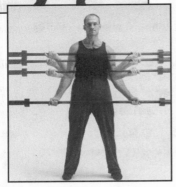

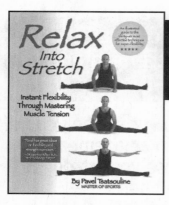
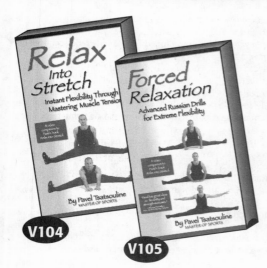

"The Do-It-Now, Fast-Start, Get-Up-and-Go, Jump-into-Action Bible for High Performance and Longer Life"

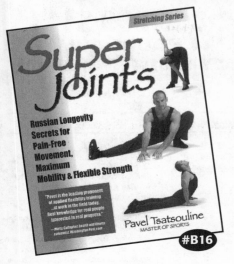

Stretching Series

Super Joints

Russian Longevity Secrets for Pain-Free Movement, Maximum Mobility & Flexible Strength

"Pavel is the leading proponent of applied flexibility training ...at work in the field today. Real knowledge for real people interested in real progress."
— Marty Gallagher health and fitness columnist, WashingtonPost.com

Pavel Tsatsouline
MASTER OF SPORTS

#B16

Super Joints
Russian Longevity Secrets for Pain-Free Movement, Maximum Mobility & Flexible Stength

With Pavel Tsatsouline
#B16   **$34.95**
8 1/2" x 11" Paperback
130 pages - Over 100 photos
and illustrations

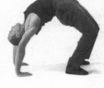

You have a choice in life. You can sputter and stumble and creak your way along in a process of painful, slow decline—or you can take charge of your health and become a human dynamo.

And there is no better way to insure a long, pain-free life than performing the right daily combination of joint mobility and strength-flexibility exercises.

In *Super Joints*, Russian fitness expert Pavel Tsatsouline shows you exactly how to quickly achieve and maintain peak joint health—and then use it to improve every aspect of your physical performance.

Only the foolish would deliberately ignore the life-saving and life-enhancing advice Pavel offers in *Super Joints*. Why would anyone willingly subject themselves to a life of increasing pain, degeneration and decrepitude? But for an athlete, a dancer, a martial artist or any serious performer, *Super Joints* could spell the difference between greatness and mediocrity.

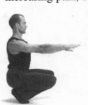

Discover:

- The twenty-eight most valuable drills for youthful joints and a stronger stretch
- How to save your joints and prevent or reduce arthritis
- The one-stop care-shop for your inner Tin Man— how to give your nervous system a tune up, your joints a lube-job and your energy a recharge
- What it takes to go from cruise control to full throttle: The One Thousand Moves Morning Recharge—Amosov's "bigger bang" calisthenics complex for achieving heaven-on earth in 25 minutes
- How to make your body feel better than you can remember— active flexibility fosporting prowess and fewer injuries
- The amazing Pink Panther technique that may add a couple of feet to your stretch the first time you do it

ORDERING INFORMATION

Customer Service Questions? Please call us between 9:00am–11:00pm EST Monday to Friday at 1-800-899-5111. Local and foreign customers call 513-346-4160 for orders and customer service

100% One-Year Risk-Free Guarantee. If you are not completely satisfied with any product–for any reason, no matter how long after you received it–we'll be happy to give you a prompt exchange, credit, or refund, as you wish. Simply return your purchase to us, and please let us know why you were dissatisfied–it will help us to provide better products and services in the future. *Shipping and handling fees are non-refundable.*

Telephone Orders For faster service you may place your orders by calling Toll Free 24 hours a day, 7 days a week, 365 days per year. When you call, please have your credit card ready.

1·800·899·5111
24 HOURS A DAY
FAX YOUR ORDER (866) 280-7619

Complete and mail with full payment to: Dragon Door Publications, P.O. Box 1097, West Chester, OH 45071

Please print clearly

Sold To: A

Name_____

Street_____

City_____

State_____ Zip_____

Day phone*_____
* Important for clarifying questions on orders

Please print clearly

SHIP TO: *(Street address for delivery)*   B

Name_____

Street_____

City_____

State_____ Zip_____

Email_____

Warning to foreign customers:
The Customs in your country may or may not tax or otherwise charge you an additional fee for goods you receive. Dragon Door Publications is charging you only for U.S. handling and international shipping. Dragon Door Publications is in no way responsible for any additional fees levied by Customs, the carrier or any other entity.

Warning!
This may be the last issue of the catalog you receive.

If we rented your name, or you haven't ordered in the last two years you may not hear from us again. If you wish to stay informed about products and services that can make a difference to your health and well-being, please indicate below.

Item #	Qty.	Item Description	Item Price	A or B	Total

Name_____

Address_____

City_____ State_____

Zip_____

HANDLING AND SHIPPING CHARGES • NO COD'S

Total Amount of Order Add:

$00.00 to $24.99 add $5.00	$100.00 to $129.99 add $12.00
$25.00 to $39.99 add $6.00	$130.00 to $169.99 add $14.00
$40.00 to $59.99 add $7.00	$170.00 to $199.99 add $16.00
$60.00 to $99.99 add $10.00	$200.00 to $299.99 add $18.00
	$300.00 and up add $20.00

Canada & Mexico add $8.00. All other countries triple U.S. charges.

Total of Goods	
Shipping Charges	
Rush Charges	
Kettlebell Shipping Charges	
OH residents add 6% sales tax	
MN residents add 6.5% sales tax	
Total Enclosed	

Do You Have A Friend Who'd Like To Receive This Catalog?

We would be happy to send your friend a free copy. Make sure to print and complete in full:

Name_____

Address_____

City_____ State_____

Zip_____

METHOD OF PAYMENT ☐ Check ☐ M.O. ☐ Mastercard ☐ Visa ☐ Discover ☐ Amex

Account No. *(Please indicate all the numbers on your credit card)*   EXPIRATION DATE

☐☐☐☐ ☐☐☐☐ ☐☐☐☐ ☐☐☐☐   ☐☐/☐☐

Day Phone ( )_____

SIGNATURE_____ DATE_____

NOTE: We ship best method available for your delivery address. Foreign orders are sent by air. Credit card or International M.O. only. For rush processing of your order, add an additional $10.00 per address. Available on money order & charge card orders only.

Errors and omissions excepted. Prices subject to change without notice.

DDP 03/02